Integrative Chinese Herbal Therapy

The Correspondences of

Dr. Lee Chen-Yu and **Dr. Juno Yang**

Volume II

Surfaces in Motion

Respiratory, Gastrointestinal, Neurological, Dermatological, and Other Conditions

Compiled, Translated, and Authored by
Scott L. Herbster, OMD, LAc

Edited by Marc Wasserman, PhD, LAc

The teacher should never be concerned that a student might surpass him in ability; rather, the teacher should only worry that he doesn't guide the student well enough.

The process of learning is the root of discovery, so don't be hesitant about putting in the extra time and effort; in the end, you will realize it was worth it.

The more complex the pathocondition, the more imperative it is to provide an effective resolution. Though the etiology and pathomechanism may appear opaque at first, you must remain resolute in your efforts to accurately identify the pattern as the basis for administering the optimal treatment. That's the only way to advance the pursuit of scientific discovery and progress—continually striving to improve your fortitude and capacities in the art of medicine.

Dr. Lee Chen-Yu (李政育)

Dr. Lee Chen-Yu (李政育), OMD, LAc, PhD

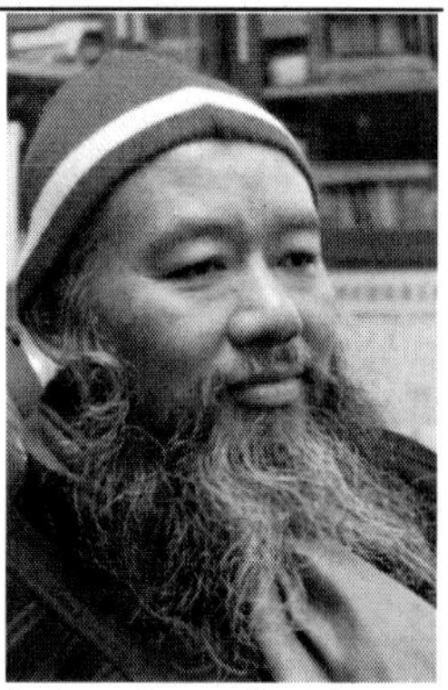

Dr. Lee Chen-Yu is an acclaimed traditional Chinese medicine physician who has practiced and conducted research for over 40 years. Renowned as a pioneering innovator at the forefront of integrative medicine, he is actively engaged in all specializations of clinical medicine. However, he is best known for his seminal research on neurology and oncology, receiving numerous U.S. patents for Chinese medicine formulas that promote nerve tissue regeneration and inhibit cancer cell growth. Dr. Lee is currently the Director of Yu Sheng Chinese Medicine Clinic (founded in 1980), and also serves as the Honorary Chairperson of the Taiwan Chinese-Western Medicine Neurology Association and Honorary PhD Advisor for Liaoning University of Traditional Chinese Medicine. He has authored more than 30 books, coauthored 10 others, written hundreds of professional papers, and been the subject of many masters and PhD dissertations. Dr. Lee has personally instructed hundreds of students from around the world and inspired the pursuit of new vistas in the applications of Chinese medicine.

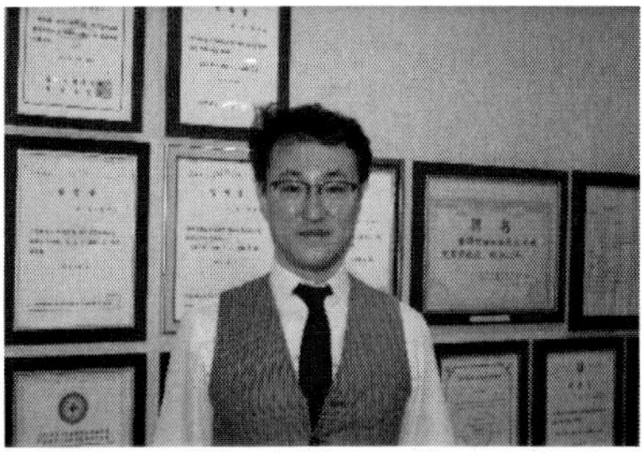

Dr. Juno Yang (梁珠勞), OMD, LAc, PhD

Dr. Juno Yang graduated from the prestigious College of Oriental Medicine at Kyung Hee University in 1998. He later went on to complete his Master of Science in Traditional Korean Medicine Pathology in 2003, and earned a PhD in Radiation Oncology from Ajou University in 2008. After his early years studying with Dr. Lee Chen-Yu, he has been very active writing innumerable professional papers, engaging in experimental research on integrative medicine, and presenting case studies at oriental medicine conferences worldwide. He has also authored three books titled Traditional Korean Medicine Therapies for Miscellaneous Diseases Vol. I (2008), Vol. II (2013), and Vol. III (2017). Dr. Yang is now the director of his own successful medical practice, Kyungheeyedang Oriental Medicine Clinic in Suwon City, near Seoul, South Korea.

ISBN: 978-0-9600303-1-6

TABLE OF CONTENTS

LIST OF CASE STUDIES

I. Respiratory Tract Disease

Section 1: Tearing on Exposure to Wind

Section 2: Reversal Cold Cough and Asthma

Section 3: Nose Piles (Nasal Polyp), Nosebleed (Epistaxis), and Chronic Sinusitis

Section 4: Other Respiratory Disorders

II. Vertigo

III. Liver Disease

Section 1: Hepatitis – Primary Cause of Liver Disease

Section 2: Hepatitis, Cirrhosis, and Liver Cancer

IV. Gastrointestinal Disorders

V. Musculoskeletal Disorders

VI. Neurological Disorders

Section 1: Facial Palsy and Trigeminal Neuralgia

Section 9: Paralysis

Section 10: Neuropathy of the Upper and Lower Extremities

VIII. Head Disorders

Section 1: Eye Disorders

Section 3: Periodontal Disease

IX. Male Genitourinary Disorders

X. Skin Disorders

Section 1: Rashes

Section 5: Blood Desiccation Itchy Skin

Section 6: Other Skin Diseases

ACKNOWLEDGEMENTS

Immeasurable appreciation and gratitude must be afforded to Dr. Lee Chen-Yu (李政育), whose unwavering guidance and dedication to his student's Dr. Juno Yang (梁珠勞), the compiler, translator, and author and editors of this series, and thousands of other aspiring traditional Chinese medicine (TCM) scholars and practitioners, has made this project possible.

Dr. Lee's nearly 40 years of clinical practice; clinical and laboratory research endeavors in both TCM treatment and integrative TCM and Western medicine; extensive affiliations and cooperation with Western medicine physicians; countless lectures, presentations, and papers; numerous books (both academic and mainstream); and health advocacy radio broadcast programs have reached out to touch the lives of millions of people worldwide. Much gratitude and respect must be given to Dr. Juno Yang, whose quest for knowledge and commitment to the clinical practice and research of TCM has made it possible for us to compile, translate and elucidate this invaluable material.

Further gratitude goes out to these fellow students and preceptees of Dr. Lee's: Frank Delaigue (an accomplished TCM practitioner with over 20 years of clinical experience) and Cyril Oswald (an aspiring TCM educator and practitioner), who together compiled and translated excerpts of this material for a French language book they co-authored titled *Les Hommes de l'Art*, which served as a valuable reference for this three-volume series; Dan Altschuler, EAMP, PhD (an acclaimed TCM educator and clinical practitioner with over 25 years of experience and currently a faculty member at the Seattle Institute of Oriental Medicine and Bastyr University), whose *Neuropathy: Traditional Chinese Herbal Treatment in a Modern Medical Environment* (English edition) served as a reference and inspiration for this book; and Chen, Ching-Hui (陳璟徽), OMD, MSc (aka "Big Brother Hui"), who has studied and served as an assistant of Dr. Lee's for nearly 30 years and has been an inexhaustible source of clarifying details about the clinical application of both TCM and integrated TCM and Western medicine.

Finally, a special thanks to Paulo Fonte, a talented physiotherapist and TCM practitioner, now practicing at Estoril Wellness Center in Estoril, Portugal, whose professionalism and optimism is always a motivating influence on everyone around; and Matthew Stampe, a massage therapist and TCM student at the Virginia University of Oriental Medicine, for providing critical analysis for these books.

FOREWORD

"The teacher should never be concerned that a student might surpass him in ability; rather, the teacher should only worry that he doesn't guide the student well enough." As a pupil of Dr. Lee's, this is something you hear him say often. He doesn't keep secrets and he'll gladly share all of his wisdom with those willing to make a sincere effort.

This book is an extension of his mission to spread knowledge and healing. Readers will face the same challenges as those traveling thousands of miles to study in his clinic. The knowledge available from the case studies in this collection provides limitless opportunity for gaining clinical experience and opens ongoing opportunities for the practical application of integrated traditional Chinese medicine (TCM) and Western medicine in our modern medical environment.

The familiar nature of the correspondences, the focus on difficult cases, the meticulous translation of source text, and the scrupulous compilation of supplemental material all make for an ideal ongoing learning companion. You'll find it challenging, often getting stuck with questions of your own. This is part of the learning process; it allows for exploration of concepts and growth of new ideas. Anyone who has studied and worked with Dr. Lee has gone through it. Be patient, clarify questions in your mind, and continually search for answers both in this text and beyond.

TCM has always been a system that grows and evolves with each generation. This book will give you a substantive framework to build upon and find your own ways to innovate. You'll see the way Dr. Lee has updated classical prescription formulas to serve as effective treatments for the severe and intractable diseases of our current times. The balance between classical wisdom and adapting to modern medical trends is his expertise.

If you were to step foot in his clinic, you'd see someone who has mastered his craft. You'd see his ability to diagnose and treat difficult cases. You'd see the comfort and guidance he provides to patients. And you'd see smiles on the faces of patients and staff. The brightness of his work compared to the gloominess of many medical settings speaks for itself.

I'm excited that this three-volume series makes a small part of the Yu Sheng Chinese Medicine Clinic available for everyone to experience.

Marc Wasserman PhD, LAc
September 2019

PREFACE

TCM Applications and Acceptance

Traditional Chinese medicine (TCM) continues resonating with potential—through a diversity of therapeutic modalities and vast pharmacopoeia, there are few limitations for its efficacy. The starkest limitations are from the institutional confines of academia and modern medicine in step with the pharmaceutical and insurance industries that seem more than often to be holding the reins. Of course, cultural factors also play a role in the acceptance of so-called "alternative" therapies, but based on the perpetual exchange of ideas, adaptation of peoples, and acculturation of societies throughout history, the viability and resounding efficacy of TCM has the persuasive power to overcome.

TCM Education and Status in Societies of Chinese (Han) Cultural Heritage

In societies influenced by Chinese culture (such as China, Taiwan, and South Korea) certified TCM (referred to as traditional Korean medicine (TKM) in South Korea) physicians are required to complete formal TCM medical school programs and pass national licensure examinations authorized by the respective nation's education oversight agency.

In China, 5- and 7-year bachelor's, master's, and doctoral programs are designed for students to receive a doctor of clinical medicine and doctor of integrated medicine, with the option of practicing both Western medicine and TCM and eligibility to take the respective national licensure examinations. In Taiwan, a 5-year post-baccalaureate and an 8-year bachelor's program are designed for students to receive a TCM degree in the former and the option of a dual degree in Western medicine and TCM in the latter, and eligibility to take the respective national licensure examinations. In South Korea, a 4-year post-baccalaureate and a 6-year bachelor's degree program are designed for students to receive a TKM degree and eligibility to take the national licensure examination.

The dual Western medicine and TCM degrees in China and Taiwan require students to fulfill all basic coursework in biomedicine and Western medicine specializations along with clinical internships in both Western medicine and TCM. For TCM (TKM) programs in Taiwan and South Korea, two-thirds of the curriculum focuses on coursework in basic biomedicine and specializations, comparative to the requirements for students in dentistry programs, and one-third on TCM, along with a clerkship in a Western medicine hospital and a clinical internship in the TCM department of a Western medicine hospital.

The relative emphasis on modern biomedicine and Western medicine specializations in the coursework load is balanced out by an intensive TCM curriculum that includes the classics and contemporary texts and their clinical applications. Based on my TCM academic pursuits in Taiwan and relationships with many TCM students, practitioners, and scholars, who have either received TCM educations or are educators themselves in countries such as China, South Korea, the United States, Australia, New Zealand, Israel, France, England, Switzerland, and Canada, I am confident that the depth and breadth of TCM curriculums in East Asian university TCM programs (at least in Taiwan, China, and South Korea) go far beyond that of TCM programs in other countries. To a large extent, this is due to an inherent cultural affinity that accepts this traditional medicine heritage as viable and effective.

There is no question that the institution of modern medicine is synonymous with Western medicine, but despite the enormous amount of funding and energies devoted to research and development, there are still glaring deficiencies. In Taiwan, China, and South Korea, this has opened up the opportunity for TCM to play a role as part of a unified medical system. Just as a major hospital may have dentistry and physiotherapy departments, they also have a TCM department. Indeed, this inclusion within the mainstream institution of modern medicine has in some ways been a boon, ensuring the perpetuation of this form of traditional medicine. However, there has been a price to pay with TCM serving a subservient role—recognized as more of a neoadjuvant, adjuvant, complementary, or palliative therapy—as opposed to primary and secondary care and first-line treatment.

There are still a few TCM physicians with clinical practices outside of the institutional healthcare system, who embrace the powers of integrated TCM and Western medicine, and have been able to achieve success at providing primary and secondary care and first-line treatment beyond the roles of adjuvant, complementary, and palliative therapy. Physicians such as Dr. Lee Chen-Yu (李政育), who have been dedicated to a lifetime of research, clinical practice, and educating, have gained due respect and elevated status within the medical community.

Backed by clinical experience and a thorough understanding of the advantages and disadvantages of Western medicine drugs and procedures, in certain cases Dr. Lee may advise patients to consult with their Western medicine physician about gradually reducing the dose and eventually discontinuing a given drug, or holding off on surgery if the side effects and potential complications outweigh the benefits—particularly if TCM offers a better therapeutic solution. Dr. Lee may also advise patients admitted to the hospital to receive a decocted TCM formula through their nasogastric (NG) tube, which requires both the consent of the patient (and/or family members) and the physician in charge.

Obviously, this type of consent and coordination requires a high degree of trust and communication. This poses significant challenges even in East Asian societies, with the legal ramifications that may arise if something unexpected happens. There is still a lot of work that needs to be done in establishing protocols and fostering universal acceptance. Evidence-based medicine research involving integrated TCM and Western medicine treatment is still sparse. However, based on both the results of evidence-based medicine studies and thousands of years of empirical clinical evidence, there is growing impetus towards recognizing the efficacy of TCM and integrated TCM and Western medicine in the treatment of a broad spectrum of diseases.

Know Your Medicinals and Define Your Paradigm

There is no single TCM medicinal or formula that *must* be administered for a specific symptom, pathocondition, or disease pattern. Classical and contemporary texts and the experience of mentors provide the foundations for the practitioner to clinically apply methodologies, but it is only through experience that dedicated physicians may develop their own paradigm. Medicinals of various properties and chemical constituents are grouped together in pairs and combinations—opposing and complementing, restraining and empowering, accentuating and corresponding—to form a formula composition whose overall action will resolve symptoms and promote the return and/or maintenance of homeostasis. In addition to personal preference based on clinical experience, a variety of factors may influence a TCM physician's selection of medicinals for a formula composition, such as availability, quality, price, storage, legal regulations, and patient preferences (taste, religion, customs, diet, etc.).

Medicinal processing plays an integral role in procuring the intended action, storage life, and mitigation of toxicity. If preparation methods are not tightly monitored and controlled, there could be potentially severe side effects (possibly even fatal). In times of antiquity, it was standard practice for TCM physicians to have their own raw medicinal processing facilities (or a close cooperative relationship with a licensed medicinal dispensary that specialized in preparing and processing medicinals) and dispensaries stocked with decocting pieces of their choice.

Nowadays, even in China, Taiwan, South Korea, and other Asian nations where TCM is a part of mainstream culture, the majority of physicians do *not* have their own processing facilities, and many do *not* even have onsite herbal dispensaries stocked with medicinal decocting pieces. Their medicinal dispensaries are more commonly stocked with medicinal extract powders/granules for the sake of convenience and regulatory oversight. In Taiwan, this is particularly prevalent, in part due to the National Health Insurance program (a single-payer system) that for the most part provides only *nominal* coverage for TCM treatment.

Dr. Lee is among the remaining TCM physicians who carry on the original spirit of the tradition, believing that you have to really "know your medicinals like the back of your hand" in order to fully utilize their best qualities, enhance their weaknesses, temper their volatilities, and harness the extent of their capacity for providing therapeutic efficacy.

Throughout the years, Dr. Lee's relationship with his pharmacopoeia has evolved as he continues to fine-tune his craft, modifying traditional formulas and designing his own to provide the optimal therapeutic regimen for his patients in Taiwan and across the globe. These formulas are referred to throughout the text, either explicitly or implicitly, as "(Yu Sheng)" formulas. Yu Sheng (育生 yù shēng)—literally meaning "the cultivation of life"—simply refers to the name of Dr. Lee's clinic.

Perspectives on the Four Examinations

The four examinations—*inspection*, *listening and smelling*, *inquiry*, and *palpation*—were first recorded in the Warring States period (475–221 BCE) nearly 2,500 years ago. Patient examinations are conducted to determine the correlation of all four examinations and then used to identify the pattern as the basis for determining treatment.

Depending on the type of symptoms, injury, and pathocondition, the four examinations are generally conducted in the following order: *inspection*—including the observation of skin, gait, mannerisms, complexion, color of stool and urine, and the tongue—offers an initial "look" at the patient and is the natural first step; *listening and smelling*—including the sound of speech and breath and the smell of the body, breath, and excretions—provides additional information and is the next natural step; *inquiry*—including patient history, chief complaint, diagnostic images, and lab test results—allows the physician to collect subjective and objective information and data about the patient's condition, which may often be the most valuable; and *palpation*—including touching and feeling the body to determine the presence of heat, tenderness, and accumulations, and also taking the pulse—enables the physician to get a "feel" for the patient's condition and is the last step.

As is often the case with experienced physicians, over the years Dr. Lee has developed a refined application of the four examinations with a keen sense for observing mannerisms, gait, skin manifestations, temperament, disposition, speech, and odor; discerning the nuances of history taking, performing abdominal palpation, and elucidating the significance of pulse.

Early on in Dr. Lee's clinical practice, he would rely on tongue examination much more, but throughout the years this reliance has diminished. He explained that the "natural" variations in size, color, texture, and fur among individuals, and the intake of food and beverages that stain the tongue and alter the appearance of the fur, make tongue examination an unreliable reference. In fact, if one observes Dr. Lee's patient interviews during consultations, you will notice that he rarely examines the tongue except for cases in which patients have pathology of the tongue or mouth proper.

Pulse-taking remains a hallmark of TCM examination and diagnostic protocol, and early on in Dr. Lee's clinical practice he authored a reputable academic book on this topic titled *Illustrated Traditional Chinese Medicine Pulse Reading* (圖解中醫脈學 *Tu Jie Zhong Yi Mai Xue*). Indeed, in its historical context pulse-taking is a vital source that opens up vistas into the discrete inner workings of the human body, revealing information about blood flow, volume, and viscosity; heart rate, cardiac output, and vascular patency; and the organs and physiological systems (endocrine system, autonomic nervous system, and central nervous system) of the entire body.

However, since the advent of modern biomedicine's diagnostic imaging and lab tests, which offer once unimaginable detail in its tangible images and quantitative data, the significance of pulse examination has in many regards been supplanted. This is compounded by the absence of a set, definable and quantifiable standard for interpreting the quality and nature of the pulse, with each individual potentially defining the *feeling* of a pulse differently. Though many well-intended TCM pratictioners and devout patients who still cling to the nostalgia may disagree with this assessment, in my opinion pulse-taking is a relatively ambiguous *art* to practice. It is even more difficult to communicate with others, as one pulse-taker's description of a particular pulse may not be the same as another's, even though they may actually be *feeling* the same pulse! However, this doesn't entirely relegate its usefulness for the individual practitioner as a reference for conducting pattern identification, but its subjectivity does limit its function as conveyed to other individuals.

Yet another factor is the widespread administration of Western medicine therapeutic agents for patients with established illnesses and as preventive care. Many of these drugs have a direct affect on the autonomic nervous system and endocrine system, which regulate cardiovascular blood flow and the feedback mechanisms affecting vasoconstriction and vasodilation. The near ubiquitous administration of pharmaceuticals in our modern society makes the "drug pulse" (藥脈 yào mài) phenomenon that much more of a challenge to objectively discern the *feeling* of a pulse.

That said, just as it was applied traditionally, Dr. Lee takes each patient's pulse, records the reading in the patient's medical record, and uses these readings as a baseline for subsequent patient examination. In certain cases where the pulse reading is noticeably inconsistent with the other examination results—presenting signs and symptoms, lab tests, and diagnostic imaging findings—then the pulse may play a vital role in pattern identification (e.g., accurately discerning true and false and complex patterns).

TCM Terminology and Usage

Readers familiar with TCM may know that there are several commonly used terminology systems employed in the translation and explanation of TCM concepts.

I began studying Chinese contemporary and classical texts on subjects such as literature, philosophy, and religion in 1991. Since 2001, I have been focusing energies on studying and practicing TCM. These pursuits have led me through a five-year postbaccalaureate program at a prominent Taiwanese medical teaching college with an affiliated hospital, pursuing studies of classical and contemporary texts in Chinese and English on my own, and also working professionally as a translator of Chinese language TCM texts.

Through these experiences, I have explored the use of the various 'systems,' mixed and matched various 'systems,' and created my own complementary interpretations. At first, this 'trial and error' approach seemed innocuous enough; after all, the objective is simply to get the idea across, right? Well, the more I began to analyze and realize the seamless congruity and irrefutable underlying logic of Prof. Nigel Wiseman's TCM terminology "system," the more I became persuaded to get on board and adopt this lexicon.

Prof. Wiseman's TCM lexicon is the only comprehensive, standardized "system" to date. I find that this system most accurately articulates the original meaning of the source text. Perhaps this particular system appeals to my bilingual sensibilities, providing insight into the underlying historical usage and context of classical terms and expressions used to explain and describe this traditional medical science throughout the millennia.

Naturally, there are limitations in any system, and I admit that some of the usage may seem awkward or unorthodox for those not familiar with the system. But as stated above, the advantages of congruity far outweigh the occasional ambiguity and archaic flavor. It is the comprehensive nature of this system that I believe is the best format to convey and advance the valuable medical insights and scientific methodology of TCM. It may require a bit of getting used to and looking up some terms at first, but in the end, I am confident you will discover the "rhyme to this reason."

INTRODUCTION

This book comprises the collection of fax and e-mail correspondence between Dr. Lee Chen-Yu (李政育), recognized as one of Taiwan's most accomplished and prominent traditional Chinese medicine (TCM) physicians, and his dedicated student Dr. Juno Yang (梁珠勞) from South Korea. Nearly 40 years of clinical experience and insights are made readily available through these clear and concise interactions, offering practical antidotes for the clinical application of integrated TCM and Western medicine.

In 2000, Dr. Yang came to study under the mentorship of Dr. Lee Chen-Yu at Yu Sheng Chinese Medicine Clinic in Taipei, Taiwan (ROC). Following this period of immersed clinical study, he returned to South Korea where he started his own TCM clinical practice, gradually honing his capacities over the years until becoming confident and competent in treating patients with complex and severe pathoconditions.

At the onset, Dr. Yang lacked experience and thus had a lot of questions about accurately diagnosing and effectively treating the broad scope of pathoconditions for which patients sought consultation. Thus, the student would correspond with his mentor by fax or e-mail seeking advice and guidance. Dr. Lee enjoyed sharing the knowledge gained from decades of study, research, and clinical experience, and further imparted the necessity for maintaining "a balance between prudence and confidence" and the importance of continuing education and developing professional capacities to make a positive impact on the lives of those depending on your medical assistance.

This regular correspondences between Dr. Lee (mentor) and Dr. Yang (student) took place from 2001 up until 2008, and consequently these interactions formed the content and outline for the conception of this book. Rather than presenting this correspondence in its original chronological order, the author has sorted and collated the material by grouping follow-up correspondences of specific patient's cases and associated pathological conditions together as well as modifying some of the letter formatting, making the presentation of each case study concise and informative. It contains troves of information on TCM pattern identification as the basis for determining treatment; clinical application of TCM medicinals, formulas, and acupuncture regimens; classical TCM pathologic terms and their correlating Western medicine pathological nomenclature; background information on symptoms, diagnostic tests, and treatment modalities; and keys to differential diagnosis and prognosis.

The sheer magnitude of this material warranted division into a three-volume series, of which, this is the second volume compiled and translated into English. *Volume II Surfaces in Motion* includes chapters on disorders of the lower respiratory tract (asthma, bronchitis, chronic obstruction pulmonary disease), upper respiratory tract (tearing on exposure to wind, sinusitis, nose piles), liver (hepatitis, cirrhosis, cancer), gastrointestinal tract (duodenal ulcers, appendicitis, constipation), musculoskeletal system (trigger finger, heel pain, osteoarthritis), nervous system (facial palsy, trigeminal neuralgia, herpes zoster, paresis, paresthesia, neuropathy, paralysis, vertigo), thyroid (hypothyroidism, hyperthyroidism, Hashimoto's thyroiditis, Graves' disease), eyes (Sjogren's syndrome, uveitis, conjunctivitis, epiphora, glaucoma), ears (tinnitus, chondritis, hearing impairment), gums (gingivitis, periodontitis, pyorrhea), male genitourinary system (erectile dysfunction, benign prostatic hyperplasia), and skin (urticaria, pompholyx, warts, seborrheic dermatitis, atopic dermatitis, xerosis).

A wide range of other pathological conditions were presented in *Volume I Beyond the Being* and more will be published in the upcoming *Volume III Roots of Life* of this series. The compilation of case studies in this three-volume series covers the gamut of pathologies: oncology, neurology, orthopedics, pulmonology, dermatology, gastroenterology, hepatology, nephrology, endocrinology, cardiology, rheumatology, gynecology and obstetrics, urology, pediatrics, otorhinolaryngology, ophthalmology, hematology, metabolic disorders, proctology, palliative care, infectious diseases, and psychological and psychiatric conditions.

By no means does this book attempt to present a comprehensive analysis of all the pathological conditions TCM is capable of treating, either independently or through Western medicine integration. Its precept stems from the candid correspondence and guidance between a promising TCM physician (student) and an innovative spirit at the forefront of integrative TCM and Western medicine development (mentor). The scope of the pathological conditions and the descriptions of the cases presented here are simply derived from the questions a dedicated student has asked seeking guidance from his mentor.

The reader should not expect an unabridged, pedagogical explanation for all of these pathoconditions. However, the compiler, translator, and author has made extensive efforts to insert further details and descriptions, including etiology, pathomechanisms, pattern identification, underlying theoretical concepts, medicinal actions, pharmaceuticals, and therapeutic procedures, of topics discussed in these correspondences in hopes of providing more informative and authoritative content.

This material will serve as a valuable reference source for practical application—a catalyst that inspires the TCM practitioner to continue applying and integrating the classical traditions within our modern biomedical environment—and an insightful medium for those interested in learning about the vast potential for both the clinical applications of TCM and integrative TCM and Western medicine therapeutic approaches.

UNIT CONVERTER

In this text, doses of medicinals are given in the traditional Chinese units (fen/qian/liang/jin). This measuring system may be initially less familiar to the Western reader than the metric system commonly used nowadays. Despite this initial learning curve, I have chosen to preserve this element of the text with the consideration of honoring the traditional way still practiced in the East. This unified system also provides a simple reading experience and avoids the need for in-text conversions or decimal points.

The gram (g) equivalencies are as follows:

1 fen = 0.375 g
1 qian (10 fen) = 3.75 g
1 liang (10 qian) = 37.5 g
1 jin (16 liang) = 600 g

I. RESPIRATORY TRACT DISEASES

Cases involving lung cancer and its complications were introduced in Volume I: *Beyond the Being* of this series and thus will not be addressed here. This chapter will focus on the most common ailments presenting in TCM clinical practice including tearing on exposure to wind, reversal cold cough, asthma, nose piles (nasal polyp), and tuberculosis (TB).

Section 1: Tearing on Exposure to Wind

Case Study #1: Sneezing, Runny Nose, and Nasal Congestion

Q: A mother brought in her 12 y/o son who has suffered from severe nasal congestion (especially in the left nostril) since he was only 2 years old. This appeared to be a classic case of tearing on exposure to wind (rhinitis). He has been through the gamut of various Western medicine treatments (oral medication, injections, and surgery), but nothing has proven effective. I prescribed a heavy dose of Ma Huang (6 qian) adding Rou Gui (1 liang), and Fu Zi and Gan Jiang (3 qian each) without significant improvement.

This case confuses me because I have effectively treated many tearing on exposure to wind cases similar to this using the same approach. Do you have any ideas why this formula wouldn't be effective for this youngster? I suspect there may be more to this case than meets the eye. Since the patient only complains of chronic congestion in the left nostril, I am wondering if this could be caused by deviated nasal septum or nasal polyps. Please help me resolve this conundrum.

A: In addition to sneezing and runny nose (nasal discharge), tearing on exposure to wind (迎風落淚 yíng fēng luò lèi) also presents with nasal congestion. But obviously nasal congestion can present in many different conditions, such as olfactory nerve palsy, allergic reactions resulting in engorgement (hyperemia) and mucosal hypertrophy of the nasal membranes, and nasal polyps or deviated nasal septum that blocks drainage from a sinus into the nasal cavity. It's common for a person even without any nasal problems to alternate nostrils when breathing through the nose. A deviated nasal septum and nasal polyps would have been clearly diagnosed by an otolaryngologist. It sounds to me like your patient has simply gotten used to relying on his right nostril to breathe, so you need to find a way to break through the barrier in order to resolve his condition.

As for treatment, you can prescribe You Gui Yin adding medicinals such as Ma Huang, Xi Xing, Xing Yi, Sang Bai Pi, Cang Er Zi, and Chuan Xiong along with Ren Shen/Chuan Qi Powder and Yu Sheng Wan. Additionally, I would examine the color of the nasal membrane using a small flashlight, and if it is bright red or purplish red, then this indicates hyperemia which can be identified as blood heat with exterior pattern, requiring the addition of Huang Qin (large doses) to the main formula.

Perform acupuncture on the acupoints Feng Chi (GB20), Ying Xiang (LI20) joining Jing Ming (UB1), Wan Gu (GB12), Feng Fu (DU16), and Shang Xing (DU23). Determination of needle manipulation technique, warm needling (moxa cones applied on needle handle), and/or application of adhesive moxa cubes applied directly on the skin should be based on presenting signs, symptoms and pattern identification. For the congested left nostril, you can also consider performing massage adjacent to the base of the nostril ipsilaterally and needling the acupoint Ju Liao (ST3) perpendicularly at a depth of approximately 5 fen. You should achieve effective results by applying this approach.

Case Study #2: What is Tearing on Exposure to Wind?

Q: Many of my patients present with symptoms of chronic rhinitis. I know you often diagnose this type of pathocondition as tearing on exposure to wind. Can you explain your reasoning for this?

A: My use of the term tearing on exposure to wind (迎風落淚 yíng fēng luò lèi) is based on the classical TCM pathologic term that describes a condition in which exposure to cold air induces sneezing, nasal discharge, and post-nasal drip, which can further irritate the lacrimal drainage system apparati. Upstream, the lacrimal ducts may become lax and lose the capacity to regulate the flow of tears produced by the lacrimal gland; and downstream, the lacrimal puncta of the superior and inferior lacrimal canals may become clogged and lose the capacity to let the tears flow out. Both of these scenarios will result in profuse tearing (epiphora).

These are the classic symptoms of rhinitis (both nonallergic and allergic types) and can also present in other pathoconditions of the sinuses such as sinusitis, nasoseptal deviation, and nosebleeds. Many people experience the symptoms encompassing tearing on exposure to wind upon sudden exposure to cold air or in cold environments.

In addition to the classical presentation of tearing on exposure to wind symptoms, allergic rhinitis is often accompanied by conjunctivitis and itchy eyes. Long-standing nasal congestion may cause headaches that affect concentration and memory and negatively impact academic and work efficiency. Long-standing rhinorrhea and post-nasal drip can irritate the throat leading to complications of chronic pharyngitis, tonsillitis, bronchitis, and otitis media.

Prevention involves keeping warm, and most importantly, protecting your nasal membranes from direct exposure to cold air with a scarf or hygienic mask. Get out in the sunshine, especially the morning and late afternoon when the UV rays aren't so intense. You can also eat acrid (cool acrid, warm acrid, and hot-spicy acrid) and aromatic foods such as onions, ginger, garlic, chili, basil, mint and pepper. And of course, getting plenty of sleep so the body can sufficiently restore and replenish itself will also be helpful in alleviating symptoms.

Case Study #3: Prescribe You Gui Yin Instead!

Q: A 38 y/o female patient has a 15-year history of tearing on exposure to wind. Recently, exposure to even a slight breeze will induce tearing. There is no external contraction (common cold) presenting. I prescribed Bu Zhong Yi Qi Tang along with Xiao Qing Long Tang. Do you think this is the right approach?

A: Tearing on exposure to wind is more prevalent in northern regions with cold climates. South Korea has cold temperatures and it snows a lot in the winter so there will inevitably be many of these types of patients. Yes, you can prescribe the spleen-fortifying qi-supplementing yang-upbearing formula Bu Zhong Yi Qi Tang combining the exterior-resolving rheum-eliminating formula Xiao Qing Long Tang. But based on my experience, a kidney yang-warming and -supplementing formula variant such as You Gui Yin will be more effective!

According to classical TCM theory, north is associated with the kidney, so regardless of the formula you choose, make sure to include The Three Great Yang-Supplementers, Ma Huang, Bai Zhi, Xi Xin, Ban Xia, and Wu Wei Zi. Another possibility would be to prescribe Xiao Qing Long Tang adding Fu Zi and Huang Qin or Ma Huang Fu Zi Xi Xin Tang variant.

Case Study #4: Tearing on Exposure to Wind – Purulent Nasal Discharge

Q: This patient has a 10-year history of intermittent tearing on exposure to wind with profuse purulent discharge every time an episode occurs. I prescribed (Yu Sheng) Tearing on Exposure to Wind Formula adding Zi Yuan, Kuan Dong Hua, Fu Zi, Cǎng Er Zi, and Xin Yi. The treatment was effective at first, but then it seemed to level off without further progress towards fully remedying the condition. Please offer your advice and guidance.

A: Typically, if the Tearing on Exposure to Wind Formula (boosts qi and fortifies the spleen, moves qi and transforms phlegm, resolves the exterior and frees the nasal orifices, and dispels wind and dissipates cold) shows initial efficacy, but then levels off, you can consider adding large doses of the The Three Great Yang-Supplementers (incrementally increasing the doses up 5 to 8 qian each), Bai Zhi (8 qian), and large doses of Ma Huang (incrementally increasing the dose up until it affects the patient's sleep, and then bring it down a bit, to where sleep is unaffected – that's the maximum optimal dose!).

However, for this type of tearing on exposure to wind patient presenting with profuse purulent discharge, you must also consider chronic infection of the sinus cavities (chronic sinusitis). You can continue prescribing your original formula variant, subtracting Zi Yuan and Kuan Dong Hua and adding Huang Qin (large dose), Lai Fu Zi, Sang Bai Pi, and He Ye. Or, you could change the formula to a heat-clearing phlegm-transforming formula such as Wen Dan Tang or a Shao Yang-harmonizing and resolving formula such as Xiao Chai Hu Tang (both including large doses of Huang Qin) adding Ma Huang, Bai Zhi, Lai Fu Zi, Sang Bai Pi, and He Ye.

Remember! The presentation of purulent discharge indicates heat pattern, so regardless of the formula chosen, you should include heat-clearing medicinals such as Huang Qin, Lai Fu Zi, Sang Bai Pi, and He Ye.

Case Study #5: Dilated Vessels on Cheeks – Is Gui Ma Ge Ban Tang Effective?

Q: At the age of 3 years old, this girl, who is now 10 years old, initially began having extended episodes of tearing on exposure to wind symptoms after being outdoors in the cold wind. In addition to presenting with nasal congestion and discharge, frequent exposure to cold wind during the winter months results in extended episodes of reddish cheeks (i.e., dilated blood vessels in the outer layer of her skin (windburn)) and slightly swollen hands (i.e., inflammation of small blood vessels in the skin (chilblains)). I prescribed Gui Ma Ge Ban Tang variant. Do you think this is a good approach?

A: Prescribing a fleshy exterior-harmonizing and evil-expelling itch-relieving formula such as Gui Ma Ge Ban Tang variant is one option; and if it's not effective at first, then try adding Gan Jiang, Fu Zi, Huang Qin, Bai Zhu, and Ze Xie. You could also consider changing to a blood-nourishing network vessel-freeing and cold-dissipating counterflow-downbearing formula such as Dang Gui Si Ni Jia Wu Zhu Yu Sheng Jiang Tang adding Gan Jiang, Fu Zi, Bai Zhu, Fu Ling, and Ze Xie; or a kidney yang-warming and -supplementing formula such as You Gui Yin adding Ma Huang, Bai Zhu, and Ze Xie. The problem with Wu Zhu Yu is that many people find it unpalatable, and if this is the case, then you can use Shan Zhu Yu instead.

Case Study #6: Auricular Acupuncture – It's Effective!

Q: I have been experimenting with various acupuncture methods for the treatment of tearing on exposure to wind and have found that auricular acupuncture consistently offers better efficacy with faster results. Shortly after insertion the symptoms of runny nose begins to resolve and the nasal passages open up. This approach has also proven effective for insomnia, plum-pit qi (梅核氣 méi hé qì), and external contraction (the common cold) in children, with results manifesting more quickly than needling body acupoints.

The downside is that in some patients symptoms may relapse soon after removing the auricular intradermal needles (ear press tacks), and there is also the uncertainty about just how many ear press tacks should be inserted and at which points. Overall, auricular acupuncture offers a simple and effective method and may be the best option for those patients who don't feel comfortable having acupoints, such as

Ying Xiang (LI20), needled on the face. Maybe you can give it a try and see how it works for you!

A: Congratulations on your clinical discoveries! I will give auricular acupuncture for the treatment of tearing on exposure to wind, plum-pit qi, insomnia, and the common cold in children a try.

The easiest way I have found for improving tearing on exposure to wind is advising the patient to simply wear a hat and get healthy doses of sunlight and exercise (especially under the mild rays of the sun). It is also important to get enough sleep (ideally 8–10 hours/day) and best if the room you sleep in gets sunlight.

As for TCM formula treatment, you must differentiate between exterior wind-heat and exterior wind-cold pattern. For *exterior wind-heat* pattern, you can prescribe sweat-effusing exterior-resolving and lung-diffusing wind-dispelling formula variants such as Da Qing Long Tang, Ma Huang Tang, Gui Zhi Tang, and Yang Dan Tang; or a heat-clearing phlegm-transforming formula such as Wen Dan Tang adding Ma Huang, Xi Xin, and Lai Fu Zi. For *exterior wind-cold* pattern, you can prescribe either Tearing on Exposure to Wind Formula adding The Three Great Yang-Supplementers; or You Gui Yin adding Ma Huang, Bai Zhi, Xi Xin, Ban Xia, and Wu Wei Zi. For male patients in particular, You Gui Yin has proven the most effective in my clinical experience.

Section 2: Reversal Cold Cough and Asthma

Case Study #1: Chronic Dry Cough – "Has Lingered on Forever"

Q: A 48 y/o female beautician explained that 3 years ago exposure to cold wind resulted in catching a common cold (external contraction), which she said "has lingered on forever" without being completely remedied. Every time she washes her hands in cold water or works with customers she coughs (a dry cough absent of heat or phlegm). Thus, I decided to harmonize the center, relax tension, move qi, and downbear counterflow by prescribing Gan Mai Da Zao Tang Combining Ban Xia Hou Po Tang. Unfortunately, this approach has not been very effective. Do you have any suggestions?

A: It sounds to me like this patient may have developed asthma, which in this case can be identified as reversal cold (厥冷 jué lěng) cough with yin vacuity pattern. I would consider prescribing a qi-boosting spleen-fortifying and qi-moving phlegm-transforming formula such as (Yu Sheng) Asthma Formula, Xiao Qing Long Tang, or She Gan Ma Huang Tang adding Gan Jiang, Fu Zi, Wu Zhu Yu, Qing Hao, Zhi Mu, Di Gu Pi, and Huang Qin. Personally, I think (Yu Sheng) Asthma Formula would be the most effective, and considering that Ren Shen is so widely available in Korea, I might also prescribe Ren Shen (powder) for the patient to take along with the decoction.

Case Study #2: Asthma Attacks – "I Can't Lie Down Flat!"

Q: A 53 y/o female patient has a 20-year history of asthma with severe aversion to heat. She frequently drinks cold beverages, and in recent years, has put on weight, which she says has seemed to exacerbate her asthma symptoms. She has shortness of breath (dyspnea) and wheezing (no sound of phlegm), and the worst part is not being able to get a good night's sleep because, as she explained, "I can't lie down flat!"

Over the years, she has tried various treatment methods (TCM, Western medicine, folk remedies), but none have been effective at ultimately remedying her condition and preventing asthma attacks. When flare-ups do occur, her only option has been relying on bronchodilators and steroids. What do you think is the best therapeutic approach for this patient?

A: The best approach for this patient with a 20-year history of asthma is to prescribe formula variants such as (Yu Sheng) Asthma Formula or You Gui Yin, making sure that you include Gan Jiang, Fu Zi, Ma Huang, Xing Ren, Bai Guo, Huang Qin, Zi Yuan, and Kuan Dong Hua. If this approach isn't effective, then add Hu Tao, Bu Gu Zhi, Mai Men Dong, and Wu Wei Zi; and if her condition still doesn't improve, then add Ha Jie, The Three Great Yang-Supplementers (incrementally increasing the doses over time), and Ren Shen (powder).

Typically, for this type of patient, I would start out with a 3 qian dose of Ma Huang, incrementally increasing the dose up until it affects the patient's sleep, and then bring it down a bit, until sleep is unaffected—that's the maximum optimal dose! If aversion to heat presents, then you can add Sheng Shi Gao, which together with the other medicinals will equip your formula with the lung-diffusing heat-discharging actions of Ma Xing Gan Shi Tang.

As for your patient's wheezing, this is likely due to the narrowing of airway passages resulting from either fibrosis (scarring) or hypertrophy (thickening). Inability to lie down flat could simply result from the extra pressure on the lungs from the distribution of gravity on the chest, causing the patient to cough and be more susceptible to flare-ups. At the onset, an integrated TCM and Western medicine therapeutic approach should be employed. Once the condition stabilizes, gradually reduce the use of inhaled corticosteroids, eventually progressing towards complete discontinuation. Next, gradually reduce the dosage and eventually discontinue the use of bronchodilators.

Remember! This treatment entails a gradual process that takes time and patience with results appearing as the regimen progresses. Magical results just won't pop up overnight. You must make sure the patient understands this!

Case Study #3: Lingering Cough Producing White Frothy Phlegm – Clinical Perspectives

Q: About 3 years ago, a 43 y/o male patient developed a cough with white frothy phlegm (sputum) that persists to this day. There were *no* abnormal sounds on auscultation and urine and stool were normal. Previously, he had been taking Western medicine drugs for several years without effective results. I prescribed (Yu Sheng) Asthma Formula variant, but the results weren't very effective either, so I added yang-supplementing medicinals, which still hasn't produced noticeable results. How would you approach this case?

A: In the treatment of lingering cough, you must distinguish when the cough occurs and whether there are any precipitating factors that increase the severity of the cough. Is the cough more severe in the daytime or at night when the patient is lying down? Do fumes from cooking or tobacco smoke precipitate coughing?

If cough is more pronounced in the daytime and induced by smoky odors, then you should consider prescribing a qi-boosting spleen-fortifying and qi-moving phlegm-transforming formula such as (Yu Sheng) Asthma Formula (including slightly larger doses of Ma Huang) adding yin vacuity heat-clearing and yin-enriching dryness-moistening medicinals like Qing Hao, Zhi Mu, and Di Gu Pi. If cough is more pronounced at night and night sweating presents, then you should prescribe an yin-enriching lung- and stomach-nourishing and counterflow-downbearing qi-precipitating formula variant such as (Yu Sheng) Mai Men Dong Tang. If sticky phlegm presents, then prescribe a heat-clearing phlegm-transforming formula variant such as Wen Dan Tang.

If white frothy phlegm presents, such as in the case of your patient, you must consider phlegm resulting from psychosomatic disorder (e.g., stress, anxiety) or water flood (水泛 shuǐ fàn). For psychosomatic disorder, you may consider prescribing a qi-moving counterflow-downbearing and stagnation-dissipating phlegm-transforming formula variant such as Gan Mai Da Zao Tang Combining Ban Xia Hou Po Tang or Ban Xia Tian Ma Bai Zhu San. For water flood, you can prescribe an exterior-resolving rheum-eliminating and cough-suppressing panting-calming formula such as Xiao Qing Long Tang or She Gan Ma Huang Tang in combination with either Xiang Sha Liu Jun Zi Tang (boosts the stomach and supplements the center, for spleen yang vacuity water flood pattern) or Shen Qi Wan (supplements the kidney and assists yang, for kidney yang vacuity water flood pattern).

Remember! Don't overlook the possibility of pulmonary tuberculosis (TB). During South Korea's cold winters people keep their windows sealed tight and spend most of their time indoors making it easier to contract TB from others. TB typically presents with signs and symptoms of late afternoon tidal heat (fever), night sweating, tidal reddening of the cheeks, and red lips; however, in some cases, there aren't any discernible symptoms, just an occasional cough. If your patient has contracted TB, then you can consider prescribing an yin-enriching fire-downbearing steaming bone-eliminating formula variant such as Zhi Bo Di Huang Tang, Ba Xian Chang Shou Wan, Bai He Gu Jin Tang, or Qin Jiao Bie Jia San, making sure to include Qing Hao, Zhi Mu, Di Gu Pi, Chai Hu, Xuan Shen, Tian Men Dong, and Mai Men Dong.

Case Study #4: Hemoptysis – Interstitial Pneumonia or Pulmonary Tuberculosis?

Q: A 36 y/o male patient explained that 4 years ago he began coughing up small amounts of bright red blood-streaked sputum, prompting him to get examined at a hospital that resulted in inconclusive results. Since the initial onset, he has had occasional episodes of profuse phlegm and phlegm containing streaks of blood, and has been taking antibiotics, bronchodilators, and hemostatic drugs prescribed by a pulmonologist. On one occasion when his symptoms suddenly worsened, he had a CT scan and endoscopy performed, revealing bronchiectasis in the lower segments of both lungs and a 2 cm opacity at the center of the left lung that was diagnosed as benign.

Showing no improvement despite long-term treatment, last year his doctors discontinued the previous medication and prescribed an anti-tuberculosis drug instead. In February this year, the patient began expectorating increased amounts of sputum and every morning he would cough up a clot of blood the size of a thumbnail. Two weeks ago, while lying down in bed he noticed the smell of blood and then coughed up 10 cc of fresh blood. A CT scan performed two days later did not reveal any signs of bleeding. The patient explained he has a family history of lung disease with his grandfather dying from complications of emphysema and asthma. Recently, the patient has occasionally experienced night sweating in the upper half of his body, has lost weight (5 kg), feels like there is more congestion in both lungs, and worries that he may have pulmonary tuberculosis (TB). I suspect interstitial pneumonia. Please offer your guidance and advice on this case. Thank you!

A: Chronic cough with hemoptysis and the patient is only 36 y/o, it must be a result of either pneumonia or pulmonary tuberculosis (TB), scarring lung tissue over time and leading to pulmonary fibrosis.

As for TCM treatment, you can consider prescribing a vacuity-heat clearing yin-enriching and lung-moistening phlegm-transforming formula such as Bai He Gu Jin Tang or Ba Xian Chang Shou Wan adding combinations of yin-nourishing vacuity heat-clearing, steaming bone-eliminating, blood-cooling, and blood-stanching medicinals such as Qing Hao, Zhi Mu, Di Gu Pi, Chuan Qi, Bai Ji, Ou Jie, Ce Bo Ye, Mu Dan Pi, and Zhi Zi. And since South Korea grows a lot of Bei Sha Shen (Coastal Glehnia Root, Radix Glehniae) you can advise the patient to consume at least 1 liang of fresh Bei Sha Shen daily (if accessible and economically feasible, 3–5 liang would be even better!). Also, if traditional Si Gua Luo (Loofah, Loofae Fructus Retinervus) and Ju Luo (Tangerine Pith, Citri Reticulatae Fructus Fasciculus Vascularis) can be obtained, advise him to boil them in water and drink as a beverage; or simply eat tangerines including the pith. This therapeutic regimen will effectively remedy hemoptysis.

Once the bleeding has been stanched, the patient should continue taking TCM medicinals up until he either incurs 2–3 common colds (external contraction) or gets through an entire winter free from cough with blood-streaked sputum. That's when you know it is time to gradually discontinue administration of TCM medicinals and the patient has been cured.

The patient should not worry too much about a family history of emphysema. Some people may have a genetic predisposition to emphysema and other associated diseases (e.g., cirrhosis) due to alpha-1-antitrypsin (AAT) deficiency. However, this autosomal recessive pathocondition is exceedingly rare, and if necessary, the patient can be tested to rule this out. If you are concerned about longstanding lung disease leading to complications of interstitial lung disease or emphysema, then you can also add Qin Jiao and Chai Hu to your formula.

Case Study #5: Pulmonary Tuberculosis Presenting with Lumbar Pain

Q: A 33 y/o female patient was diagnosed with a lumbar herniated disc 6 years ago. This condition has still not been adequately remedied and now she has a noticeable postural shift to the left in her lumbar region. One year ago, she became infected with *Mycobacterium tuberculosis* and was administered anti-TB medication for 7 months without any improvement in her symptoms. Recent follow-up tests still indicated TB (+) and her lower back pain has persisted. Do you think this lumbar pain is simply a result of previous physical injury or could it be spinal tuberculosis? What should the focus of treatment be?

A: Hum!...pulmonary tuberculosis (TB) presenting with lumbar pain and lateral shift to the left. You cannot rule out the possibility of tuberculosis of the spine (TB may cause deviated eyes and mouth (facial palsy) as well!).

The focus of treatment should definitely be on TB, selecting an array of yin vacuity heat-clearing steaming bone-eliminating and yin-nourishing dryness moistening medicinals. I would consider prescribing a formula such as Zhi Bo Di Huang Tang, Ba Xian Chang Shou Wan, Xiao Chai Hu Tang, Mai Men Dong Tang, or Bai He Gu Jin Tang adding combinations of medicinals such as Huang Bo, Zhi Mu, Qing Hao, Di Gu Pi, Xuan Shen, Sha Shen, Sheng Du Zhong, The Three Insects, and possibly Huang Qi. The key medicinals here are Huang Bo, Zhi Mu, Qing Hao, and Di Gu Pi (large doses of each), which will provide effective treatment for both TB and herniated disc (as well as facial palsy resulting from TB).

You can also consider administering acupuncture treatment. For the lumbar pain and lateral shift (as well as deviated eyes and mouth (facial palsy)), it's best to apply warm needling (adhesive moxa cubes applied directly on the skin in the case of facial palsy). To treat the *Mycobacterium tuberculosis* infection proper, it's best to select the acupoints San Yin Jiao (SP6), Tai Chong (LV3), Yin Ling Quan (SP9), Fei Shu (UB13), Shen Men (HT7), Chi Ze (LU5), and Shen Shu (UB23), while applying neutral supplementation and drainage manipulation. Through this dual approach, the patient can anticipate a complete cure within 3–6 months.

Remember! For patients with TB, it would be perfectly fine for the patient to consider taking Western medicine drugs (especially if administered at the onset), with this concomitant therapeutic regimen likely providing even better overall efficacy.

Case Study #6: Recurrent Tuberculosis and Sequelae

Q: Eight months ago a 50 y/o female patient began experiencing frequent night sweating, crackling sounds in the chest when lying down, persistent bouts of coughing, and occasionally coughed up blood-streaked sputum. After undergoing an examination, she was diagnosed with bronchiectasis and administered Western medicine drugs for a long period of time without much improvement. That's when she decided to give TCM a try.

The patient provided the following medical history: She was infected with pulmonary tuberculosis (TB) about 30 years ago. At that time, she had symptoms of night sweating and phlegm-heat, was diagnosed with TB, took anti-TB drugs for 3 years, and discontinued the drug treatment once the follow-up TB test was confirmed negative. Do you think the diagnosis of bronchiectasis is accurate? Could it be recurrent tuberculosis?

A: Frequent night sweating and coughing up blood-streaked sputum suggests that the patient may suffer from either recurrent tuberculosis (TB), reinfection with a new strain of *Mycobacterium tuberculosis*, or manifestations of TB sequelae such as fibrosis, bronchostenosis, and bronchiectasis. From your description of the patient's history and symptoms, it sounds more like a case of recurrent TB to me, but the same TCM therapeutic approach will apply for either of these possibilities.

I would consider prescribing a formula variant such as Zhi Bo Di Huang Tang, Ba Xian Chang Shou Wan, Bai He Gu Jin Tang, Qin Jiao Bie Jia San, or Mai Men Dong Tang. Regardless of which formula you choose, it is essential to include yin vacuity heat-clearing and yin-nourishing dryness moistening medicinals such as Zhi Mu, Huang Bo, Qing Hao, Di Gu Pi, Tian Men Dong, Mai Men Dong, Xuan Shen, and Sha Shen. For blood-streaked sputum, add Ou Jie and Ce Bo Ye; and if the patient has loose stools, add Fu Ling and Cang Zhu. Of course, you could also consider performing acupuncture as well, needling acupoints such as San Yin Jiao (SP6), Tai Chong (LV3), Yin

Ling Quan (SP9), Fei Shu (UB13), Shen Men (HT7), Chi Ze (LU5), and Shen Shu (UB23).

After administering this therapeutic regimen for a period of time, if a severe cough persists, then add Ma Huang (a small dose initially, incrementally increasing if necessary) and Xing Ren. Prescribed in combination with large doses of yin-nourishing medicinals Ma Huang's acrid flavor and warm nature will not counteract the formula's overall action of effectively remedying yin vacuity lung dryness and night sweating.

Remember! You must administer the yin vacuity heat-clearing and yin-nourishing dryness-moistening medicinals for a minimum of 6 months to 1 year. Even when the patient's condition has been completely remedied, it is prudent to administer TCM medicinals for a period of time during the autumn each year as a way of regulating the constitution (dry weather increases susceptibility for cough!). The only way to ensure that the *Mycobacterium tuberculosis* infection has been relegated to an inactive state is to administer TCM medicinals for a long duration. Don't fool yourself or let the patient fool herself into thinking that just because symptoms have resolved TCM medicinals can be abruptly discontinued!

Case Study #7: Spontaneous Pneumothorax

Q: A 23 y/o male patient explained that 2 years ago he suffered from spontaneous pneumothorax while serving his compulsory military service and subsequently has incurred symptoms of chest pain and shortness of breath, which fluctuate in severity. Most TCM etiology and pathomechanism textbooks and case study material I have referenced identify pneumothorax as qi vacuity pattern. Why do you identify this condition as yin vacuity pattern?

A: Primary spontaneous pneumothorax occurs due to the formation of small air pockets in lung tissue called blebs that rupture and result in air leaking into the pleural space. Secondary spontaneous pneumothorax is caused by brittle alveoli that have lost their elasticity and thus can be identified as lung yin vacuity pattern. A simple analogy is a ping pong ball that is made from two interfacing halves of a sphere: if these two halves aren't hermetically sealed and air gets inside the ball, then the ball either loses its bounce or will not bounce as high.

Spontaneous pneumothorax most commonly occurs in patients with damaged lung tissue resulting from either previous or existing lung disease (e.g., pulmonary tuberculosis (TB), chronic obstructive pulmonary disease (COPD), cystic fibrosis, and pneumonia), people with a history of spontaneous pneumothorax or hemothorax, and in patients who have undergone surgery, chemotherapy, or radiotherapy for lung cancer. Even if an underlying condition may appear to have been completely cured, years later when the patient gets older and tissues lose their elasticity, spontaneous pneumothorax could occur again.

If the pneumothorax is mild, with only a small amount of air leaking into the pleural space, and there are merely symptoms of chest distention and/or aching pain, then you can prescribe a heat-clearing phlegm-damp-transforming water-disinhibiting formula such as Chai Ling Tang or Xiao Chai Hu Tang adding Qing Hao, Zhi Mu, Di Gu Pi, Ma Huang, Xuan Shen, and Xing Ren. Even if the patient's condition is more serious, with large amounts of air building up in the pleural space, but it still is *not* necessary to insert a chest tube or the facilities for inserting a chest tube are *not* available, then you can prescribe a formula variant such as Chai Ling Tang or Ling Gui Zhu Gan Tang.

Remember! For pneumothorax, add large doses of Fu Ling; and for hemothorax, add large doses of Bai Ji, Chuan Qi, and The Three Yellows. You can also take advantage of the abundance of homegrown Bei Sha Shen in South Korea by advising your pneumothorax patients and those whom have suffered lung tissue damage to use Sha Shen like a fresh vegetable, cooking it up with other foods in tasty dishes!

Case Study #8: Chronic Obstructive Pulmonary Disease – Emphysema and Bronchiectasis

Q: I have a male elderly patient who explained that he has had symptoms of cough with production of sputum for many years, and laying down flat results in shortness of breath (panting) and cough. I suspect the patient suffers from chronic obstructive pulmonary disease (COPD). Can I prescribe yang-supplementing medicinals for this condition? Do you think prescribing She Gan Ma Huang Tang combining Wen Dan Tang is a good approach?

A: Wen Dan Tang can be prescribed for treating patients with yellow, sticky phlegm, which can be identified as phlegm-heat with repletion heat or residual heat pattern, whereas She Gan Ma Huang Tang treats watery phlegm and frog rale in the throat (喉中水雞聲 hóu zhōng shuǐ jī shēng), which can be identified as cold rheum lying depressed in the lung (寒飲鬱肺 hán yǐn yù fèi). You must differentiate the consistency and color of the patient's phlegm. How about appetite? Is there edema? And if edema presents, then add The Four Lings for best results. Does the patient wheeze or cough up blood?

Typically, COPD starts out as chronic bronchitis and may progress to *emphysema* (irreversible bronchial narrowing and alveolar hyperinflation that may lead to loss of diffusion area) or possibly *bronchiectasis* (irreversible dilation in the bronchioles caused by inflammation that leads to mucous plugging and progressive airway destruction).

If the patient presents with chronic cough, severe dyspnea, mucupurulent sputum, and wheezing, then you must consider *emphysema*; and if the patient presents with chronic cough, copious amounts of thick purulent sputum, crackles, rhonchi and wheezing, and possibly chest pain and hemoptysis, then you must consider bronchiecstasis. For *bronchiecstasis*, I would consider prescribing a lung-diffusing phlegm-transforming and cough-relieving panting-calming formula such as She Gan Ma Huang Tang combining Wu Ling San and adding Gan Jiang, Fu Zi, Huang Qin, Ting Li Zi, and Ren Shen (powder). For *emphysema* (or *obstructive pneumonia*), I would consider prescribing either a qi-boosting spleen-fortifying and qi-moving phlegm-transforming formula such as (Yu Sheng) Asthma Formula or a kidney yang-supplementing formula such as You Gui Yin adding Ma Huang, Xing Ren, Ma Huang (larger dose), Hu Tao, Bu Gu Zhi, Mai Men Dong, Wu Wei Zi, and Ren Shen (powder). And during cold weather months make sure to add The Three Great Yang-Supplementers and Huang Qin (as a counterbalance), or even Ge Jie (powder) if the condition is severe. As long as the patient presents with watery (mucoid) sputum upon expectoration, then it is a good idea to administer the yang-supplementing approach.

Case Study #9: Kidney Failing to Absorb Qi

Q: Recently a 78 y/o male visited my clinic for consultation. He explained that since having an argument with his wife about 2 years ago, he has frequently experienced shortness of breath, difficulty breathing (dyspnea), and dry cough. These symptoms are more severe when walking even short distances or going upstairs. He took Western medicine for 1 1/2 years in attempts to treat this condition, which didn't have noticeable results. Now, he wants to try TCM in hopes of regulating his constitution and getting healthy once again. I prescribed (Yu Sheng) You Gui Yin adding Ma Huang (large dose), Zi Yuan, Kuan Dong Hua (1 liang), and Xing Ren (3 qian). However, up to now, he has only shown slight improvement. Please offer your advice and guidance.

A: Based on your description of this patient's condition, it sounds like emphysema to me. Chronic airway inflammation that leads to obstruction of the small airways (bronchioles and alveoli) such as in emphysema, chronic obstructive pulmonary disease (COPD), and severe persistent asthma correlate with the classical TCM pathomechanism of kidney failing to absorb qi (腎不納氣 shèn bù nà qì).

People with a history of smoking, air pollution exposure, pneumothorax, hemothorax, pulmonary tuberculosis (TB), and severe pneumonia, as well as those undergoing partial surgical resection, chemotherapy, and radiotherapy, have a higher risk of developing emphysema. Over time (especially in old age!) damaged lung tissue, chronic airway inflammation, and pulmonary fibrosis leads to destruction of the alveolar walls, expiratory airway collapse, and obstruction, which inhibits the exchange of oxygen and carbon dioxide on the alveoli surface. An increasing amount of alveoli over a larger area of lung tissue become affected, resulting in panting and short, hasty breathing (dyspnea) to the point where the slightest physical activity (even speaking or a temper flare) will induce rapid panting.

Emphysema patients often present with the characteristic sign of a protruding vein located near Yin Tang (EX-HN-3) (or other veins throughout the body) and neck arteries. Chronic inflammation causes white blood cell accumulation and metabolic waste build up in the airways that result in mucus hypersecretion and expectoration of mucopurulent sputum. Patients with kidney failing to absorb qi (e.g., emphysema, COPD, chronic persistent asthma) are also more susceptible to external contraction (common colds) that may result in severe, acute exacerbations. My mentor Tan Qin (覃勤) (style name: Xing Qun (醒群))—a former R.O.C. (Taiwan) legislator, founder of China Medical University (Taichung, Taiwan), and the inaugural Chairperson of the National Union of Chinese Medical Doctor's Association (R.O.C.)—had emphysema with these classic accompanying signs and symptoms.

For patients with emphysema, Western medicine will typically just prescribe bronchodilators and expectorants and provide supportive treatment (e.g., postural drainage) to relieve symptoms. In addition to acute exacerbations of COPD, other common complications are pulmonary hypertension, cor pulmonale, pulmonary cachexia, or secondary spontaneous pneumothorax. Regardless of the Western medicine treatment approach, there really is no definitive cure that can ultimately prevent exacerbations or complications in the future. The focus of treatment is on slowing down the rate of deterioration. The best patients can hope for is to reduce the severity of symptoms, enabling them to move around independently and take care of themselves. As the disease progresses, if the patient experiences severe dyspnea or respiratory failure (i.e., low blood oxygen levels (hypoxia) or both hypoxia and high blood carbon dioxide levels (hypercapnia)), then supplemental oxygen must be administered to relieve symptoms.

Here are several TCM approaches for the treatment of kidney failing to absorb qi that manifests in pathoconditions such as emphysema, COPD, and chronic persistent asthma:

In the absence of concomitant pulmonary tuberculosis (TB), you can prescribe formulas such as (Yu Sheng) Asthma Formula adding The Three Great Yang-Supplementers, Zi Yuan, Kuan Dong Hua, He Tao, Bu Gu Zhi, Huang Qin, and Ren Shen/Chuan Qi Powder; or a kidney yang-supplementing formula such as You Gui Yin or Shen Qi Wan (if the patient also has an enlarged prostate, then it would be optimal to prescribe Shen Qi Wan!) adding Ma Huang, Xing Ren, Wu Wei Zi, Bai Guo, Huai Shan, Gan Jiang, Zi Yuan, Kuan Dong Hua, He Tao, Rou Gui, Huang Bo, Mai Men Dong, and Bu Gu Zhi (make sure to crush prior to decocting).

If severe panting presents, then prescribe Ge Jie (ground into powder) mixed into Ren Shen/Chuan Qi Powder, and possibly even Lu Rong (powder). If this isn't effective, then you can consider adding Hai Long (Syngnathus acus, Pipefish) and Hai Ma (Hippocampus,

Seahorse); and if this still doesn't provide effective relief, then prescribe Hei Xi Dan combined with Western medicine expectorants and antiasthmatics, and consider advising the patient to receive supplemental oxygen.

Is the exacerbation of symptoms the result of depressed accumulation (鬱積 yù jī) of static blood in the lung, pulmonary embolism, or pulmonary hypertension? Is there pericardial effusion, pleural effusion, or pulmonary edema? Has the patient already entered the renal failure stage? For patients with depressed accumulation of static blood in the lung, you should add large doses of The Four Lings along with blood-quickening stasis-dissolving medicinals such as Dang Gui, Chuan Xiong, Chi Shao, Dan Shen, and Chuan Qi. If there is excessive water accumulation (pericardial effusion, pleural effusion, or pulmonary edema), then add Ting Li Zi, Fang Ji, Fu Ling, and Ze Xie; if the heart is enlarged, prescribe (Yu Sheng) Bu Yang Huan Wu Tang; and if liver and kidney failure is present, then you should add Ding Shu Xiu, Ren Dong Teng, Pu Gong Ying, Da Huang, Xi Lu Rong (powder), Rou Gui, and Chi Shao (very effective at treating vasospasm!) along with large doses of Fu Ling and Ze Xie.

The formula you prescribed should be fine. But remember! It is common for this type of patient to have poor stomach intake (poor appetite) and no pleasure in eating (dulled taste bud senses) as a result of dampened submucosa plexus (Meissner's plexus) receptors in the small intestine. Since (Yu Sheng) You Gui Yin already contains Cang Zhu, Fu Ling, and Shan Yao, you just need to add Shan Zha and Ji Nei Jin to increase appetite and promote digestion, and of course, large doses of Ma Huang (promotes sweating and resolves the exterior, diffuses the lung and calms panting, disinhibits water and disperses swelling, and frees the nasal orifices). The climate in South Korea is very cold during the winter, so for most people you should be able to add anywhere from 3–5 qian of Ma Huang without affecting sleep. This will make the patient feel warm and mitigate shortness of breath and the severity of panting.

Section 3: Nose Piles, Nosebleed, and Chronic Sinusitis

Case Study #1: Chronic Rhinosinusitis – Postsurgical Complications

Q: A 33 y/o female patient had suffered from chronic rhinosinusitis with purulent nasal discharge, repeated sneezing, nasal congestion, and tenderness on the face for many years. It got to the point where the discomfort was such a distraction in her life that she couldn't stand it anymore, so she decided to go ahead with a surgical procedure.

She never imagined that the surgical procedure would result in olfactory nerve damage resulting in loss of her sense of smell (anosmia) and a persistent low-grade fever with yellow nasal discharge and cough producing yellow sputum. After receiving treatment from another TCM physician without effective results, she decided to visit my clinic. What is your opinion about this case? How should I approach treatment?

A: There are three possible causes for this patient with chronic sinusitis incurring postsurgical complications of persistent low-grade fever with yellow nasal discharge and cough producing yellow sputum:

1) It's possible that during the surgical procedure paranasal microbes might have entered the blood stream and affected the nervous system, thus resulting in further infection.
2) The patient may have contracted a secondary microbial infection (external contraction) not directly related to surgery.
3) The olfactory nerve was manually damaged by the surgical procedure.

From your description, it sounds like a secondary microbial infection to me. But regardless of the cause, you should consider prescribing a heat-clearing phlegm-transforming formula such as Wen Dan Tang adding Ma Huang, Bai Zhi, Xin Yi, and Xi Xin. At first, remember to include large doses of Huang Qin and Lai Fu Zi to abate heat and resolve inflammation and eliminate phlegm and nasal discharge. As her condition begins to improve and the exterior phlegm-heat symptoms resolve, then you can also add Di Long (frees the channels and quickens the network vessels) and The Three Great Yang-Supplementers (promote nerve innervation) for her anosmia. This approach should provide effective results.

Case Study #2: Nose Piles Correlate with Nasal Polyps and Papillomas

Q: In my clinical practice, I have begun to notice that many of my patients with persistent tearing on exposure to wind also have nasal polyps and papillomas. I have heard that after resection (polypectomy) it is very common for the polyps and papillomas to grow back again. Some traditional Korean medicine (TKM) physicians say that the pulverized powder of Chan Chu (Dried Toad, Venenum Bufonis) and Xiong Huang (Realgar) effectively remove and eliminate these types of growths. What is your approach to treating this condition?

A: Nasal polyps correlate with nose piles (鼻痔 bí zhì) in classical TCM pathologic terminology. Usually, you just need to focus on remedying the tearing on exposure to wind and the nose piles will spontaneously shrink, thus alleviating the need for Western medicine drugs and surgical intervention. Many exterior-resolving TCM medicinals such as Ma Huang, Bai Zhi, Xi Xin, and Man Jing Zi all have the action of shrinking nose piles, so in the great majority of cases there really is no need for risking potential complications of surgery, which could damage the sinuses and intracranial membranes and lead to "brain leak" (i.e., cerebrospinal fluid leaks into the sinuses) or olfactory nerve palsy.

In my opinion, using Chan Chu and Xiong Huang by TKM physicians to remove and eliminate these growths is even more dangerous! If you wanted to administer a topical application, a much safer and effective method would be a rub-on medicinal formula such as (Yu Sheng) Athlete's Foot/Pompholyx Infusion, which I commonly prescribe for the treatment of athlete's foot and pompholyx, but can also be rubbed on these types of nasal growths. All you need to do is mix the key medicinals—Xiong Huang, Da Huang, Ru Xiang, Hua Shi, Gan Shi, and Qing Fen—together and you will have a formula that effectively resolves inflammation, abates heat, and erodes nasal polyps.

Case Study #3: Epistaxis – Frenetic Movement of Hot Blood

Q: A 35 y/o male explained that he began having nosebleeds (epistaxis) about 3 months ago after overexerting himself at work. Since then he has experienced spontaneous nosebleeds that produce a substantial amount of blood flow, making both the patient and the people around him quite uncomfortable and concerned. He was diagnosed with a deep vessel rupture by an otolaryngologist, but due to its location it wasn't possible to perform cauterization to stanch the bleeding. Blood tests and liver ultrasound revealed *no* abnormal findings. Do you think Huang Lian Jie Du Tang is a good formula for this patient?

A: A patient presenting with spontaneous nosebleeds for 3 months clearly indicates frenetic movement of hot blood (血熱妄行 xuè rè wàng xíng) to the head. For this condition, you can prescribe Ru Mo Si Wu Tang adding large doses of Mu Dan Pi, Zhi Zi, Huang Qin, Huang Lian, Ou Jie and Ce Bo Ye along with Chuan Qi (powder) and Zhu Sha (powder). If bleeding persists, then consider further adding Long Gu, Mu Li, Niu Xi, and Dai Zhe Shi. Remember! The secret for best results in treating this condition is making sure to include the combination of Chuan Qi and Zhu Sha in your formula.

Section 4: Other Respiratory Disorders

Case Study #1: Tuberculous Pleurisy with Pleural Effusion – Don't Prescribe Shi Zao Tang!

Q: A 38 y/o female patient explained that 4 months ago she suddenly experienced short, hasty breathing and dry cough. Following a hospital examination, she was diagnosed with tuberculous pleurisy (TBpl) and administered Western medicine drugs that proved effective in alleviating symptoms. However, subsequent follow-up examination revealed the presence of pleural effusion. I am confident that Chai Ling Tang is the right approach, but I was also considering combining Shi Zao Tang as well to resolve the symptoms of water-rheum collecting internally. Do you think this formula will be effective?

A: A heat-clearing phlegm-damp-transforming water-disinhibiting formula such as Chai Ling Tang will most certainly provide effective treatment for TBpl with pleural effusion. The formula will be even more effective if you add large doses of Fu Ling, Ze Xie, Ting Li Zi, and Fang Ji along with Qing Hao, Zhi Mu, and Di Gu Pi.

However, I do not recommend prescribing Shi Zao Tang for several reasons:

First, it would appear that the patient's TBpl has not completely resolved yet, and based on your description of this patient's history and current condition, it doesn't sound like her condition is severe enough to warrant such a drastic water-expelling (峻下逐水 jùn xià zhú shuǐ) approach. The essential medicinals in this formula all have high toxicity and are processed by steeping in salt water for long periods to further intensify their offensive precipitation (攻下 gōng xià) potency.

Second, even if she was in a critical condition, modern medicine's drainage tubes offer such a convenient, minimally invasive solution to pleurisy (water accumulation in the pleura) that it is unnecessary to prescribe these types of TCM medicinals.

Remember! You should only consider prescribing Shi Zao Tang when the patient has a relatively healthy physical constitution in the presence of water accumulation (水蓄 shuǐ xù) inside the intestines, ascites, or thoracic cavity perfusion that severely compresses surrounding structures and causes urinary and fecal stoppage, propped breathing (倚息 yǐ xī), and panting when lying down. Based on my clinical experience, I have determined that it's best not to prescribe Shi Zao Tang unless absolutely necessary, thus averting the potential for adverse effects and complications resulting in possible malpractice disputes.

Case Study #2: Non-Tuberculous Pleurisy – Wu Ling San (Nephritis Formula)

Q: Yesterday an interesting patient visited me. Western medicine doctors diagnosed the patient with pleurisy not associated with tuberculosis (TB). Massive pleural effusion (accumulation of pleural fluid in the pleural cavity) and fullness in the chest and hypochondria (胸脅苦滿 xiōng xié kǔ mǎn) have caused extreme discomfort. Thoracentesis (insertion of a needle into the pleural cavity to drain the accumulation of pleural fluid) has been performed every 2 months for the past 2 years for symptomatic treatment of refractory pleural effusions. The patient has had chemical pleurodesis (a chemical (e.g., talc) inserted into the pleural space that leads to inflammation and fibrosis of the pleura and adhesion of the pleural space) performed on 2 separate occasions without success.

The patient doesn't want to go through with this toilsome and painful procedure anymore, so he decided to try TCM instead and visited me for consultation and treatment. At first, I prescribed Chai Ling Tang (including 1 liang of Fu Ling and Ze Xie each) adding Qing Hao, Zhi Mu, and Di Gu Pi. After taking this formula, the severity of fullness in the hypochondriac region increased, so I changed the formula to Wu Ling San. I don't have a lot of experience treating this type of condition. Please share your experiences and knowledge with me.

A: Indeed, in cases of recurrent pleural effusion and fullness in the chest and hypochondria like this that require regular drainage (thoracentesis), prescribing Wu Ling San (Nephritis Formula) would be the optimal choice. However, you must include large doses of Fu Ling, Huang Qi, and Ren Shen (powder); and if the patient experiences shortness of breath, then add Ma Huang and Xing Ren. In some cases, you may consider prescribing a kidney yang-warming and -supplementing formula such as You Gui Yin or Shen Qi Wan instead, including a large dose of Fu Ling and adding Ze Xie, Ting Li Zi, and Fang Ji.

Don't worry too much about the presentation of repeated effusions; just continue to administer the TCM formula and advise the patient to have thoracentesis performed if necessary, which will facilitate a gradual reduction in the amount of pleural effusion (e.g., from 500 cc gradually down to 300 cc). Over time, this integrated approach will prolong the periods necessitating drainage (e.g., from 1x/every 2 months down to 1x/every 3–4 months), control symptoms, and eventually alleviate the need for drainage altogether.

Case Study #3: Chemical Vapors Irritate Throat

Q: A 50 y/o male auto mechanic accidentally inhaled a potent lead-based chemical while on the job 2 months ago and has subsequently experienced itchy throat, cough, and sneezing. He immediately sought medical assistance and has been taking Western medicine without any improvement. Follow-up tests and scans have revealed *no* significant findings. Initially, I approached this like a case of tearing on exposure to wind and prescribed Mai Men Dong Tang variant, which wasn't very effective. What do you think about the idea of changing the formula to Mai Men Dong Tang combining Huang Lian Jie Du Tang or Ma Huang Jia Zhu Tang variant?

A: First, if this were a classic case of tearing on exposure to wind, then you could simply prescribe You Gui Yin adding Ma Huang, Wu Wei Zi, Bai Guo, Xi Xin, Ban Xia, Bai Zhi, and Ren Shen (powder) along with encouraging the patient to get out in the sunshine, or even better, to exercise in the sunshine. Symptoms would rapidly improve with this approach.

Second, in this case, the patient presented with a history of accidentally inhaling chemical vapors of a volatile substance resulting in irritation of the mucous membranes (epithelial cells) of the throat. After more than 2 months, the body's natural regenerative capacities should have resolved the damage to the epithelium caused by the chemical substance by now. Thus, I would also strongly consider the possibility of either psychosomatic origins or tearing on exposure to wind.

Third, before you prescribe any formula, you must first accurately identify the signs, symptoms, and pattern. Is it a dry or productive cough, what color is the phlegm, and at what time is the cough most prevalent (daytime or nighttime)?

In light of the patient's history, I would be tempted to suggest prescribing (Yu Sheng) Asthma Formula adding Huang Qin, Qing Hao, Zhi Mu, Di Gu Pi, and Ren Shen (powder); and if there is profuse yellow nasal discharge, then I would add large doses of Huang Qin and Lai Fu Zi.

Case Study #4: Trachael Hemorrhage Leads to Persistent Vegetative State

Q: One year ago, a 64 y/o patient in a persistent vegetative state (PVS) was brought by family members to my clinic. They explained that the patient had suffered tracheal hemorrhage with too much time elapsing prior to receiving treatment, thus resulting in the current vegetative state.

Over the past year, I have continued administering Bu Yang Huan Wu Tang adding The Three Great Yang-Supplementers (1 qian each), Ban Xia, Zhu Ru, Zhi Shi, and Huang Qin (3 qian each), Ren Shen (2 qian), Ma Huang (1 qian), Chuan Qi (3 qian), and Di Long (5 qian). Recently, examination of the patient has shown intense deep tendon reflexes (brisk and hyperactive with clonus). Do you think it is possible for the patient to regain consciousness? What signs should I look for that may indicate improvement?

A: That is an excellent formula for treating PVS patients. Continue administering this formula and the patient has a good chance of improving, but recovery from a vegetative state is a very slow process. You must pay attention to the slightest changes in the patient's body and behavior, particularly response to stimuli (e.g., pain, touch, palpation, light, and sound), bowel movements and urine secretion, and whether or not unassisted penile (or clitoral) erection occurs spontaneously. Also, carefully observe the patient's limb movements, eye opening, response and tracking of light source, head rotation, signaling, guttural vocalizations, and pupil and motor reflexes. All of these are reliable signs indicating improvement in the patient's condition.

Remember! If a nasogastric (NG) or nasojejunal (NJ) tube has been inserted, the patient must not orally ingest any liquids (even decocted medicinals!) until adequate recovery has been established and the NG (or NJ) tube has been taken out. Long-term NG (or NJ) tube insertion makes these patients susceptible to esophageal and gastric bleeding and ulcerations, thus you could consider advising the patient to go ahead with a gastrostomy (or jejunostomy).

Case Study #5: Papillomatosis of the Vocal Cords

Q: A 38 y/o female patient who visited my clinic explained that every time she goes singing at KTVs after recovering from the common cold she gets a hoarse voice. Recently, hoarseness has lingered on for even longer than normal, prompting her to get it checked out with a specialist. Endoscopy revealed the presence of pseudomembranous tissue on her vocal cords and her doctor recommended that she have surgery. Please offer your opinions and advice regarding this case.

A: The pseudomembranous tissue you mention most likely refers to the presence of either papillomatosis, polyps, or nodules on her vocal cords that produce the symptom of hoarseness. To treat this condition, I would prescribe the following formula: Jie Geng, He Zi, and Ban Xia (8 qian each), Gan Cao (5 qian), Gan Jiang, Fu Zi, and Huang Qin (3–5 qian), and Yu Sheng Wan (1 pill/day). This approach will rapidly improve her condition. In fact, I have also prescribed this formula to effectively treat patients suffering from dysphonia and aphonia resulting from surgical complications of thyroid cancer (e.g., recurrent laryngeal nerve swelling and damage).

You can leave the decision about surgery for papillomatosis, polyps, or nodules up to the patient. If the patient is undecided, then you can administer the above formula for 2–3 weeks and see how the patient feels. If you don't want to get involved in the acute stage treatment of this condition or the patient decides right away to have surgery, then following surgery you can prescribe Bu Zhong Yi Qi

Tang adding Huang Qin, Jie Geng, and He Zi. If this approach doesn't enable her to completely regain her natural voice, then add Gan Jiang and Fu Zi. This approach will gradually provide effective results.

II. VERTIGO

Dizziness (頭暈 tóu yūn) is a broad term used to describe the feeling of spinning, tilting, or possibly even being about to pass out (syncope). Common causes of dizziness are anemia, nervousness, and orthostatic (postural) hypotension. Vertigo (眩暈 xuàn yūn) is a specific type of dizziness that refers to an intensified spinning, swaying or tilting dizziness in which the person may feel a sensation of rotating around in space (subjective vertigo), or of having objects rotate around the individual (objective vertigo). Common causes of vertigo are benign paroxysmal positional vertigo (BPPV), Meniere disease, vestibular neuritis, head injury, medications, and cerebrovascular accident (CVA).

Case Study #1: Vertigo Feels "Like There Is a Tight Band Wrapped Around My Head"

Q: A 43 y/o female patient has a 6-year history of vertigo and has been treated by numerous TCM and Western medicine doctors without effective results. In the past couple of years, she has also been taking Western medicine drugs to control hypertension.

Recently, the patient has suffered from migraine headaches, saying that when attacks occur she feels "like there is a tight band wrapped around my head." That's when she decided to visit my clinic for treatment. I prescribed Ban Xia Tian Ma Bai Zhu San (including a large dose of Tian Ma (1 liang)) adding Yu Sheng Wan (3 pills/day), but there hasn't been any noticeable improvement. Please offer your advice and guidance on this case.

A: This patient with vertigo, hypertension, and migraine can be classified as spinning head and painful brain (頭旋腦痛 tóu xuan nǎo tong) in classical TCM pathologic terminology. First, you must determine the status of blood pressure.

If the patient has been taking antihypertensive medication, but blood pressure still doesn't come down, then you can prescribe an yin-enriching fire-downbearing formula such as Zhi Bo Di Huang Tang, a blood-quickening qi-supplementing formula such as Bu Yang Huan Wu Tang, or a liver-settling wind-extinguishing and yin-enriching yang-subduing formula such as Jian Ling Tang. Just make sure to include Tian Ma, Huang Bo, Gan Cao, and Long Yan Gan in your formula selection.

If blood pressure is already under control within a normal range, then you can consider prescribing a heat-clearing phlegm-transforming formula such as Wen Dan Tang or a Shao Yang-harmonizing and -resolving formula such as Xiao Chai Hu Tang adding Long Gu, Mu Li, and Tian Ma.

If administration of antihypertensive medication causes too rapid of a decrease in blood pressure, then you can prescribe Ban Xia Tian Ma Bai Zhu San (including a slightly larger dose of Tian Ma) adding Gan Cao, Chuan Xiong, Wu Zhu Yu, Long Yan Gan, and Yu Sheng Wan.

Including acupuncture in your therapeutic regimen is also a good idea. I would needle acupoints such as Feng Chi (GB20), Bai Hui

(DU20), Tai Chong (LV3), San Yin Jiao (SP6), Shen Men (HT7), and He Gu (LI4). Regardless of the specific condition or pattern, make sure to advise the patient to get 8–10 hours of sleep a night.

Case Study #2: Twitching Eyelid, Dizziness That Threatens Collapse, Heavy Head As If Swathed

Q: In the past, I have prescribed Ban Xia Tian Ma Bai Zhu San variant to successfully treat a number of patients presenting with a constellation of symptoms, including twitching eyelids brought on by nervousness, headache that feels like a tight band wrapped around the head, paroxysmal bouts of vertigo that nearly produces sudden collapse, and pronounced shoulder and back pain. But recently I have prescribed this formula for two patients with similar symptoms and have not seen any improvement at all. Do you think changing the formula to Wen Dan Tang combining Xiao Chai Hu Tang adding Tian Ma would be a good approach?

A: Prescribing the spleen- and stomach-supplementing, phlegm-damp transforming, and wind-stabilizing formula Ban Xia Tian Ma Bai Zhu San for twitching eyelid (blepharospasm) (胞輪振跳 bāo lún zhèn tiào), head heavy as if swathed (頭重如裹 tóu zhòng rú guǒ), and dizziness that threatens collapse (眩暈欲仆 xuàn yūn yù pū) is a good choice for patients with peripheral causes (e.g., vestibular neuritis, Meniere disease, benign paroxysmal positional vertigo (BPPV)). However, I recommend including large doses of Tian Ma (at least 8 qian) and Huang Qi (2–3 liang) and adding Gan Cao, Long Yan Gan, The Three Insects, Ren Shen/Chuan Qi Powder, and Yu Sheng Wan.

For patients whose symptoms result from central causes (e.g., basilar artery stenosis, vertebrobasilar ischemia, cerebellar stroke), you should prescribe a blood-quickening qi-supplementing formula such as Bu Yang Huan Wu Tang adding large doses of Ge Gen and Chuan Xiong (8–10 qian each), The Three Great Yang-Supplementers, Tian Ma, Huang Qin, The Three Insects, Ren Shen/Chuan Qi Powder, and Yu Sheng Wan. Ge Gen and Chuan Xiong are essential medicinals for pathoconditions involving compromised cerebrovasculature, with their capacity to dilate coronary arteries, increase coronary, cerebral, and peripheral blood flow, and reduce peripheral vascular resistance.

It would be best to perform acupuncture as well, which will help to relieve symptoms and remedy the condition more quickly and effectively. I would consider selecting acupoints such as Feng Chi (GB20), Tian Zhu (UB10), He Gu (LI4), Zu San Li (ST36), and Tai Chong (LV3); Zan Zhu (UB2) and Si Zhu Kong (SJ23) (needle transversely joining above the eye), and Zan Zhu (UB2) (needling transversely towards Cheng Qi (ST1) below the eye); and starting at a point directly below the zygomatic arch near Xia Guan (ST7), transversely needle three radiating points towards Si Zhu Kong (SJ23), Quan Liao (SI18), and Jia Che (ST6) respectively (corresponding with the three main pathways of the facial nerves (CN7) and trigeminal nerves (CN5)).

Case Study #3: Vertigo, Nystagmus, Nausea, and Diarrhea – Yang Ming Channel Pattern

Q: Three weeks ago a 36 y/o male patient began experiencing vertigo accompanied by nystagmus, stiffness and pain in the nape and neck, and occasional severe episodes of vertigo with nausea, vomiting and diarrhea. The only way to relieve these symptoms is to lie down flat on his back. He has been taking Western medicine drugs with only slight improvement. Sometimes all it takes to elicit an attack is to simply stair at a stationary object. Do you think this is a classic case of vertigo?

A: As I discussed during my presentation on vertigo at the Traditional Korean Medicine Symposium in 2001, there are many potential causes of vertigo. The most common are inner ear disorders (e.g., vestibular system, infection), concussion, ocular disorders (e.g., glaucoma, cataracts, and anisometropia), stomach heat pattern, and Yang Ming channel pattern. The vertigo caused by concussion typically resolves once the initial injury from trauma subsides.

The two most common types of inner ear disorders that cause otogenic vertigo are benign paroxysmal positional vertigo (BPPV) and Meniere disease. Both of these conditions can present with symptoms of throat irritation, stuffiness in the chest, painful distention in the chest and hypochondrium, frequent urination, abdominal urgency and rectal heaviness (tenesmus) (裡急後重 lǐ jí hòu zhòng), and stiffness and pain in the nape of the neck (頸項強痛 jǐng xiàng qiáng tòng). Diarrhea is not a classic symptom of inner ear disorders. Typically, diarrhea presents in stomach heat pattern and Yang Ming channel pattern. For this patient, the key here is to clearly differentiate between tenesmus and diarrhea. Does the patient feel a burning sensation in the anus during defecation (loose stool or watery consistency)? Is there a sulfurous odor (like rotten duck eggs)?

Based on your description of this patient's history and symptoms, it sounds to me like Yang Ming channel pattern resulting from exterior evil entering the interior with water collecting in the stomach and intestines. You should prescribe a formula that focuses on treating Yang Ming channel heat such as Qing Wei San, Ge Gen Qin Lian Tang, or Huang Lian Jie Du Tang adding Bai Zhu, Fu Ling, Ze Xie, and Tian Ma. If the vertigo is severe or the patient is in the midst of an acute episode, then you can prescribe a large dose of Tian Ma (at least 1 liang); and if the patient endures long durations of vomiting and/or diarrhea, has a reduced food intake, or completely abstains from eating, then you should add Gan Cao, Da Zao, and Long Yan Gan to supplement the center, boost qi, and nourish the blood.

Once gastrointestinal heat has resolved, then you can prescribe a spleen- and stomach-supplementing, phlegm-damp transforming, and wind-stabilizing formula such as Ban Xia Tian Ma Bai Zhu San variant as explained before. And if there is residual heat, add large doses of Huang Qin and Huang Bo.

Case Study #4: Headache, Vertigo, and Heel Pain

Q: A 46 y/o female patient explained that ever since going on a hike this summer she has had a headache with a sensation of heat on the top of her head, stiffness and pain in the nape and neck, and pain in both heels. Sometimes the headache is so bad it brings on dizzy spells in which the room around her starts spinning. The strange thing is that all of these symptoms are more severe in the morning and decrease after midday, and the intensity of the headache can be dampened by applying pressure.

A: It sounds to me like this patient with headache and vertigo most likely incurred summerheat strike (heat stroke) during her summer hike that resulted in the manifestation of visceral agitation and psychosomatic symptoms brought on by menopausal transition.

As for treatment, I would first focus on the heel pain and vertigo by prescribing an yin-enriching fire-downbearing formula such as Zhi Bo Di Huang Tang adding Tian Ma, Qing Hao, Di Gu Pi, Huo Luo Dan (dispels wind and eliminates dampness, transforms phlegm and frees the network vessels, and quickens the blood and relieves pain), and Yu Sheng Wan; bleed at the site of pain on the heel; and needle Cheng Shan (UB57), Kun Lun (UB60), Feng Chi (GB20), and Bai Hui (DU20). Once the heel pain is remedied, then change to a heat-clearing phlegm-transforming formula such as Wen Dan Tang adding Qing Hao, Zhi Mu, Di Gu Pi, Tian Ma, Niu Xi, and Yu Sheng Wan; or a center-harmonizing tension-relaxing, qi-moving counterflow-downbearing, and stagnation-dissipating phlegm-transforming formula such as Gan Mai Da Zao Tang Combining Ban Xia Hou Po Tang adding Qing Hao, Di Gu Pi, Tian Ma, and Yu Sheng Wan.

III. LIVER DISEASE

Liver disease used to be referred to as the "national disease of Taiwan." This chapter will guide the reader through an accurate interpretation of the laboratory test data and explain how to apply the integrated TCM and Western medicine approach in the treatment of liver disorders such as hepatitis, cirrhosis, and hepatic cancer.

Section 1: Hepatitis – Primary Cause of Liver Disease

Case Study #1: Chronic Hepatitis B Infection

Q: I have a 33 y/o friend who is a heavy alcohol drinker. About 10 years ago, a regular health check up revealed that he had been infected with the hepatitis B virus (HBV) via mother-to-child (perinatal/vertical) transmission. Relevant lab tests are as follows: AST 40 (0–40 u/L), ALT 70 (1–30 u/L), T-Bil 2.2 (normal range 0.2–1.2 mg/dL), and HBeAg (+).

Is it possible for HBeAg to return to (-)? Last year at a TCM Warm Disease Conference a doctor from Macao made a presentation claiming that he had treated a patient whose HBeAg had transitioned from (+) to (-).

A: In my opinion, as long as AST and ALT are within a normal range, for the time being you don't have to be too concerned. As for (+) and (-), the only difference is that if its (+), it's transmittable; and if it's (-), it isn't. Regarding radio immunoassays (RIA) that detect the half-life decay rates of HBeAg radioactive isotopes, a lot of it depends on the habits and choices the patient makes. For instance, if the patient leads a healthy lifestyle, results may show (-); but if the patient eats poorly, doesn't get enough sleep, drinks excessive amounts of alcohol, or takes medication that compromises the liver, then HBeAg may test (+).

For this case, you can prescribe a depressed steaming damp-heat-draining and liver- and gallbladder-clearing and draining formula such as Zhi Zi Bo Pi Tang variant, and advise the patient to get to bed early (best to be asleep by 11 p.m.) and awake early, getting at least 8 hours of sleep every day. Through this therapeutic regimen and sensible lifestyle modifications, the patient should be able to stay free of troublesome symptoms.

Case Study #2: Cholestatic Hepatitis

Q: I have another good friend who has recently been diagnosed with cholestatic hepatitis. I prescribed Xiang Sha Liu Jun Zi Tang adding Da Huang and Zhi Zi, but the results have been poor with the liver function indices remaining elevated. This makes me suspect that mild cirrhotic change may have already occurred. Do you think adding Gan Jiang and Fu Zi to my original formula would be effective?

A: The best approach for treating cholestatic hepatitis is by coursing the liver and disinhibiting the gallbladder and maintaining a healthy diet and lifestyle. Prescribing Xiang Sha Liu Jun Zi Tang adding Da Huang and Zhi Zi is a good formula. Continue prescribing this formula for a period of time, and if liver function indices still do not decrease, then yes you should add Gan Jiang, Fu Zi, and a large dose of Huang Qin (counterbalances the heat of the yang-supplementing medicinals).

Case Study #3: Autoimmune Hepatitis

Q: A male patient with a history of autoimmune hepatitis recently visited my clinic. His most recent lab test results are as follows: AST 70 (0–40 u/L), ALT 110 (1–30 u/L), and T-Bil 3.02 (normal range 0.2–1.2 mg/dL). The patient continues to take oral corticosteroids (2 pills/day), but without any noticeable improvement. That's why he decided to try TCM. He has 2–3 bowel movements (loose stools) per day.

Based on the patient's history and presenting symptoms, I prescribed Xiang Sha Liu Jun Zi Tang adding Da Huang (8 qian) and Rou Gui and Gan Jiang (5 fen each). There has been some marginal improvement, but very slow. Do you think I am on the right track?

A: Remember! Regardless of the type of hepatitis, if the patient has received corticosteroids over long periods of time the condition can be identified as exhaustion of the liver and kidney (肝腎衰竭 gān shèn shuāi jié) pattern. If corticosteroids are abruptly discontinued, this could rapidly evolve into fulminant hepatitis, hyperbilirubinemia, or hepatorenal syndrome (HRS); and in severe cases, hepatic encephalopathy (HE) or even death.

Prior to initiating treatment you must carefully determine whether or not your patient's condition is idiopathic or associated with another autoimmune disease (e.g., SLE, type 1 diabetes mellitus, Hashimoto's thyroiditis, celiac disease). For instance, if there is an association with systemic lupus erythematosus (SLE), then you should consider prescribing a qi-boosting spleen-fortifying and qi-moving phlegm-transforming formula such as Xiang Sha Liu Jun Zi Tang adding Huang Qi, Tu Si Zi, The Three Great Yang-Supplementers, Huang Qin, and Ren Shen/Chuan Qi Powder; or a kidney yang-warming and supplementing formula such as You Gui Yin adding heat-clearing water-disinhibiting and jaundice-resolving medicinals. If AST and ALT levels are increased, then add Da Qing Ye and Ban Lan Gen; and if T-Bil is increased, then add Zhi Zi and Da Huang. Naturally, if the autoimmune hepatitis is associated with another autoimmune disease, then you may need to consider prescribing other formulas that specifically address the pathomechanisms of those respective pathoconditions.

While administering these formulas, you should also advise the patient to consult with his Western medicine physician about the possibility of gradually reducing the dosage of corticosteroids, and eventually discontinuing administration altogether. Then, 1–2 weeks after discontinuation, you should change to a heat-clearing toxin-resolving and yin vacuity-heat clearing yin-enriching formula such as (Yu Sheng) Hyperactive Immune Formula, which will put you back on the track of treating the root!

Case Study #4: Fulminant Hepatic Failure from Drug-Induced Hepatotoxicity

Q: South Korea has a high prevalence of liver disease. Recently, I have been carefully reading through your book *TCM Treatment of Common Liver Diseases*, and have found the part on fulminant hepatic failure (FHF) that discusses hepatic encephalopathy (HE) difficult to understand. Could you further elaborate on your treatment approach for these complex conditions?

A: Excellent! It just so happens that recently I have been treating a patient with FHF caused by drug-induced hepatotoxicity and complicated by hepatic encephalopathy. Her history is as follows: The patient developed drug-related skin and mucous membrane eruptions (suggestive of Stevens-Johnson syndrome) after taking Western medicine drugs and was referred to a dermatologist. Subsequently, the patient continued taking the medication and this time she developed FHF, with AST and ALT soaring to unbelievable levels! In all my years of practicing medicine, this was the only time I have ever treated a patient with PLT of only 30,000–40,000, AST and ALT over 7,000, and ammonia at nearly 100 (reference range < 35). Administration of Western medicine drugs were discontinued, except for intravenous immunoglobulin (IVIG), and I prescribed the heat-clearing phlegm-damp-transforming water-disinhibiting formula Chai Ling Tang adding large doses of The Three Yellows and Da Huang. On the third day, after being administered only 2 days (approx. 600 cc/day) of TCM decoction along with IVIG, the ammonia level returned to normal, AST dropped to below 1,000, and the patient regained consciousness.

Just take your time and read through the explanations and case studies. Providing effective treatment for liver disease is not an easy process. The best way to learn is by gaining clinical experience and referencing successful case studies. Remember! Significant achievements come from ongoing dedication and commitment. Never rest on your laurels: you must continue striving to elevate your clinical capacities. There will be times when you feel alone, but there will also be joy in the accomplishment of breakthroughs.

Case Study #5: Chronic Hepatitis in Pregnancy

Q: Three years ago, a 29 y/o female patient with chronic HBV incurred mild classic symptoms and was administered a regimen of the antiviral drug Lamivudine for 5 months. At first, this medication was effective in reducing AST/ALT levels, but 3 months into the treatment, levels began increasing again. Her doctors switched to the antiviral drug Adefovir, which was also ineffective and thus discontinued, and then to regular interferon alfa-2a injections.

Now, she is in her seventh month of pregnancy and her most recent lab test results are as follows: AST 350 (0–40 u/L), ALT 420 (1–30 u/L), and HBV DNA > 20,000 (> 200,000 IU/mL at high risk of infecting newborn). After having her child, she plans to begin TCM treatment. Can administration of TCM medicinals effectively reduce these hepatitis indices? And if these levels can be reduced, will AST and ALT levels rebound once again?

A: For patients who are pregnant with chronic active hepatitis, it would be best to begin administering TCM medicinals immediately, otherwise the patient is at risk of developing fulminant hepatic failure. In fact, long-term administration of these antiviral class of drugs (i.e., -vir, -dine, interferon-α) pose the risk of hepatic failure. Typically, if liver enzyme indices (i.e., AST, ALT) do not spike back up within 6 months of discontinuing these antiviral drugs, then levels will most likely remain normal.

Administering the right TCM medicinals during pregnancy will not harm the fetus in any way; on the contrary, Huang Qin is known as a fetus-quieting sacred medicinal in the TCM pharmacopoeia! The most common causes of spontaneous abortion and intrauterine fetal death (IUFD) (aka stillbirth) are birth defects, placental complications, and infections. The TCM medicinals Huang Qin, Huang Lian, Huang Bo, Ma Huang, Rou Gui, and Lian Qiao all have anti-inflammatory, antibacterial, and antiviral actions that will benefit pregnancy. After roughly three months of pregnancy, fetal cell differentiation will have been completed, and at that time, not even Western medicine drugs will harm the fetus. So you really don't need to worry about TCM medicinals having any type of deleterious effect.

Remember! Prescribing the appropriate TCM medicinals will quiet and nourish the fetus and calm the liver.

Section 2: Hepatitis, Cirrhosis, and Liver Cancer

Case Study #1: Jaundice – Sign of Liver and Gallbladder Disease

Q: A 41 y/o female patient has a longstanding history of chronic autoimmune hepatitis and has been taking immunosuppressants and corticosteroids for many years in efforts to treat her condition. She had previously incurred biliary duct obstruction with jaundice, prompting an endoscopic retrograde cholangiopancreatography (ERCP) procedure that opened up the duct (duct dilation).

Last July, she incurred a severe episode of jaundice and further inspection revealed the presence of 3 cysts, prompting her doctors to immediately perform cholecystectomy to remove the gallbladder, cysts, and bile duct and insert a stent for drainage. Following surgery her liver function tests were as follows: T-Bil as high as 20 eventually dropping down to 8 (normal range 0.2–1.2 mg/dL), AST 100 (0–40 u/L), and ALT 70 (1–30 u/L). And the patient still has jaundice over the entire body. What approach should I take in the treatment of this patient's condition?

A: This is a relatively simple case. You will see positive results if you prescribe a Shao Yang-harmonizing and -resolving formula such as Xiao Chai Hu Tang adding Zhi Zi, Da Qing Ye, Ban Lan Gen, and Da Huang (increasing the dose incrementally until the patient maintains approx. 3 stools/day). If the patient is still being administered corticosteroids, then advise her to begin gradually reducing the dosage and eventually discontinuing altogether. Remember! Don't abruptly discontinue!

If T-bil decreases, but still remains at elevated levels and jaundice is still present, then you can add The Three Great Yang-Supplementers (1.5 qian each). After administering this formula for a period of time, once signs and symptoms begin to improve you can begin gradually reducing the amount of the The Three Great Yang-Supplementers down to 1 qian and then 5 fen each. Administer this formula up until the T-Bil level and skin discoloration (jaundice) return to normal.

Case Study #2: Chronic Hepatitis Progresses to Cirrhosis and Splenomegaly

Q: A 50 y/o female patient with chronic hepatitis developed progressive hepatic fibrosis that led to cirrhosis. The most recent liver function tests are as follows: AST 27 (0–40 u/L), ALT 10 (1–30 u/L), and increased levels of AFP. An ultrasound scan revealed hepatic atrophy and splenomegaly. Depressed and worried about following in the footsteps of her father who died prematurely from complications of cirrhosis, she has repeatedly "pleaded" with me to help cure her illness.

Since her liver enzyme levels were within normal range and she only had slightly elevated AFP, it didn't appear to me that her condition was very serious. After treating this patient for a period of time, it became clear that the extent of her liver disease was quite mild. The problem was that she was just stressed out and worried too much. She has been very compliant in taking her TCM medicinals and goes for monthly Western medicine follow-up tests and examinations. However, this overwhelming concern for her health is verging on obsessive and also putting a lot of pressure on me. What do you think is the best approach for treating this patient?

A: Indeed, it sounds like her condition has stabilized. All you need to do is try reassuring her that everything will be fine, and if she insists on receiving treatment, then simply prescribe a qi-boosting spleen-fortifying and stomach-harmonizing dampness-percolating formula such as Shen Ling Bai Zhu San adding Long Yan Rou and Yu Sheng Wan or a liver-coursing depression-resolving and spleen-fortifying blood-nourishing formula such as Xiao Yao San adding Da Zao, Long Yan Rou, and Yu Sheng Wan. These formulas will regulate her constitution, ensure her condition remains stabilized, and most importantly, calm her nerves and quiet the spirit!

In patients who do present with signs of hepatocyte destruction (e.g., elevated AST, ALT, ALP, ammonia), signs of impaired hepatic synthesis (e.g., decreased T. Pro, A/G, Hb, and PLT levels), jaundice (e.g., elevated T-Bil), or even mild hepatic encephalopathy (HE), you must typically differentiate between the three patterns of spleen qi vacuity, liver blood vacuity, and liver and kidney yin vacuity as the basis for determining treatment. The following are recommended formula variants for each pattern:

- Spleen qi vacuity—Xiang Sha Liu Jun Zi Tang, Shen Ling Bai Zhu San, Bu Zhong Yi Qi Tang, and Wu Wei Yi Gong San variants.

- Liver blood vacuity—Sheng Yu Tang, Qi Bao Mei Ran Dan, Xue Ku Fang, and Bu Yang Huan Wu Tang variants.
- Liver and kidney yin vacuity—Zhi Bo Di Huang Tang, Ba Xian Chang Shou Wan, Bai He Gu Jin Tang, Dang Gui Liu Huang Tang, and Zuo Gui Yin variants.

If T-Pro is low, then add Ren Shen (or Dang Shen), Huang Qi, Bai Guo, Huai Shan, Fu Ling, and Bai Guo. If T-Pro still remains low after adding the above medicinals, then add The Three Great Yang-Supplementers and Ren Shen (powder); or possibly even Xi Lu Rong (powder), Zhu Jie Qi, Mo Han Lian, and Tu Si Zi. If T. Bil and D. Bil are high, then add Da Huang (increasing the dose incrementally until the patient maintains about 3 stools/day) and Zhi Zi (or possibly Huang Shui Qie (Sodom Apple, *Solanum coagulans* Forsk.)). If AST and ALT are increased, then add Fu Ling, Da Qing Ye, and Ban Lan Gen. These therapeutic approaches will enable the patient to achieve gradual and sustained improvement.

Case Study #3: Cirrhosis – Portal Hypertension, Esophageal Varices, and Splenomegaly

Q: This patient's cirrhosis has caused portal hypertension resulting in esophageal varices and splenomegaly. Ultrasound scans reveal fine nodules diffusely dispersed over the surface of the liver, AST 20 (0–40 u/L), ALT 20 (1–30 u/L), and AFP 200 (< 10 ng/mL). What is the best approach for treating this patient?

A: For the treatment of portal hypertension caused by cirrhosis resulting in esophageal varices and splenomegaly, I refer to fullness and distention in the chest and hypochondriac region (胸肋滿脹 xiōng lē mǎn zhàng) and hard glomus (痞硬 pǐ yìng) in the *Treatise on Cold Damage and Miscellaneous Diseases* and mother-of-malaria (lump glomus occurring in malaria) (瘧母 nüè mǔ) in *On the Essential Prescriptions of the Golden Coffer*. In this case, elevated alpha-fetoprotein (AFP) levels most likely result from a slowed metabolism caused by hepatocellular damage, not hepatocellular cancer (HCC). You just need to add appropriate doses of yang-supplementing medicinals and these levels will gradually decrease. Once the liver function has returned to normal, the splenomegaly will also gradually resolve.

Remember! You must also closely monitor the patient's T/D Bil, T-Pro, BUN/CR, Hb, and PLT levels. You can prescribe a qi-boosting spleen-fortifying and qi-moving phlegm-transforming formula such as Xiang Sha Liu Jun Zi Tang or heat-clearing phlegm-damp-transforming water-disinhibiting formula such as Chai Ling Tang adding The Three Great Yang-Supplementers, Huang Qin and/or Huang Lian (3 qian for every 1 liang of the combined total to counterbalance the heat), Da Huang (increasing the dose incrementally until the patient maintains about 2–3 stools/day), and Ren Shen/Chuan Qi Powder.

If ascites and extensive lower leg edema presents, then add large doses of Fu Ling and Ze Xie; if low T-Pro levels present, then add large doses of Fu Ling, Bai Guo, Huai Shan, Yi Yi Ren, and Ren Shen (powder); if T-Bil levels spike again, then add slightly larger doses of Zhi Zi and Da Huang; and if PLT levels fall to 80,000–90,000 (normal range 150,000–400,000 uL), then you should subtract Chuan Qi (powder) and add Zhu Jie Qi and Xi Lu Rong (powder).

If the patient presents with cirrhosis with hemolysis or esophageal varices, then add Dan Shen, Ren Shen (powder), The Three Great Yang-Supplementers, Huang Qin, Da Huang, Xi Lu Rong (powder), and Zhu Jie Qi; if elevated BUN and CR levels present, then add Ding Shu Xiu, Ren Dong Teng, Pu Gong Ying, and Da Huang; and if water amassment presents, then prescribe a kidney yang-warming qi transformation-promoting and dampness- and water-disinhibiting by bland-percolation formula such as (Yu Sheng) Wu Ling San (Nephritis Formula) or a spleen- and stomach-supplementing phlegm-damp transforming formula such as Ban Xia Tian Ma Bai Zhu San.

These approaches will provide effective treatment for your patient's condition.

Traditionally, many TCM doctors use Gui Pi Tang variant to treat this condition, and this is another possible approach, but you must take into consideration ascites and blood test results. If elevated ammonia levels present, then you should incrementally increase the dose of Da Huang up until the patient maintains $\geq$ 3 stools/day; and for elevated BUN and CR, add Pu Gong Ying, Ren Dong Teng, and Xi Lu Rong (powder). Once the cirrhosis improves, splenomegaly will also resolve.

I once treated an HCC patient presenting with AFP levels of > 30,000 and hepatomegaly so severe that the abdominal mass extended down to the navel. Through TCM treatment the patient gradually improved and eventually stabilized. So you can see that with some patience and effort the TCM pharmacopoeia offers ample medicinals to effectively treat hepatitis, cirrhosis, HCC, hepatic encephalopathy (HE), and hepatorenal syndrome (HRS).

Case Study #4: Hepatitis B Virus – May Develop into Severe Complications!

Q1: Three years ago, a 42 y/o female patient discovered that she had been infected by the hepatitis B virus (HBV). Both AST and ALT levels were > 100, but after being administered the antiviral drug Adefovir, these levels dropped back down to normal. However, later in autumn of that year she developed ascites, prompting the discontinuation of Adefovir and the administration of diuretics instead, along with follow-up CT scans every 2 months.

The most recent lab test results are as follows: T-Bil 2.0 (0.2–1.2 mg/dL), AST 38 (0–40 u/L), ALT 45 (1–30 u/L), and ALB 43 (normal range 35–55 g/L). And the patient's bowel movements and appetite are normal. Do you think it is necessary for me to administer treatment for this patient? Please offer your advice and guidance. Thank you!

A: Hmm…a cirrhotic patient presenting with ascites, normal levels of AST, ALT, and ALB, and only slightly elevated levels of T-Bil. I would consider prescribing a qi-boosting spleen-fortifying and qi-moving phlegm-transforming formula such as Xiang Sha Liu Jun Zi Tang or Shen Ling Bai Zhu San adding Dan Shen, Dang Shen, and Da Huang (small dose); or a heat-clearing phlegm-damp-transforming water-disinhibiting formula such as Chai Ling Tang adding Zhi Zi and Da Huang (small dose). And if ascites is severe, then make sure to include large doses of The Four Lings.

This therapeutic regimen will bring T-Bil back down to normal and resolve ascites, and then the patient can begin gradually reducing the dose and finally discontinuing Western medicine drugs altogether. If this approach is not taken, the condition could readily develop into a smorgasbord of severe complications such as cirrhosis, liver failure, fulminant hepatitis, hepatic encephalopathy (HE), and hepatorenal syndrome (HRS).

Q2: I followed your advice on this patient. After 3 weeks of administering the TCM formula, ascites has completely resolved, bitter fullness in the chest and hypochondriac region no longer presents, and urine and stools are both normal. However, elevated T-Bil levels remain, the patient said that she *feels* "heat" after taking the TCM medicinal decoction, and at night her lower legs feel heavy and distended. Why do you think this is?

A: Congratulations! Your patient's ascites has already resolved. The symptoms you have described are normal, so don't fret and get overanxious. Just continue administering your formula adding Zhi Zi, Da Huang (small dose), Dang Shen, Dan Shen, and combinations of other blood-quickening stasis-transforming medicinals such as Chuan Xiong, Chi Shao, Xian Zha, Gu Sui Bu, and Xu Duan. This approach will gradually bring T-Bil back down to normal.

The feeling of heaviness and distention in the lower legs at night suggests restless leg syndrome, for which these blood-quickening stasis-transforming medicinals will also remedy. As for the *feeling* of "heat" after taking the TCM formula, I attribute this to psychosomatic Shao Yang phantom heat; and if this symptom really troubles the patient, then you can add Qing Hao, Zhi Mu, and Di Gu Pi into your formula.

Case Study #5: Ascites – Common Symptom of Cirrhosis

Q: A 62 y/o female patient with cirrhosis was hospitalized 2 months ago due to severe ascites. She was administered diuretics resulting in 6–7 stools per day and received albumin (ALB) infusions to get ALB and total protein (T-Pro) levels back up to normal range.

Right now she does not have ascites, but her gastroenterologist told her that she needed a liver transplant in order to survive. Her most recent lab test results are as follows: AST 67 (0–40 u/L), ALT 54 (1–30 u/L), ALP 117 (44–147 IU/L), AFP 44 (< 10 ng/ml), T-Bil 2.7 (0.2–1.2 mg/dL), T-Pro 6.8 (5.6–8.4 g/dL), PLT 100,000 (150,000–400,000 uL), PTT 40 (30–45 sec.), and normal levels of BUN, CR, and ammonia.

I want to prescribe Chai Ling Tang variant (including large doses of Cang Zhu, Fu Ling, and Ze Xie) adding Xu Duan, Gu Sui Bu, Ren

Shen (powder), Jin Ying Zi, and The Three Great Yang-Supplementers. What do you think about this approach?

A: A common side effect of diuretics is constipation and *not* diarrhea. Thus, I doubt that the 6–7 stools per/day is a result of the diuretic medication. Typically, to promote bowel movements of that extent, sennosides (the main active constituents in Fan Xie Ye (Senna Leaf, Folium Sennae)) would normally be prescribed since it functions as a stimulant laxative. There is no correlation between ALB dropping from 3.2 to 2.6 and the administration of diuretics. Remember! Don't get confused about this!

The patient's lab test results clearly show normal ammonia, BUN, and CR levels; T-Bil (only slightly elevated) and PLT (only slightly decreased) are both within an acceptable range; and there are not any abnormalities involving coagulation or hemolysis. In fact, there is *no* sign whatsoever of liver failure. So why would her gastroenterologist recommend having a liver transplant? Why is it necessary to frighten the patient with this radical procedure? All this patient needs is to maintain adequate nutritional supplementation and immediately begin a TCM therapeutic regimen (the formula you mentioned will be effective!). Through this approach she will be on the path towards gradual improvement and recovery.

Case Study #6: "Sweating Liver" – Chai Ling Tang Variant

Q: I have read in *Harrison's Principles of Internal Medicine* that there are three theories explaining the accumulation of ascitic fluid developing from cirrhosis. I have also seen where some physician's have used the metaphor "sweating liver" to describe this physiological mechanism (or phenomenon). Do you think this description more accurately correlates with ascites or hepatorenal syndrome?

A: Based on the theories proposed in *Harrison's Principles of Internal Medicine*, I would say that "sweating liver" refers to ascites developing from cirrhosis, most likely resulting from portal vein hypertension along with a concomitant decrease in circulating blood volume and low levels of protein and albumin in the blood.

I have treated a hepatocellular carcinoma (HCC) patient that had undergone transcatheter arterial embolization (TAE) who presented with this type of phenomenon as well. The patient's routine blood tests and ultrasound were normal, but refractory ascites led to repeated drainage with therapeutic paracentesis. Eventually, exploratory surgery was performed discovering that fluid was continuously permeating the surface of the liver—as if the liver were sweating!

At first, I prescribed great yang-supplementing medicinals in attempts to return yang and bolster right qi, thus inhibiting the proliferation of cancer cells. But this approach resulted in exacerbating the fluid build-up on the liver, requiring the patient to undergo additional repeated drainage. Then, I decided to change the focus of treatment and prescribed the heat-clearing phlegm-damp-transforming water-disinhibiting formula Chai Ling Tang variant. This formula proved very effective in remedying the refractory ascites ("sweating liver") and stabilizing the patient's condition.

Case Study #7: "Hemolytic" Cirrhosis

Q: A 60 y/o female patient has a more than 30-year history of chronic hepatitis. Last year, after returning from a trip to Europe, she noticed her abdomen was enlarging (ascites). However, an overshadowing optimism (or *subconscious denial*!) impelled her to disregard this sign and she continued going about life as normal. Finally, 3 months later, a pronounced sagging distention (墜脹 zhuì zhàng) sensation in her abdomen prompted her to visit my clinic. I wanted to prescribe a TCM medicinal decoction, but she refused. She was only willing to receive acupuncture, which did prove effective in providing *temporary* relief of the aching pain in her lower extremities and abdominal discomfort caused by ascites, but the patient's ascites continued getting worse.

Eventually, she went in for a thorough hospital examination, with the lab test results as follows: T-Pro 6.2 (5.6–8.4 g/dL), ALB 2.4 (3.4–5.6 g/dL), T-Bil 4.3 (0.2–1.2 mg/dL), BUN 12.7 (8–25 mg/dL), CR 0.5 (0.5–1.5 mg/dL), HB 10.1 (F, 12–16 g/dL), HCT 27.5 (F, 37–47%), and PLT 38×10^3/l (150–400 $x10^{3}$ /uL). What would you do for this patient? blood- and qi-supplementing, blood-cooling stasis-dispelling, and yin-enriching

A: This is a case of what I call "hemolytic" cirrhosis presenting with hemolytic manifestations and anemia (e.g., HB↓, HCT↓, and PLT↓). Obviously, it would be wise for this patient to begin taking a TCM medicinal decoction as soon as possible.

I would consider prescribing a qi-boosting spleen-fortifying and qi-moving phlegm-transforming formula such as Xiang Sha Liu Jun Zi Tang, a blood- and qi-supplementing stasis-dispelling formula such as Sheng Yu Tang combining Wu Ling San (Nephritis Formula) (including large doses of Fu Ling and Ze Xie), or a heat-clearing phlegm-damp-transforming water-disinhibiting formula such as Chai Ling Tang variant. Regardless of the formula you choose, make sure to add Da Huang (increasing the dose incrementally until the patient maintains 2–3 stools/day), Zhi Zi, The Three Great Yang-Supplementers (starting out with 2 qian each, gradually increasing the dose), Ren Shen (powder) (3 qian), Xi Lu Rong (powder), Bai Guo, Huai Shan, Yi Yi Ren, Qian Shi, and Huang Qin.

Remember! As long as T-Pro, ALB, and PLT increase back up to normal levels, then the ascites will gradually resolve. You must also pay attention to electrolyte levels, making sure that Na+ remains within normal range, because as you know, hyponatremia will also cause edema!

Case Study #8: Malignant Liver Tumors – Why Yang-Supplementing Medicinals?

Q: You often use yang-supplementing medicinals to treat malignant liver tumors. Is the reason to accelerate the generation of hepatocytes and prevent immunosuppression that may result from Western medicine surgical procedures and drug administration?

A: I use the yang-supplementing method for liver cancer patients whom have already been administered Western medicine drug treatment (i.e., chemotherapeutic agents, immunosuppressants). In these types of patients, the liver cancer tumor marker alfa-fetoprotein (AFP) decreases for a period of time, but then rapidly rebounds when the malignant hepatocytes undergo necrosis and the catabolism of enzymes occurs.

The objective of this approach is to accelerate the metabolism of malignant hepatocytes that have undergone necrosis. This will result in a rapid decrease in AFP, inhibit the rate of malignant hepatocyte proliferation, and eventually lead to shrinking and calcification of the tumor, which effectively renders the tumor *inactive*.

The root or "essential state" of liver cancer can typically be identified as stasis heat pattern, if the patient hasn't been administered Western medicine drug treatment, then the standard TCM therapeutic approach is to prescribe large doses of cold and bitter heat-clearing toxin-resolving medicinals. And if this approach fails to provide effective results, then you must add yang-supplementing medicinals into the mix to boost the metabolism and immune system and bolster right qi.

Case Study #9: TCM Medicinals Prevent Hepatic Cirrhosis Deterioration and Development into Hepatocellular Cancer

Q: I have a patient with hepatic cirrhosis who has already begun TCM medicinal treatment. Based on your clinical experience, what are the chances of this condition developing into hepatocellular cancer (HCC)?

A: It seems everyone has their own hypothesis of how cirrhosis evolves into HCC. The way I see it is that cirrhosis causes hepatocytes to shrink and undergo necrosis, a process that the brain interprets as a cellular insufficiency, thus inducing a feedback mechanism to increase the production of hepatocytes and resulting in an overcompensated state with excessive amounts of potentially "renegade" (neoplastic) hepatocytes.

Malignant liver cells (neoplastic hepatocytes) can be classified into two types: "old" cells that are metabolized too slowly and "new" cells that are produced too quickly. "New" cells that are produced too quickly can be identified as heat pattern, and "old" cells that have undergone necrosis and are being metabolized too slowly can be identified as yang vacuity pattern.

The liver cancer tumor marker alfa-fetoprotein (AFP) is produced whenever liver cells are regenerating and can be referenced to differentiate the following 5 stages:

1) Post-resection cell regeneration stage
2) Acute diffuse hepatocellular necrosis stage

3) Iatrogenic hepatocyte damage stage
4) Malignant hepatocyte proliferation stage
5) Post-embolization, post-ethanol injection, or post-ablation therapy malignant hepatocellular necrosis stage

As long as you accurately identify the pattern as the basis for determining the appropriate treatment, in the great majority of cases hepatic cirrhosis will *not* deteriorate and develop into malignancy.

Case Study #10: Why Does Liver Cancer Relapse Following Liver Transplant?

Q: I have read that a substantial percentage of patients who receive liver transplants will have a relapse of liver cancer. Is there any way for TCM to effectively treat these patients?

A: If hepatocellular cancer relapses following a liver transplant, you must first determine the exact location of the neoplasm. Administration of immunosuppressants (i.e., corticosteroids) following transplant is imperative in order to prevent organ rejection, but the downside is that it makes the patient more susceptible to recurrence with rapid proliferation. In most cases, I would advise the patient to undergo either radiofrequency ablation (RFA), transcatheter arterial chemoembolization (TACE), selective internal radiation therapy (SIRT), or percutaneous ethanol injection (PEI) accompanied by the administration of TCM medicinals.

At this stage, I view the condition as reverting back to the "essential state" and will prescribe a formula such as Chai Ling Tang (clears heat, transforms phlegm-damp, and disinhibits water), Ru Mo Si Wu Tang (nourishes and quickens the blood and dispels stasis), or Tong Jing Fang (quickens the blood and dissipates stasis, warms and supplements the liver and kidney, and frees the channels) adding The Three Yellows, Bai Zhu, Fu Ling, Ze Xie, Chuan Qi (powder), Qing Hao, Zhi Mu, Wan Ling Dan, and Yu Sheng Wan. You can also add Ren Shen (powder) starting out with a small dose and gradually increasing.

This formula will facilitate transplant acceptance, reduce the risk of malignant recurrence, and improve the overall prognosis. It should be prescribed up until there are no signs of organ rejection (graft-versus-host disease (GvHD)) or other complications.

Case Study #11: Cirrhosis – Qi-Boosting Spleen-Fortifying Approach

Q: I have just begun treating a new patient diagnosed with cirrhosis. Originally, I thought about prescribing Sheng Yu Tang adding Zhi Zi to increase the blood supply to the liver, but then I remembered you recommended Xiang Sha Liu Jun Zi Tang adding Zhi Zi and Da Huang. Is your reasoning for prescribing this formula based on the compromised capacity of cirrhotic liver tissue to receive an influx in blood supply or is it because the increased blood supply will stimulate the hepatitis virus?

A: The main reason I recommend a qi-boosting spleen-fortifying and qi-moving phlegm-transforming approach (e.g., Xiang Sha Liu Jun Zi Tang) instead of a blood-supplementing blood-regulating, blood-cooling stasis-dispelling, and yin-nourishing qi-supplementing approach (e.g., Sheng Yu Tang) is because patients with cirrhosis often have esophageal varices and poor appetite. This typically results in reduced enzyme secretions in the liver, spleen, gallbladder and stomach and compromised nutrient absorption capacity of the small intestines (if severe, malabsorption), which makes the patient susceptible to low T-Pro levels (hypoproteinemia). Sheng Yu Tang includes a relatively large dose of Huang Qi (up to 2 liang), which increases the risk of esophageal varices and rupture in these susceptible patients. The reason is *not* because Sheng Yu Tang poses a risk of stimulating replication of the hepatitis virus in patients with cirrhosis.

However, for patients with a good appetite, pronounced darkened skin and low platelet levels (thrombocytopenia) or severely compromised blood supply due to hepatic artery obstruction that leads to hepatic atrophy, I would indeed consider prescribing Sheng Yu Tang adding Zhi Zi. This approach will promote hematopoiesis and increase platelet levels, thus preventing potential complications of vomiting blood (hematemesis) and bruising (purpura) that may arise from thrombocytopenia.

Remember! Cirrhotic patients are susceptible to malabsorption, which can be identified as spleen vacuity pattern and requires administration of a qi-boosting spleen-fortifying and qi-moving phlegm-transforming formula such as Xiang Sha Liu Jun Zi Tang. As a general rule, I will only prescribe blood and qi-supplementing formulas such as Sheng Yu Tang or Bu Yang Huan Wu Tang if the patient has a good appetite and strong physical constitution and/or is in the very early stage of cirrhosis.

Case Study #12: Can TCM Medicinals Increase T-Pro and ALB in Cirrhotic Patients?

Q: Today I served as a guest speaker at a university. A Western medicine physician who attended the lecture asked me if a CT scan image would reveal visible changes on the surface of the liver following successful TCM treatment of cirrhosis. I said of course it would. I explained that a wide range of astringing and kidney yang-supplementing medicinals (e.g., Bai Guo, Jin Ying Zi, Tu Si Zi, She Chuang Zi) can be administered to increase the concentration of serum total protein (T-Pro) and albumin (ALB) in the blood. And sweet and neutral astringing, spleen-supplementing stomach-fortifying and bland-percolating dampness-disinhibiting medicinals (e.g., Yi Yi Ren, Fu Ling, Lian Zi, and Qian Shi) will increase the absorption capacity of the small intestine and thus directly increase the concentration of T-Pro and ALB in the blood. Is this an accurate way to explain the pharmacodynamics?

A: That's right! Administering those medicinals will definitely be effective in increasing T-Pro and ALB in patients with cirrhosis. However, I would also add Gan Jiang and Fu Zi (2 qian each) and Ren Shen (powder) (1–2 qian) for best results, and you can also add large doses of The Three Yellows to lower AST and ALT levels.

Qian Shi has an astringing, kidney-boosting, and spleen-fortifying dampness-disinhibiting by bland percolation action that increases T-Pro and ALB concentrations. Other medicinals such as Lian Xu, Huang Bo, Zhi Zi, Fu Ping, Che Qian Cao, He Ye, He Geng, and Yu Mi Xu have a heat-clearing dampness-disinhibiting and inflammation-reducing action that increases T-Pro and ALB concentrations in the serum. Fu Ling, Ze Xie, and Zhu Ling disinhibit dampness by bland percolation and Fang Ji and Ting Li Zi disinhibit water and urine to increase T-Pro and ALB. Fu Ling, Bai Zhu, Yi Yi Ren, Shan Yao, Lian Zi, Qian Shi, Dang Shen, Ren Shen, and Huang

Qi supplement spleen qi and nourish the spleen and stomach to increase T-Pro and ALB. Jin Ying Zi (Da Jin Ying and Xiao Jin Ying), Bai Guo, Long Gu, Mu Li, Shan Zhu Yu, and all types of "seed" medicinals have an astringing action that increases T-Pro and ALB. The Three Great Yang-Supplementers (Gan Jiang, Fu Zi, and Rou Gui), Lu Rong, Hua Jiao, Rou Cong Rong, Suo Yang, and Tu Si Zi supplement kidney yang to increase T-Pro and ALB. All of these medicinals with their various flavors, nature, and actions can increase T-Pro and ALB. You just need to accurately identify the pattern to determine the right ones for your patient!

Da Huang, Pu Xiao, Gan Sui, and Yuan Hua drastically expel water amassment (fluid accumulation) from the inside and outside of the intestines to remedy constipation caused by intestinal dysmotility and increased abdominal compartment pressure (intra-abdominal hypertension (IAH)) that may lead to abdominal compartment syndrome (ACS) and exacerbation of ascites. All of these medicinals have the action of draining excess water (fluid) via the intestines at a much faster rate than possible through the bladder.

For the treatment of short, hasty, discontinuous breathing, rapid panting, ascites, and pleural effusion caused by cirrhosis, Ban Xia, Zi Su Zi, Hou Po, Lai Fu Zi, Shi Di, Mu Xiang, and Sha Ren can be prescribed to relax the diaphragm and promote a fluid "convection" downwards. If pulmonary embolism or pleural effusion presents, then prescribe Ting Li Zi, Fang Ji, Ma Huang, Xing Ren, Jiang Pi, and Sang Bai Pi. All of these medicinals through their specific actions will promote increased T-Pro and ALB in cirrhotic patients.

Remember! For the treatment of cirrhosis with TCM medicinals, you must start out with small doses and gradually increase the amount. If too large of a dose is prescribed at the onset, this may lead to increased portal venous pressure (portal hypertension) that induces the flow of transudate and/or blood from the surface of the liver and results in exacerbation of ascites. If severe edema presents, you can advise the patient to concomitantly take small doses of Western medicine diuretics at first to expedite the resolution of ascites and generalized edema, while gradually increasing the dose of The Three Great Yang-Supplementers and Ren Shen (powder) and incrementally increasing the dose of Da Huang up until the patient maintains 3 stools/day. This approach will prevent intestinal dysmotility caused by abdominal pressure from ascites (a phenomenon much like external pressure on a worm rendering it incapable of squirming!) and severe abdominal distention.

When prescribing TCM medicinals you must seek a mutually complementary balance between the actions of *opening* (開 kāi) and *closing* (闔 hé). This concept resonates throughout the duality of nature. For example, supplementing also requires some draining, astringing also requires freeing, and closing also requires opening. The pathomechanism of disease can be seen as a complex gestalt of factors. You cannot *lock* in too tightly on a singular aspect; otherwise, you run the risk of overcompensating on that one aspect. If you determine it's necessary to prescribe *"locking"* medicinals (e.g., drastic supplementation, drastic water-expelling, great cold heat-draining, toxin-resolving insect-killing, great heat yang-supplementing), then it should be processed into either pill or powder form, and only administered in small, incrementally increasing doses.

Regarding a CT scan image revealing visible changes on the surface of the liver following successful TCM treatment of cirrhosis, you must first understand that there are two main types of cirrhosis: 1) *atrophic* liver (60% of cases) and 2) *hypertrophic* liver (40% of cases). For the *hypertrophic* type, I would prescribe Xiang Sha Liu Jun Zi Tang (boosts qi and fortifies the spleen and moves qi and transforms phlegm). Once the symptoms have resolved, the liver will return to its normal size. For the atrophic type, I would prescribe Blood Desiccation Formula (nourishes the blood, enriches yin, and emolliates the liver), Qi Bao Mei Ran Dan (supplements and boosts the liver and kidney and nourishes blood and replenishes essence), or possibly Sheng Yu Tang (supplements qi and nourishes blood). However, I would be cautious about over-supplementing qi due to the risk of excessive blood perfusion that may lead to congestion, stagnation, and depression. Even after the symptoms have resolved, it will take some time for the liver to gradually regain its normal size. For both types you can prescribe a formula variant such as,.

For the *atrophic* type, the ultrasound image may reveal a thickened appearance during the therapeutic regimen, which should *not* be misinterpreted as already having regained normal size. This "halo" phenomenon simply results from increased blood perfusion to the liver and the rapid regeneration of hepatocytes that create a haze of accelerated metabolic frequencies. After administering this formula for a period of time, the "halo" will resolve and the coarse, nodular texture on the surface will also appear smoother and suppler. Blood perfusion and hepatocyte regeneration are concentrated in the parenchyma and takes time to work its way up to repair the surface. Remember! For the *atrophic* type, AFP levels may increase during the regeneration process.

Case Study #13: Chronic Hepatitis B (HBV) – AFP Levels Spike Following Administration of Western Medicine Drugs

Q: A 41 y/o male patient with chronic hepatitis B virus (HBV) presented with increased levels of alpha feto-protein (AFP). After receiving treatment with the -vir and -dine classes of antiviral drugs, liver function test levels dramatically increased—AST 192 (0–40 u/L), ALT 170 (1–30 u/L), AFP 1031 (< 10 ng/mL), T-Bil 2.01 (0.2–1.2 mg/dL), and ALP 220 (44–147 IU/L)), but the CT scan did not reveal a tumor. Why would AFP spike like this?

A: AFP is a protein produced whenever liver cells are regenerating as a result of liver damage (e.g., hepatitis, cirrhosis) or cancer (e.g., hepatocellular, testicular, ovarian). For HBV patients who have a flare-up following administration of the -dine and -vir classes of antiviral drugs, you can prescribe a heat-clearing toxin-resolving formula such as Huang Lian Jie Du Tang variant to lower the AST and ALT levels. This will eventually bring AFP levels back down to 200–300 (though there may be fluctuations during this process up to as high as 2000!). If several weeks go by and these levels still do not fall back down to near normal levels, then add The Three Great Yang-Supplementers (starting out with small doses and gradually increasing), which will drive AFP levels back down to normal.

In HBV patients, normally once AST and ALT levels drop back down, AFP will follow suit. HBV patients who are administered the -dine or -vir classes of antiviral drugs or interferon injections, prompting a spike in AFP or ferritin levels without increases in AST and ALT, can be identified as kidney yang vacuity pattern.

Typically, if the condition does not progress to fulminant hepatic failure, and AST and ALT levels remain at mildly elevated levels of 100–200 and AFP ≥ 1000, then you can consider prescribing Huang Lian Jie Du Tang adding The Three Great Yang-Supplementers from the onset. If convenient, have the patient get his HBV DNA (viral load) tested; and if results show viral copies of ≥ 100,000 up to 1 billion per milliliter, this indicates rapid viral replication. In this case, you should change to a blood-nourishing liver-emolliating formula such as Xue Ku Fang, Qi Bao Mei Ran Dan, or Sheng Yu Tang adding Wu Wei Zi, Huang Qin, and Mu Dan Pi. If increased AFP levels still present, then add The Three Great Yang-Supplementers.

Case Study #14: Congenital Hepatomegaly – TCM Medicinals Reduce AFP Levels

Q: In your book *TCM Treatment of Common Liver Diseases*, why do you add such large doses of The Three Great Yang-Supplementers (Gan Jiang, Fu Zi, and Rou Gui) in the treatment of congenital hepatomegaly for infants? Also, do you have any suggestions on what advice I can give these families to calm the cries and discomfort of these infants?

A: You are referring to the special case of that 1 y/o child with AFP $\geq$ 30,000. Why would I prescribe such high doses of The Three Great Yang-Supplementers? A thorough examination that included blood tests, biopsy, ultrasound, and CT scan could find *no* evidence of a precipitating factor or cause. And despite having a slightly reduced appetite and a swollen and distended liver (hepatomegaly), the child had a strong constitution with normal energy levels (trotting around and exploring everything!).

This suggested to me that the problem involved the feedback mechanism between the brain (control panel) and the viscera (indivisible parts). Thus, in order to "boost" the metabolism and recalibrate the system, I simply prescribed The Three Great Yang-Supplementers. After administering the TCM formula, AFP decreased and the hepatomegaly subsided. The child's appetite was normal and everyone was happy!

Case Study #15: Chronic HBV – Increased T-Bil Levels

Q: I have a 35 y/o female patient with a history of chronic hepatitis B infection (HBV) that she was diagnosed with in her youth.

She has been taking Lamivudine and Adefovir for many years without effectiveness. Her lab test results are as follows: AST 150 (0–40 u/L), ALT 200 (1–30 u/L), T-Bil 1.8 (0.2–1.2 mg/dL), and PLT 100,000 (150,000–400,000 μL).

I prescribed Huang Lian Jie Du Tang adding Da Huang, Xu Duan, and Gu Sui Bu. The patient's AST and ALT dropped down to between 50–60 and T-Bil increased to 2.5. Why would T-Bil increase despite reduced liver enzyme levels?

A: In this case where T-Bil increases after administration of cold bitter medicinals in a chronic HBV patient, I would continue prescribing the same formula and monitoring the patient. It's very well possible that this increase is a reflection of the residual hepatitis infection along with concomitant cholangitis. You should consider adding Xian Zha, Dan Shen, and Chi Shao to your original formula. If this still doesn't bring T-Bil down, then add small doses of Gan Jiang and Fu Zi to boost the metabolism and immune system and bolster right qi

Once the T-Bil levels have stabilized, this indicates that the inflammation has subsided, so you can reduce the dose of The Three Yellows and add larger doses of Gan Jiang and Fu Zi to promote blood perfusion and healing of damaged tissue. Prolonged administration of high doses of bitter flavor and cold nature medicinals such as The Three Yellows may exacerbate liver blood stasis, resulting in the vicious cycle of residual heat (i.e., hepatitis and cholangitis). This approach circumvents the potential for this problem arising.

Case Study #16: Can TCM Medicinals Effectively Treat Hepatitis and Cirrhosis?

Q: A 47 y/o male patient visited my clinic simply to *regulate the constitution* with supplementing medicinals. I had him do a routine blood workup that revealed the presence of active HBV infection with T-Bil 1.3 (0.2–1.2 mg/dL), AST 350 (0–40 u/L), and ALT 480 (1–30 u/L). It is a Korean custom to take supplementing medicinals during the spring and autumn, but considering this patient's condition, it was obvious that the last thing he needed was more heat from supplementing, so I prescribed Huang Lian Jie Du Tang adding Pu Gong Ying and Lian Qiao. This was very effective in improving both liver function and enzyme levels and treating the inflammation.

A: This is a good example of how TCM doctors need to provide patients with accurate information about taking supplementing medicinals. Acute hepatitis with elevated liver enzyme and function levels can be identified as heat pattern, thus, you would naturally want to administer heat-clearing toxin-resolving and blood-quickening blood-cooling medicinals such as Huang Lian Jie Du Tang adding Dan Shen and Mu Dan Pi.

However, for chronic hepatitis or cirrhosis, you might consider prescribing a formula such as Xiang Sha Liu Jun Zi Tang (boosts qi and fortifies the spleen) or Sheng Yu Tang (nourishes yin and supplements qi); for patients with hypertension, you could administer Bu Yang Huan Wu Tang (supplements qi and the blood), Ru Mo Si Wu Tang (nourishes and quickens the blood), or Sheng Yu Tang (supplements blood and qi and nourishes yin); and for patients with diabetes, you could administer Zhi Bo Di Huang Tang (enriches yin and downbears fire) adding Sang Bai Pi.

You can see here that the concept of *supplementing* varies depending on pattern identification and should be strategically administered within the parameters of treating pathogenic conditions and disease prevention.

Case Study #17: Autoimmune Hepatitis – TCM Medicinals Supplant Corticosteroids

Q: Recently, I have been writing a medical case report about an autoimmune hepatitis (AIH) patient. The details are as follows:

[07/31] after undergoing resection of a hepatic cyst, T-Bil spiked to 27.3 (0.2–1.2 mg/dL)

[08/03] began immunosuppressant treatment (Prednisolone)

[09/07] T-Bil dropped down to 14.1 and AST 69 (0–40 u/L) and ALT 83 (1–30 u/L)

[10/10] T-Bil dropped down to 8.2 and AST 85 and ALT 122 increased

[11/14] T-Bil increased slightly to 8.9 and AST 114 and ALT 161 continued increasing

[12/02] T-Bil dropped down again to 8.2 and AST 249 and ALT 165 continued increasing

That's when I began administering TCM medicinals and having the patient gradually reduce the dosage of corticosteroids. After one year, the patient had completely discontinued Western medicine drugs as well as TCM medicinals. The most recent lab test results show T-Bil 0.9, AST 29.4, and ALT 33.9. The patient has remained healthy without relapse and has not taken any medication.

I have mixed feelings about this case and wonder whether immunosuppressant **treatment** (corticosteroids) alone would have been just as effective. What is the purpose of TCM treatment in this case? Without TCM treatment, would other complications arise? I found a medical paper reporting on the efficacy of immunosuppressants in the treatment of autoimmune hepatitis, advising the administration of small doses of corticosteroids for the prevention of cirrhosis. In this patient's case, T-Bil dropped from 27 down to normal levels in 1 month, but the patient had been taking small doses of corticosteroids for nearly his entire life.

A: You should publish this medical case report. The title could be *Integrative TCM and Western Medicine Treatment of Autoimmune Hepatitis and Hyperbilirubinemia.* How can you prove that the integrated treatment approach was truly effective? Well, on [11/14] T-Bil 8.9, AST 114, and ALT 161; and then on [12/02] T-Bil 8.2, AST 249, and ALT 165, which clearly indicates the condition was not under control and relapse had occurred. After taking TCM medicinals T-Bil, AST, and ALT all stabilized, and both the TCM medicinals and Western medicine drugs were eventually completely discontinued, indicating that autoantibodies are no longer attacking the immune system.

This is the same situation for systemic lupus erythematosus (SLE); Western medicine can control the condition (often requiring indefinite administration of immunosuppressant drugs), but only in very rare cases does it cure the disease. When TCM medicinals are integrated into this treatment regimen, you will see a rapid increase in C3, C4, Hb, WBC, RBC, PLT, T-Pro, and A/G; and decrease in ANA, anti-dsDNA, ESR, and CRP. Through this integrative approach, both Western medicine drugs and TCM medicinals can be gradually reduced and eventually discontinued. You can present this theoretical basis in your medical case report. As for the paper you read reporting on the use of corticosteroids reducing T-Bil from 27 down to normal, which is a unique case and gives a false impression, because after discontinuing the medication the levels will rebound. You will find many more papers reporting on this unfortunate, but more common, scenario!

Now, Western medicine can administer plasmapheresis, steroid pulse therapy, intravenous immunoglobulin (IVIG), and other immunosuppressants for the treatment of autoimmune hepatitis. However, this condition is still difficult to control, and long-term drug administration of these drugs carry the risk of toxicity on the liver, kidney, and nervous system. In the majority of patients, drug treatment is administered indefinitely up until hepatorenal syndrome (HRS), renal failure, or uremia develop, which requires renal dialysis, liver dialysis, or liver transplant, and may possibly lead to death. That case of yours is definitely the result of integrative TCM and Western medicine treatment. There is no question that administration of corticosteroids can rapidly resolve the inflammation, but once you discontinue the medication it will relapse.

Long-term administration of corticosteroids presents a higher risk of developing cirrhosis and it really isn't the best option available. If the patient is only administered a small dosage for a short period of time or maintains a regimen with a minute dosage without incurring a microbial infection (external contraction), then he/she may be just fine; but once external contraction (microbial infection) occurs, the risk of death is high.

IV. GASTROINTESTINAL DISORDERS

Some of the simplest and most practical methods of resolving common gastrointestinal disorders will be presented here. For instance, a disorder of the seven gates (七沖門 qī chōng mén) must be considered in cases of swill diarrhea with nontransformation of food (飧泄不化 sūn xiè bù huà), sesame oil treats constipation in the elderly, and for patients with difficult defecation (abnormal bowel movements) be aware of spinal stenosis.

Case Study #1: Swill Diarrhea with Nontransformation of Food

Q: A 40 y/o female patient explained that she has had diarrhea (sloppy stool (溏便 táng biàn) and sometimes thin sloppy stool (稀溏 xī táng)) every morning after breakfast for the past 10 years. Occasionally, her stools smell of the food she just ate for breakfast, especially vegetables. She passes 3–4 stools/day, has shortage of qi, a feeling of heaviness, and glomus below the heart (心下痞 xīn xià pǐ). She is a vegetarian and doesn't drink alcohol. Do you think this pathocondition can be identified as spleen qi vacuity pattern?

A: This patient's history and presenting symptoms suggests either the pattern of Li Zhong Tang (Center-Rectifying Decoction) manifesting in swill diarrhea with nontransformation of food (飧泄不化 sūn xiè bù huà) as presented in *On Cold Damage*; hypersensitivity of the central nervous system leading to disrupted regulation of the opening (開 kāi) and closing (闔 hé) mechanism (i.e., when the mouth opens during eating the anus will also open and the patient will defecate) of the seven gates (七冲門 qī chōng mén); or a vagus nerve disorder. For any of the possible etiologies above, you can treat this condition with Li Zhong Tang (aka Ren Shen Tang) adding Yu Sheng Wan. If glomus below the heart still persists following administration of this formula, then add Ji Nei Jin, Sha Ren, and Mu Xiang.

Case Study #2: Duodenal Ulcer – "There's Blood in My Stool!"

Q: A 42 y/o male patient incurred an episode of black tarry stool (melena) followed by larger amounts of red blood (hematochezia) and was rushed to the emergency room by ambulance where a CT scan, MRI, and x-ray were performed. Results revealed a duodenal ulcer and *no* abnormalities in the other segments of the small and large intestine, thus he was released from the hospital after several days. Subsequently, he incurred symptoms of dizziness, nausea, shortness of breath, and sharp pain upon palpation in the left lower abdomen parallel with the navel. Why do you think these symptoms would present?

A: Black tarry stool (melena) suggests duodenal ulcer. That's because the lesion is typically small with only miniscule amounts of bleeding, and by the time it passes all the way down through the GI tract to the stool, it has already stagnated and deoxygenated into a gooey muck. If the patient strains too much while defecating, this could irritate the lesion leading to relatively larger amounts of fresh, red blood. In actuality there really won't be that much blood. It's just that most people are so nervous about the sight of blood that they perceive the amount to be much more than there really is. The perception of *all that blood* may even lead to the sensation of dizziness, nausea, and shortness of breath as a result.

Of course, you can't completely rule out the possibility of chronic bleeding from duodenal ulcers causing anemia and resulting in dizziness, but it seems highly unlikely in this case. The sharp pain upon palpation in the left lower abdomen likely results from spasm of the celiac artery or abdominal muscle. You can prescribe a heat-clearing toxin-resolving formula such as Huang Lian Jie Du Tang combining Xiao Ban Xia Jia Fu Ling Tang and adding Lai Fu Zi, Yuan Hu, and Mu Xiang; or possibly Huang Lian Jie Du Tang adding Ban Xia, Shao Yao, Fu Ling, Tian Ma, and Ren Shen/Chuan Qi Powder. If there is persistent and pronounced bleeding, then you can consider adding blood-stanching stasis-dispelling medicinals such as Ou Jie, Ce Bo Ye, Ru Xiang, Mo Yao, Chuan Qi, and Hai Piao Xiao. This approach will stanch bleeding, heal the ulcer, and also promote blood production (hematopoiesis).

Case Study #3: Duodenal Ulcer – Black Tarry Stools

Q: A 41 y/o female patient complained of frequent glomus below the heart, black tarry stools, and feeling fatigued every day for the past 3 years. Administration of Western medicine drugs slightly improved her condition, but after she stopped taking the medication the black tarry stools appeared again. Do you think An Zhong San variant is a good formula for this patient? Or would Xie Xin Tang, Qing Wei San, or Huang Lian Jie Du Tang variants be better?

A: Duodenal ulcers presenting with black tarry stools (melena) caused by mild intestinal hemorrhage can be identified as stomach heat pattern. In my experience, I have had the best results prescribing cold and bitter heat-clearing blood-cooling medicinals, specifically Huang Lian Jie Du Tang adding Ou Jie, Ce Bo Ye, Ru Xiang, Mo Yao, Chuan Qi, and Hai Piao Xiao. This decoction should be administered either cool or at room temperature. Remember! Patients with duodenal ulcers and melena should be restricted to cold (or room temperature) foods and that goes for soups and stews as well (cook and then let it cool!). Spicy foods (e.g., chili pepper, raw garlic) and drinks that irritate the intestinal lining (e.g., tea) should be strictly avoided.

TCM medicinals should be administered up until an endoscopy confirms that the duodenum endothelium has completely grown back before you can discontinue treatment. However, the optimal approach would be administering long-term follow-up treatment with Chuan Qi (powder), Hai Piao Xiao (powder), and possibly a bit of Huang Qin (powder) as well (wash down these medicinals with cool water 4x/day before each meal and prior to going to bed). These medicinals will effectively prevent the troublesome recurrence of ulceration.

Case Study #4: Appendicitis – Ge Gen Qin Lian Tang

Q: My wife has appendicitis, so I prescribed Ge Gen Qin Lian Tang adding Da Huang. This formula was quite effective at remedying her symptoms, but she still has a mild fever and mild right lower quadrant tenderness. Do you have any suggestions about adding other medicinals?

A: Your main formula is accurate. I would continue administering this formula and you can consider adding combinations of medicinals such as Mu Dan Pi, Tao Ren, Fu Ling, Chi Shao, Yuan Hu, Mu Xiang, and Chuan Qi (powder) to effectively remedy abdominal tenderness. Naturally, if the problem recurs, then she should consider going ahead with an appendectomy.

Case Study #5: Chronic Constipation – Try TCM Extract Powder

Q: A 43 y/o female patient complained of having constipation for the past 15 years and has tried various Western medicine and folk medicine therapies without much effect. She frequently has abdominal distention and fullness and passes stool (malodorous and sticky in consistency) every 1 or 2 days. She feels too embarrassed to defecate at work because she has to go through the process of washing her sticky stool from the toilet every time. This is emotionally stressful on her. Please offer your guidance and advice on the best approach for treating this patient?

A: A female patient with a 15-year history of constipation. If she has a stout physical constitution, then prescribe the proprietary extract powder of Tao Ren Cheng Qi Tang (quickens the blood and transforms stasis and precipitates stasis heat) and Di Dang Tang (attacks and expels static blood) (2 g of each formula). Usually, the patient will pass stool within 4 hours after taking these medicinals. If the patient passes 3 or more stools, then you can reduce the dose to 1 g each; and if the patient still passes 3 or more stools, then reduce the dose to 0.5 g each.

This formula can be administered long-term to regulate the constitution. If a dose of 0.5 g of each formula is sufficient, then you can add combinations of stool-softening medicinals such as Dang Gui, He Shou Wu, Huang Jing, Sheng Di Huang, and Rou Cong Rong; and intestine-lubricating medicinals such as Tao Ren, Xing Ren, Huo Ma Ren, and Yu Li Ren (these "seed" medicinals contain oils that lubricate the intestines!). If the patient has been taking Western medicine stool softeners (emollient laxative) or bulk-forming laxatives for a long period of time, and now after switching over to the abovementioned TCM extract medicinal regimen she is unable to pass stool, then add small doses of The Three Great Yang-Supplementers (boosts the metabolism!).

If you decide to prescribe decocted medicinals, then you should add Da Huang (starting out at a small dose of 5 fen and gradually increasing the dose up to as much as 5–7 qian if necessary). If the patient still isn't able to pass stool, then add Pu Xiao, which functions as a saline laxative (starting out at 3 fen and gradually increasing to as much as 5 qian if necessary). If this still isn't effective, then add The Three Great Yang-Supplementers and Huang Qin.

If all of these methods prove ineffective, then I would advise the patient to undergo a detailed hospital examination to determine whether or not there are any physiological or structural abnormalities.

Case Study #6: Chronic Constipation (In the Elderly) – Promote Defecation and Regulate the Constitution

Q: I have a 92 y/o elderly female patient whose chief complaint is constipation. Her family explained that the patient has had problems with constipation since her youth, but the condition has gotten worse in recent years, requiring her to be hospitalized periodically in order to receive an enema. X-ray revealed the presence impacted feces (fecal impaction) in her intestines. I prescribed Zhi Bo Di Huang Tang adding Yu Li Ren (2 liang). Do you think this is a good approach?

A: This elderly woman with chronic constipation can be identified as yin vacuity constipation with cold impediment pattern. I recommend prescribing a blood-nourishing yin-enriching dryness-moistening formula such as Xue Ku Fang, Qi Bao Mei Ran Dan, or Dang Gui Yin Zi adding The Three Great Yang-Supplementers, Huang Qin, and Da Huang (incrementally increasing 5 fen or 1 qian doses until the patient maintains 2–3 stools/day). If this formula proves ineffective at maintaining 2–3 stools/day, then add larger doses of The Three Great Yang-Supplementers and Da Huang. In order to control the dosage, it may be more convenient to package the Da Huang decocting pieces separately into 5 fen packets, which the patient (family member or caretaker) can simply add into the formula for decoction.

Remember! The key here is finding the right amount of Da Huang so that the patient maintains 2–3 stools/day. If the draining precipitation action of Da Huang is too drastic (e.g., 5–8 stools/day), then reduce the dosage (1 packet/3x/2–3 days) and proceed in this manner until you eventually are able to discontinue administration of the formula altogether. Then, you can consider prescribing extract powder, choosing a simple combination of the blood-supplementing intestinal-moistening medicinals such as Dang Gui and He Shou Wu (extract powder); or if necessary, add these two medicinals into the formula combination of Tao Ren Cheng Qi Tang (quickens the blood and transforms stasis and precipitates stasis heat) and Di Dang Tang (attacks and expels static blood).

It is not uncommon for elderly people with chronic constipation to feel a sensation of insects biting the anus and suffer from depression and anxiety when they can't pass stool. This can make it particularly challenging for family members and caretakers. Thus, the treatment priority is to promote defecation while gradually regulating the constitution, which will provide long-term efficacy.

As for prescribing Zhi Bo Di Huang Tang adding Yu Li Ren, you may as well prescribe You Gui Yin adding Yu Li Ren and Da Huang instead. Yu Li Ren is grown in northern latitudes and you have a lot of this medicinal in South Korea. You should also advise patients with constipation to drink plenty of fluids and regularly eat foods high in moisture content and fiber such as bamboo shoots, red and white radish (cooked or pickled), pumpkin, sweet potato, burdock root, grapefruit, oranges, longan, litchi, seaweed, onion, garlic, leek, soybeans, brown rice, and nuts (all kinds). Oils are particularly helpful supplements for treating chronic constipation in the elderly, so for this patient I would also advise her to take 1–3 tablespoons of seed or nut oils (e.g., sesame, peanut, walnut, flax) every day.

Case Study #7: Why Does Beer Drinking Cause Soft Stools?

Q: South Korean's love to drink beer. Recently, people have been asking me: "Why do I have sloppy stools (溏便 táng biàn) and sloppy diarrhea (溏泄 táng xiè) the day after drinking a lot of beer?" Some TCM doctors identify this as interior cold pattern. What do you think?

A: The gastrointestinal tract is inundated with liquid after drinking large quantities of beer and the main ingredients (malted barley, hops, and brewer's yeast) in most beers all have water-disinhibiting (diuretic) and intestinal motility-promoting actions. Absorption of this sudden influx of fluids and its subsequent excretion from the body through perspiration or urination cannot be metabolized fast enough. The remainder of this fluid gets leftover in the large intestines and colon where it is mixed together with the chyme inside of the large intestines. It is this *brew* that often leads to what can be called compensatory or reflex soft stools.

Case Study #8: Diarrhea – Anxiety, Cold-Type Foods, Excessive Fluid Intake, Bacterial Infection, Inflammatory Disease

Q: For patients with allergic gastroenteritis, Western medicine will prescribe antibiotics to control the bacterial infection. Initially, this treatment provides effective relief, but oftentimes about 1 month later patients will experience episodes of abdominal pain and diarrhea every time they feel nervousness and anxiety. How would TCM treat this type of condition?

A: Well, to begin with, I am not sure you have your facts straight on this condition. It seems you are referring to the rare condition called eosinophilic gastroenteritis (EGE), for which Western medicine would prescribe immunosuppressants to control the inflammation. Antibiotics target bacteria and are prescribed in cases of bacterial diarrhea, which typically presents with diarrhea that has a sulfurous odor like "rotten duck eggs" and a burning sensation in the anus. Concomitant secondary bacterial infection presenting with stomach damp-heat pattern symptoms (i.e., diarrhea, abdominal pain) may occur in people with EGE, but again this condition is rare, and it should be confirmed by history, lab studies, and stool cultures.

You must also consider the possibility of generalized anxiety disorder (GAD) and hypersensitivity-related causes such as lactose intolerance, celiac disease (maladaptive immune response to gluten), irritable bowel syndrome (IBS) (non-inflammatory), and irritable bowel disease (IBD) (inflammatory and includes ulcerative colitis (UC) and Crohn's disease (CD)). People with GAD also present with sloppy stools (溏便 táng biàn) and diarrhea (瀉泄 xiè xiè) that are induced by anxiety attacks. And people who eat lots of fruits and vegetables (cold nature type foods), or drink excessive amounts of liquids without exercising or sweating much, are also susceptible to bouts of frequent sloppy stools.

In general, if a person has 2–3 sloppy stools per day, but doesn't have any pain or other discomfort, then I recommend *a wait-and-see approach*, just going about daily activities and not worrying too much about it, because the condition will likely resolve on its own. If a person feels discomfort, then I would prescribe a center-harmonizing agitation-calming and stagnation-dissipating phlegm-transforming formula such as Gan Mai Da Zao Tang Combining Ban Xia Hou Po Tang adding Cang Zhu, Ze Xie, and Yu Sheng Wan. If you determine that a bacterial infection is causing the diarrhea (i.e., sulfurous malodor and burning sensation in anus), then make sure to add Huang Qin and Huang Lian into your formula, or change the formula to Ge Gen Qin Lian Tang variant.

Remember! Decocted raw TCM medicinals are basically like soup or stew. So if the patient already has a large intake of fruits, vegetables, and liquids, and you prescribe large a volume of TCM formula decoction, then this may worsen the condition instead of help!

Case Study #9: Cholera – Leads to Intestinal Dysmotility

Q: I have a female patient who suffers from severe intestinal dysmotility (almost to the point of gastroparesis) following a cholera infection. She has already received 3 weeks of antimicrobial infusions and fluid therapy. The diarrhea is under control, but now she has constipation that can only be relieved by taking laxatives (produces soft stool). This condition is really taking its toll on her emotionally as well. Do you think this is a type of condition that will spontaneously resolve over time? Or is this something that could lead to chronic dysfunction?

A: This is a case where *Vibrio cholerae* interferes with spinal nerve function and can be classified as a "bacterium-induced palsy," resulting in anal sphincter paralysis. For this condition, I would prescribe one of the formulas in the Paralysis Formula Series based on the following considerations:

1) If the patient has not been administered corticosteroids, then this can be identified as residual heat or exterior wind-heat pattern, requiring administration of Paralysis Formula #1 (Di Long San Variant).
2) If the patient has been administered corticosteroids, then this can be identified as either spleen yang vacuity with dual blood and qi vacuity pattern, requiring administration of Paralysis Formula #2 (Shi Quan Da Bu Fang Variant); or kidney yang vacuity pattern, requiring administration of Paralysis Formula #3 (You Gui Yin Variant) adding Da Huang (incrementally increasing doses up until the patient maintains 2–3 stools/day) and The Three Great Yang-Supplementers (start out with small

doses each, gradually increasing to 5 qian and possibly even up to 7–8 qian if necessary).

Remember! You must explain to your patient that results will not appear *overnight*; she must have patience! Symptoms will be relieved and her condition will improve *over time.*

Case Study #10: Radiation Enteritis, Colitis, and Proctitis

Q: One of the research topics for my PhD program is radiation enteritis. Both my academic advisor and I would typically prescribe Xiang Sha Liu Jun Zi Tang variant for this condition. Can you share your experiences in the treatment of this condition?

A: Radiotherapy damage (e.g., enteritis, proctitis, colitis) can be a very complicated condition, especially if obliterative endarteritis develops, presenting with edema (possibly resembling elephantiasis!), sclerosis, submucosal fibrosis, abscesses, perforations, bleeding, and ischemia.

In mild cases of radiotherapy damage, I usually prescribe the kidney yang-warming qi transformation-promoting and bland-percolating dampness- and water-disinhibiting formula Wu Ling San (Nephritis Formula) (including large doses of Fu Ling, Ze Xie, Huang Qi, and The Three Great Yang-Supplementers) adding large doses of Yin Xing Ye and Da Huang (increasing incrementally until the patient maintains 2–3 stools/day). The keys to my therapeutic approach are using large doses of Yin Xing Ye (up to 8 qian), steeping the decocting pieces in 5 bowls (1,000 ml) of water along with 1 bowl (200 ml) of rice wine for at least 1/2 hour (ideally 2 hours), and then proceeding with decoction.

For cases in which there is only inflammation *without* ulceration or hemorrhage, I would typically prescribe a spleen-fortifying phlegm-transforming and center-supplementing diarrhea-checking formula variant such as Xiang Sha Liu Jun Zi Tang, Si Jun Zi Tang, Liu Jun Zi Tang, Bu Zhong Yi Qi Tang, Shen Ling Bai Zhu San, Ping Wei San, or Li Zhong Tang. Remember! It's also a good idea to add The Three Great Yang-Supplementers (boosts the metabolism and bolsters right qi) and Huang Qin (counterbalances the heat) into your main formula to avert the potential for the development of chronic complications manifesting in true cold and false heat pattern.

In cases in which there is inflammation *with ulceration* and *hemorrhage*, patients typically present with fresh blood in the stool and foul-smelling stool with clear or white lymphatic mucous (may look like nasal discharge or even have the consistency of fish brains!). In classical TCM pathologic terminology, this pathocondition can be classified as red and white diarrhea (赤白痢 chì bái lì). Red refers to the presentation of fresh blood and white to the lymph (described in classical TCM texts as resembling fish brains!). The presentation of fresh blood and pussy mucous (lymph) in the stool can be identified as gastrointestinal damp-heat pattern, requiring administration of a heat-clearing diarrhea-checking formula variant such as Huang Lian Jie Du Tang, Ge Gen Qin Lian Tang, or Qing Wei San including large doses of Cang Zhu and adding blood-quickening stasis-transforming and blood-cooling blood-stanching medicinals such as Chuan Qi, Ce Bo Ye, Ou Jie, Huai Hua, Di Yu, and Niu Xi. In cases of fecal frequency caused by excessive radiotherapy and increased intestinal motility, you can prescribe Wu Ling San (Nephritis Formula) including large doses of Cang Zhu and Ze Xie.

For patients *currently undergoing* a radiotherapy regimen who present with sloppy stools and frequent bowel movements, I may prescribe as much as 8 qian to 1 liang of Cang Zhu. For these patients, it will typically require administration of the TCM formula for 1 to 2 months following completion of the radiotherapy regimen before the sloppy stools and frequent bowel movements completely resolve. Repeated administration of radiotherapy can cause atrophy of the intestinal mucosa and dysmotility. For these patients, you should consider prescribing either a spleen-fortifying qi-supplementing yang-upbearing formula variant such as Bu Zhong Yi Qi Tang or a blood-nourishing yin-enriching dryness-moistening formula variant such as Xue Ku Fang, Qi Bao Mei Ran Dan, or Di Huang Yin Zi. Remember! Make sure to include The Three Great Yang-Supplementers, Huang Qi, Huang Qin, Da Huang, and possibly even Pu Xiao in your formula selection.

In cases in which there is inflammation *with ulceration* and *necrosis*, presenting with pussy mucous (lymph) and blood (mucosanguinous) stools, or even perforation, and the patient does *not* want to undergo surgery, you should first perform acupuncture to relieve pain, and then administer TCM medicinals.

I would consider needling acupoints such as Nei Guan (P6), He Gu (LI4), Zu San Li (ST36), Shou San Li (LI10), Bai Hui (DU20), Tai

Chong (LV4), Wei Shu (UB21), Da Chang Shu (UB25), and Ba Liao (UB31–34).

If there is no late afternoon tidal heat, then go ahead and prescribe the spleen-fortifying qi-supplementing yang-upbearing formula Ti Gang San. If you prescribe Shen Ling Bai Zhu San or Xiang Sha Liu Jun Zi Tang, then you should add Huang Qin, Huang Lian, Bai Zhi, Fang Feng, Di Yu, Huai Hua, and Sheng Chi Shao (or Sheng Bai Shao) (large dose of up to 1 liang). You could also consider adding Jin Yin Hua, Pu Gong Ying, Tian Hua, Ru Xiang, and Mo Yao.

If the patient has had severe diarrhea to the point of passing clear thin (watery) bloody stool or watery sloppy diarrhea that is odorless, then prescribe a spleen-fortifying qi-supplementing yang-upbearing formula such as Bu Zhong Yi Qi Tang, Gui Qi Jian Zhong Tang, or Shen Ling Bai Zhu San; or a dual qi- and blood-supplementing formula such as Bu Yang Huan Wu Tang or Shi Quan Da Bu Tang. Make sure to include Huang Qi and Ren Shen (powder) (large doses of each), Huang Qin, Bai Zhi, Fang Feng, and The Three Great Yang-Supplementers in your formula.

For the treatment of sloppy stools and diarrhea, some TCM doctors like to prescribe astringing medicinals such as Wu Wei Zi, Wu Pei Zi, Hai Piao Xiao, Da Jin Ying, Bai Guo, and Sheng Mu Li. In my opinion, these types of medicinals should only be prescribed for patients with odorless, watery diarrhea (水泄 shuǐ xiè) or recurrent rectal prolapse (anal desertion) who have a somber white facial complexion. If excessive amounts of astringing medicinals are prescribed at the onset, this could lead to intestinal congestion with abdominal distention and water amassment inside and outside of the intestinal lumen; and in severe cases, these medicinals could cause the inflamed mucous membrane and tissue to ulcerate, rupture, and hemorrhage, resulting in abdominal pain and red and white (mucosanguinous) diarrhea. Remember! Don't prescribe astringing medicinals too early, especially in cases presenting with heat pattern.

Case Study #11: Crohn's Disease – Intestinal Heat and Red Diarrhea

Q: A 9 y/o male patient began having periodic bloody stool (大便出血 dà biàn chū xiě) and diarrhea when he was 5 years old.

Following examination, a gastroenterologist diagnosed him with Crohn's disease (CD). Three years ago, the patient had a thorough examination performed at a large hospital revealing the presence of tens of thousands of variegated shaped and sized polyps on the mucosa of the colon. The patient's doctors and parents were surprised by the findings and at a loss on how to treat this condition. Doctors said that South Korea has only a handful of these types of cases and this condition has a low prevalence worldwide.

Recently, the patient still has had periodic bloody stools (small amounts, bright red color). I applied the method you taught me, instructing the patient to drink fresh lotus root juice, and the frequency of blood-streaked stools did indeed decline. Please advise me on what approach I should take next. Thank you!

A: Technically, the "polyps" you refer to are pseudopolyps, resulting from inflammation that leads to ulcerations which leave behind scar tissue when they heal—this is what the endoscopy reveals. The manifestation of inflammatory ulcerations in Crohn's disease can be identified as intestinal heat pattern and periodic bleeding can be classified as red diarrhea (赤痢 chì lì).

Yes, advising the patient to drink fresh lotus root juice (cools the blood, dissipates stasis, checks bleeding, and engenders flesh) is a good idea, but I would also prescribe a heat-clearing diarrhea-checking formula such as Huang Lian Jie Du Tang, Huang Qin Tang, Qing Wei San, or Ge Gen Qin Lian Tang (including large doses of Huang Qin and Huang Lian) adding Huai Hua, Di Yu, Fang Feng, Bai Zhi, Zhi Zi, Mu Dan Pi, and Chuan Qi (powder). In some cases it may be advisable to add small amounts of Wan Ling Dan (resolves toxin, disperses welling-abscesses, and dispels wind) or Xiong Huang (resolves toxin and kills insects) along with Hua Shi and Shi Gao. If bleeding continues and is pronounced, then add Ou Jie, Ce Bo Ye, and Ai Ye accordingly.

Case Study #12: Lumbar Spinal Stenosis – Gastrointestinal Abnormalities

Q: A 54 y/o female patient was diagnosed with lumbar spinal stenosis 1 year ago and began taking Western medicine. One month later, she noticed her face getting fatter (she had gained 10 kg) and felt pain and glomus under the heart (心下痞痛 xīn xià pǐ tong). Despite passing 2 stools per day, she still has abdominal fullness, and every day after eating lunch, she feels bloated and unable to pass gas up until the next morning. Endoscopic examination revealed *no* abnormalities. What do you think the cause of this gastrointestinal discomfort could be?

A: Lumbar spinal stenosis with gastrointestinal abnormalities suggests conus medullaris syndrome (spinal cord damage from T12 to L2 resulting in bowel dysfunction and anal sphincter paresis). This condition can be treated just like paralysis, by administering Paralysis Formula #2 (Shi Quan Da Bu Tang Variant) or Paralysis Formula #3 (You Gui Yin Variant) adding enough Da Huang, Pu Xiao, Gan Jiang, and Fu Zi to maintain 2–3 stools/day.

Case Study #13: Colorectal Cancer – Da Huang and Pu Xiao Improve Abdominal Distention and Fullness

Q1: I have been treating a complicated case involving a colorectal cancer patient with metastasis to the liver, and a recent scan revealed a mass in the pelvic cavity. The patient received epidermal growth factor receptor (EGFR) inhibitor target therapy without effective results and her doctors recommended partial colectomy followed by adjuvant radiotherapy as the best option.

After surgery and completion of radiotherapy, the most recent lab tests showed CEA 99 (≤ 3 ng/mL). She has difficult and ungratifying defecation, a poor appetite with mild nausea, and left-sided lower abdominal distention and fullness that worsens when lying down flat on her back. I prescribed Ru Mo Si Wu Tang adding Huang Qin and Huang Lian (8 qian each), Zhi Zi (2 qian), Fu Ling and Ze Xie (5 qian each), Wan Ling Dan (8 pills/3x/day), and Yu Sheng Wan (2 pills/day). Unfortunately, her symptoms didn't improve after taking this formula.

Fortunately, my mother doesn't have colorectal cancer, but she does have this kind of constipation: every time she takes laxatives she passes hard stool like sheep's droppings (排便如羊屎 pái biàn rú yáng shǐ) followed by sloppy stools, and when she eats a bit more than usual she feels fullness and distention below the heart. This type of constipation and abdominal discomfort is really tough to treat. How would you do it? Would it be better to add Da Huang to the formula? Please offer your guidance and assistance.

A: It is common for patients with colorectal cancer to have stasis swelling (瘀腫 yū zhǒng) in the intestinal wall. Prescribing the blood-nourishing blood-quickening, stasis-dispelling pain-relieving, and network vessel-freeing channel-regulating formula Ru Mo Si Wu Tang is a good choice, but you should also add Pu Xiao along with Da Huang, and gradually increase the dose of Wan Ling Dan by 4 pills (3x/day) each week (up to a maximum of 28 pills/3x/day). For male patients, you should gradually increase the dose of Yu Sheng Wan up until the patient starts having difficulty urinating (due to the anticholinergic effects resulting in the inhibition of parasympathetic control of the urinary bladder and urinary retention). For females, you can typically prescribe much higher doses of up to 6–8 pills/day. If the patient presents with abdominal distention and fullness, reflex vomiting, sagging distention, and rectal heaviness (tenesmus), and the feces is as thin in diameter as a chopstick, then you should incrementally increase the dose of Da Huang and Pu Xiao until the patient maintains 5–6 stools/day.

Q2: Thanks for your invaluable input. I followed your advice, but it appears that the process of decocting Da Huang together with the other medicinals in the formula may have diminished its draining precipitation (laxative) action. And the patient commented on the extremely salty flavor of Pu Xiao, saying that it made the decoction almost unpalatable. What can I do to rectify this situation?

A: If the patient refuses to take Da Huang and Pu Xiao, then you can prescribe Fan Xie Ye (Senna Leaf, Folium Sennae) or the extract powder of Tao Ren Cheng Qi Tang (quickens the blood and transforms stasis and precipitates stasis heat) and Di Dang Tang (attacks and expels static blood). Remember! The more difficult the condition is, the greater the need to provide treatment. That's the only way to gain deeper insights into pathoconditions, conduct accurate pattern identification as the basis for treatment, and continue improving your skills in the science and art of medicine.

As for your mother's constipation, you can advise her from a physician's perspective to alter her dietary habits, reminding her to take in plenty of fluids and eat a wide variety of foods such as eggs, milk, fish, meat, fruits and vegetables, and nuts and legumes in order to maintain a balanced nutritional intake. If for some reason she is unable to maintain a well-balanced diet, then taking multivitamin supplements is another option. Remember! The best way to promote healthy stools is by thoroughly chewing fibrous natural foods such as sweet potatoes, legumes, corn, and stalky green vegetables. Good luck!

V. MUSCULOSKELETAL DISORDERS

This chapter presents a broad spectrum of the most commonly presenting acute and chronic musculoskeletal disorders in the TCM clinical setting, including crane's knee-wind, lumbus wilting, trigger finger, and heel pain. As with other chapters in this series, it also introduces pathoconditions that some TCM practitioners may have never encountered, such as myositis ossificans, osteolysis, avascular necrosis, and fibrodysplasia ossificans progressiva (FOP).

Case Study #1: Professional Pianist Can't Extend Her Fingers!

Q: The patient is a 27 y/o female pianist. One morning she awoke to the disturbing realization of not being able to extend the fingers of her right hand. Obviously, for a pianist this is a devastating occupational injury. She was so distraught it brought her to tears. Not long after the initial presentation, the tips of her fingers (right hand) felt sore, a generalized malaise set in, and she couldn't sleep at night.

She underwent a full hospital examination, but they couldn't find any cause, so she decided to visit me for consultation. What could this be? Her hands are her life! Do you think my prescription of Gui Qi Jian Zhong Tang adding Ma Huang and Ren Shen is the right choice? Will she fully recover without any lasting complications?

A: There are many possible causes for this patient's condition including trigger finger, nerve compression, nerve dysfunction, compromised lymphatic return leading to stiffness and swelling, morning qi vacuity, and joint running-wind (歷節風 lì jié fēng) (correlates with rheumatoid arthritis (RA)). A thorough medical examination must be conducted to make a definitive diagnosis. However, based on your description, it sounds to me like this patient's condition can be identified as either qi vacuity or dual qi and yang vacuity pattern.

I think you have chosen the right formula in Gui Qi Jian Zhong Tang adding Ma Huang and Ren Shen (powder), but I would make sure to include large doses of The Three Great Yang-Supplementers and Ma Huang. You can also advise her to exercise at least 1 hour every day (walking or any other cardiovascular activity, preferably outdoors in the sunshine!) and make sure to keep her hands and fingers warm.

Case Study #2: Trigger Finger – Warm Needling and TCM Medicinals

Q: Recently, several trigger finger (stenosing tenosynovitis) patients have visited me for treatment. I have tried acupuncture repeatedly on these patients without much success at all. Do you have any suggestions?

A: Effective treatment of trigger finger requires administration of both acupuncture and medicinals. For acupuncture, you must needle directly into the metacarpal joint and apply warm needling (place moxa cones on needle handle and burn 3 cones/needle each session); and for medicinals, you can prescribe a flesh-resolving yang-upbearing channel-coursing formula such as Ge Gen Tang or a qi- and blood-supplementing formula such as Gui Qi Jian Zhong Tang or Shi Quan Da Bu Tang. Just make sure to include Gan Jiang and Fu Zi.

If this approach still isn't ineffective, then increase the number of moxa cones (burning 4–5 cones/session) and add larger doses of Huang Qi, Gan Jiang, and Fu Zi to your formula. If joint swelling presents, then add Fu Ling and Ze Xie; and if redness and inflammation present, then add Huang Qin and Huang Lian. This approach should provide noticeable results relatively quickly.

Case Study #3: Heel Pain – Damp-Heat Pouring Downward

Q: I have a 55 y/o female patient with a history of heel pain (left side) in the *absence* of trauma. The pain intensifies upon dorsiflexion and especially during the first couple of steps after getting up out of bed in the morning. Examination of the patient's heel revealed *no* visible abnormalities or pronounced local tenderness, and the patient does *not* have lumbar pain. Please offer your advice on this case.

A: In the great majority of cases (including plantar fasciitis, heel spurs, calcaneal stress fracture, heel pad syndrome), heel pain can be identified as urinary bladder channel or kidney channel damp-heat pouring downward (濕熱下注 shī rè xià zhù) pattern. For this condition you can prescribe an yin-enriching fire-downbearing and heat-clearing dampness-drying formula such as (Yu Sheng) Zhi Bo Di Huang Tang, Er Miao San, San Miao Wan, or Jia Wei Er Miao San adding Huo Luo Dan (dispels wind and eliminates dampness, transforms phlegm and frees the network vessels, and quickens the blood and relieves pain). In a small number of cases heel pain may be caused by gout, thus requiring the administration of Long Dan Xie Gan Tang or Huang Lian Jie Du Tang adding Long Dan Cao.

In addition to prescribing medicinals, you should also bleed locally at the site of pain, typically presenting at the center and/or along the sides of the heel; and needle acupoints along the channels that correspond with the site of pain such as Cheng Shan (UB57), Kun Lun (UB60), Cheng Jin (UB 56), Fei Yang (UB58), and Tai Xi (K3). For intractable cases involving bone spurs, you might consider a more invasive needling technique that involves inserting a 1.5 cun needle along the lateral aspect of the foot perpendicular to the site of pain. Remember! This is extremely painful so you must be stealth upon insertion!

Case Study #4: Cold Incites Sharp Pain in the Heart of the Sole

Q: A 55 y/o male patient who says he is a recreational alcohol drinker has a history of gout (no recent signs or symptoms of a flare-up) and recently experienced sharp pain in the heart of the sole in his right foot. Coming into contact with cold seems to exacerbate this condition. What do you think this could be?

A: Pain in the heart of the sole (足心痛 zú xīn tòng) can be identified as kidney channel damp-heat pouring downward (濕熱下注 shī rè xià zhù) pattern. I would prescribe a heat-clearing dampness-drying and yin-enriching fire-downbearing formula such as Er Miao San, San Miao Wan, Si Miao Wan, or (Yu Sheng) Zhi Bo Di Huang Tang adding Huo Luo Dan (dispels wind and eliminates dampness, transforms phlegm and frees the network vessels, and quickens the blood and relieves pain). In addition, I would bleed locally at the site of pain and the well points of the affected foot; and needle acupoints such as Tai Chong (LV3), Di Wu Hui (GB42), Ran Gu (K2), San Yin Jiao (SP6), Cheng Shan (UB57), and Kun Lun (UB60).

Case Study #5: Diabetes – Pain in the Heart of the Sole

Q: Ten years ago, a 78 y/o female diabetic patient began having pain in the heart of the sole of both feet. She has tried all kinds of therapies, but nothing has been effective, and in recent years the swelling and pain has been intensifying. Acupuncture temporarily relieves the swelling and pain, but the pain still comes back at nighttime. What is the best way to treat this condition?

A: Long-standing diabetes complicated by pain in the heart of the sole of both feet can be identified as damp-heat pouring downward pattern. You should consider prescribing a heat-clearing dampness-drying and yin-enriching fire-downbearing formula such as Er Miao San, San Miao Wan, Si Miao Wan, Jia Wei Er Miao San, or (Yu Sheng) Zhi Bo Di Huang Tang adding Huo Luo Dan (dispels wind and eliminates dampness, transforms phlegm and frees the network vessels, and quickens the blood and relieves pain). Another possibility is to prescribe a blood-nourishing blood-quickening, stasis-dispelling pain-relieving, and network vessel-freeing channel-regulating formula such as (Yu Sheng) Ru Mo Si Wu Tang adding Niu Xi, Huang Bo, and Huo Luo Dan.

As for acupuncture, you can needle Bei Lao Gong (located in opposition to Lao Gong (PC8) on the dorsal aspect of the hand at the V-shaped base between the 3rd and 4th metacarpal bones), Cheng Shan (UB57), Kun Lun (UB60), San Yin Jiao (SP6), Ran Gu (K2), Tai Chong (LV3), and Di Wu Hui (GB42).

Case Study #6: Gouty Arthritis

Q: Three days ago, a 40 y/o male patient with a history of gouty arthritis experienced heat and swelling in the medial aspect of his left foot just above the ankle, making it difficult to walk. I prescribed Huang Lian Jie Du Tang adding The Four Lings and Long Dan Cao, and externally wrapped his ankle in the medicinal paste Diao Fen Gao. How long does it usually take for serum uric acid (SUA) levels (hyperuricemia) to come back down to normal? How long before the patient can walk normally again? What's the best way to treat this pathocondition?

A: That's a great formula! Typically, for best results in the treatment of gouty arthritis, you can also bleed at the site of swelling and pain along with the well points on the affected foot; needle Tai Chong (LV3), Zhong Feng (LV4) and a contralateral acupoint on the opposing hand that corresponds with the channel of the affected site;

and add The Three Yellows (a total of 8–10 qian). This approach will quickly resolve inflammation, enabling the patient to be walking freely with minimal discomfort, if any, in about 3 to 5 days. For best results in patients with recurrent flare-ups of chronic gout, you should add Shan Zha, Dan Shen, Chi Shao, and Huo Luo Dan (dispels wind and eliminates dampness, transforms phlegm and frees the network vessels, and quickens the blood and relieves pain).

Remember! The active constituents in the medicinal paste degrade when it has dried. So once the Diao Fen Gao wrap has dried (usually taking about 6 to 8 hours) it must be changed. The patient can keep the premade medicinal paste wraps in the refrigerator and change 3 or 4x/day on their own at home.

The rate at which SUA levels decrease varies. I have a patient whose SUA dropped down from 9 mg/dL to 3 mg/dL (normal range 4.0 to 8.5 mg/dL) after taking just 3 packets (3 days/3x/day) of the above formula, resulting in the patient feeling sluggish and drowsy. Each patient's condition is unique and you must take this into consideration when administering treatment. If SUA drops too quickly, the patient may feel fatigued, malaise, sluggish, drowsy, clumsy, and inattentive. It takes time for the brain's feedback mechanism to recalibrate the system, so your goal should be to gradually lower SUA levels down to about 5 or 6 mg/dL. During the acute phase, the patient should have their blood tested weekly, and in the chronic stage, a blood test every 1–3 months is sufficient.

Case Study #7: Pediatric Knee Joint Swelling and Pain – Juvenile Idiopathic Arthritis

Q: A 12 y/o boy visited my clinic presenting with swelling and pain along the joint line of his left knee. There was no history of trauma and the x-rays were normal. Does this sound like a case of juvenile idiopathic arthritis to you?

A: A swollen and painful knee joint without history of trauma at such a young age; aside from juvenile idiopathic arthritis (juvenile rheumatoid arthritis), it would be prudent to also have a blood test taken to rule out syphilitic arthritis. The U.S. military has had a long-term military presence in South Korea, and partying and perusing comes with the territory so to speak. This promiscuity makes the soldiers susceptible to contracting syphilis from infected partners and then passing it on to others. That's why I would consider the possibility of this boy having syphilitic arthritis.

Regardless of the diagnosis, the TCM therapeutic approach for these two arthritic conditions is similar. You can prescribe a heat-clearing toxin-resolving formula such as Huang Lian Jie Du Tang adding The Four Lings for both pathoconditions. In the case of juvenile rheumatic arthritis, you could also consider prescribing a heat-clearing yin-enriching blood cooling formula such as Hyperactive Immune Formula or Zhi Bo Di Huang Tang adding The Four Lings. In the case of syphilitic arthritis, you should also add Tu Fu Ling (or Bi Xie) and Long Dan Cao, large doses of The Three Yellows, Wan Ling Dan, and possibly even a small dose of Xiong Huang. These approaches will effectively resolve the symptoms and stabilize the pathocondition.

Case Study #8: "Joint-Bone Lysis"

Q1: A 54 y/o female patient told me she had a history of "joint-bone lysis," explaining that radiographs taken about 10 years ago showed the base of her 4th metatarsal bone was missing (it had dissolved!). Thus, her doctors recommended surgical removal of the surrounding tissue and prescribed Western medicine drugs (unspecified) to control the condition. Recently, she began feeling pain in her 5th metatarsal joint (no swelling), the same way her 4th toe started out, and x-ray images revealed a gradual pattern of joint space narrowing and bone thinning (lysis). Doctors advised her to have surgery, but she adamantly refused. How would you go about treating this patient?

A: Based on your description, the history and presentation suggests an osteolytic lesion of infectious or inflammatory origin. Regardless if you have a definitive Western medicine diagnosis or not, your patient's history and symptoms correlate with the TCM pathoconditions of powdery bone flat-abscess (粉骨疽 fěn gǔ jū), putrefied bone flat-abscess (腐骨疽 fǔ gǔ jū), and eroding bone flat-abscess (蝕骨疽 shí gǔ jū). These pathoconditions typically manifest as an open sore with a round, pinkish induration about the size of a coat button, and once the skin is broken, a white, "chalky" suppuration (looks almost like talc) oozes from the wound. The suppuration of this bony (chalky) matter is self-limited, and once it has been completely evacuated, the open sore will quickly heal. Superficially, you may not even be able to tell there was a wound there at all, but inside, dissolution of the bone has already occurred.

If the diagnosis of powdery bone flat-abscess, putrefied bone flat-abscess, and eroding bone flat-abscess is correct, your patient may also present with late afternoon tidal heat (fever) (日晡發熱 rì bū fā rè) and night sweating, a tell-tale sign that indicates osteolytic change is indeed occurring in the 5th metatarsal bone. You should immediately administer a heat-clearing toxin-resolving and blood-cooling steaming bone-eliminating formula such as Zhi Bo Di Huang Tang, Ji Sheng Jie Du Tang, Xian Fang Huo Ming Yin, or Qin Lian Si Wu Tang. Just make sure to include Qing Hao, Zhi Bo, Di Gu Pi, Lu Jiao Jiao, The Three Insects, and Wan Ling Dan.

If vexing heat in the five hearts (五心煩熱 wǔ xīn fán rè) presents, even in the absence of late afternoon tidal heat (fever), then you can still prescribe an yin-enriching steaming bone-eliminating and essence-replenishing blood-supplementing formula variant such as Zhi Bo Di Huang Tang or Zuo Gui Yin. If the patient's face and feet have a pale complexion, then consider prescribing a kidney yang-supplementing formula variant such as You Gui Yin. Once the patient's symptoms resolve and the condition stabilizes, you should change to the great essence-marrow-supplementing formula Gui Lu Er Xian Jiao, administering over the long-term to regulate the constitution.

For the treatment of powdery bone flat-abscess, Western medicine will typically perform surgical debridement of lysed bone and decayed tissue and administer an antimycobacterial drug (to prevent the condition from exacerbating) along with calcium tablets (to supplement the loss of calcium), allicin (garlic extract), and glucosamine. Unfortunately, this treatment tends to offer less than satisfactory results.

Q2: That patient wasn't willing to accept our TCM diagnosis and therapeutic plan for "joint-bone lysis," and she is still taking Western medicine anti-arthritic drugs. Now, the cuboid bone proximal to the 5th metatarsal (near Chong Yang (ST42) on the dorsal aspect of the midfoot) is inflamed—red, swollen, hot, and painful. You can feel the heat by just putting your hand near the inflamed area. The only time the pain subsides is when she sits still; when she stands up and walks about the pain is unbearable. Her doctors advised her to have surgery, but she remains reluctant and is considering her options.

A: You really need to sit down with this patient and explain why it is imperative to begin taking TCM medicinals immediately! Our therapeutic approach has proven effective in innumerable cases similar to this one. For best results, I would personally prescribe (Yu Sheng) Zhi Bo Di Huang Tang adding Qing Hao, Zhi Mu, Di Gu Pi, and The Three Insects. The plan is to first resolve the inflammation, and once the condition has stabilized and pain resides, then you can begin to gradually add in The Three Great Yang-Supplementers. As I mentioned previously, after taking this formula for a period of time, you can start adding Gui Jiao and Lu Jiao Jiao (or Cu Lu Rong), and eventually change over to the long-term administration of Gui Lu Er Xian Jiao. This TCM approach will offer the best overall outcome!

Case Study #9: Acute and Chronic Knee Inflammation – Heat, Swelling, and Pain

Q: I have been successfully applying your therapeutic approach for knee inflammation and arthritis on many patients. My treatment principle is as follows: In the acute stage (or during flare-ups) of joint-running wind (膝關節 xī guān jié) presenting with pronounced heat and swelling, I will prescribe Huang Lian Jie Du Tang adding Fu Ling, Ze Xie, and Huo Luo Dan (and sometimes adding Yi Yi Ren, Ma Huang, Niu Xi, and Cang Zhu as well). For the chronic condition of crane's-knee wind (鶴膝風 hè xī fēng), I will prescribe Zhi Bo Di Huang Tang (including large doses of Huang Bo and Cang Zhu of up to 8 qian each) adding Huang Qin and Huang Lian. This approach has consistently produced exceptional results at quickly resolving the inflammation, swelling and pain. Can you offer more insights about treating these types of pathoconditions?

A: Congratulations! Yes, for acute heat, swelling and pain, prescribing a heat-clearing toxin-resolving formula adding bland-percolating dampness-disinhibiting, blood-quickening stasis-dispelling, and channel- and network vessel-freeing medicinals will be very effective. And for the heat, swelling and pain of chronic inflammation, prescribing an yin-enriching fire-downbearing formula that includes large doses of heat-clearing toxin-resolving and wind-damp-dispelling medicinals will be very effective as well.

There are many types of arthritis and just as many pathoconditions described in TCM classical texts that correlate with the pathologic nomenclature in modern biomedicine. For instance, *joint-running wind* encompasses early stage osteoarthritis, rheumatoid arthritis (RA), and other inflammatory arthritic conditions; *crane's-knee wind* typically denotes a pathocondition resulting from long-standing *joint-running wind*, presenting with swelling and pain in the knee joint along with atrophy of the thigh and calf muscles, and encompasses chronic stages of osteoarthritis (OA) (degenerative arthritis), RA, tuberculous (TB) arthritis, and other inflammatory arthritic conditions; *wind-damp* and *wind-damp traveling influx (moving impediment)* (風濕走注 fēng shī zǒu zhù) encompass any type of rheumatic joint pain and migratory arthritis; *pain wind* (痛風 tòng fēng), *fire flow* (流火 liú huǒ), and *fire cinnabar* (火丹 huǒ dān) encompass pseudogout and gout; *fire flow* and *fire flow traveling influx (moving impediment)* (流火走注 liú huǒ zǒu zhù) encompass syphilitic arthritis and gonococcal arthritis; and *spinal cord taxation*, *vertebral taxation*, and *bone taxation* (骨勞 gǔ láo) encompass TB arthritis.

In fact, any of these classical TCM pathologic terms mentioned above may also encompass the symptoms presenting in various stages of osteomyelitis and even bone cancer. So remember! These classical TCM pathologic terms are useful references and guidelines, providing a general description of a particular pathocondition whose etiology and pathomechanisms may either directly correlate or encompass the pathologies we see today throughout their various manifestations (signs, symptoms, pattern identification) and evolution (stages) of disease. However, a problem with using these classical TCM pathologic terms is that their meanings are open to different interpretations, which can obviously lead to confusion. To avoid confusion, you must be meticulous in identifying the pattern and Western medicine diagnosis in order to determine the optimal therapeutic approach.

The following are some tips from my years of clinical practice: Typically, *OA* presents with just pain in the absence of overt swelling and heat, especially when the weather is cold, but as long as a person walks regularly and keeps the joint warm, the pain can be controlled. If pain presents in the absence of pronounced swelling and heat, and the pain is more severe when walking up the stairs, then this indicates mild inflammation resulting from a *sprained (or torn) anterior cruciate ligament (ACL)*. If the pain is more severe when walking down the stairs, then this suggests inflammation from a *sprained (or torn) posterior cruciate ligament (PCL)*.

In cases of *OA* that present with pain in the absence of swelling and heat, you can consider prescribing kidney yang-supplementing, blood-supplementing essence-replenishing, and wind-damp dispelling formula variants such as You Gui Yin, Zuo Gui Yin, Shen Qi Qan, Du Huo Ji Sheng Tang, or San Bi Tang. For inflammatory pathoconditions inducing arthritis that can be identified as yin vacuity with blood heat pattern (e.g., gonorrhea, syphilis, AIDS, herpes I (HSV-1) and II (HSV-2), TB arthritis, RA), you should consider prescribing a heat-clearing toxin-resolving and yin vacuity-heat clearing yin-enriching formula such as Hyperactive Immune Formula. For gonorrhea and syphilis induced arthritis add Tu Fu Ling, Bi Xie, and Xiong Huang; for TB add Qing Hao, Zhi Mu, and Di Gu Pi (or Yuan Shen, Chai Hu, and Qin Jiao); and for herpes virus, change to a liver and gallbladder repletion fire-draining and lower burner damp-heat-clearing formula such as Long Dan Xie Gan Tang adding Fu Ling, Bi Xie, and Xiong Huang.

If heat presents, you can bleed locally at the affected site and distally at the well points corresponding with the channels and network vessels of the affected site; and needle acupoints above and below the affected site. Remember! Do *not* needle inside the joint space for heat pattern conditions! For cold pattern conditions, you can needle inside the joint space and warm needle (applying moxa cones on the needle handle).

Case Study #10: Knee Malalignment (Subluxation) – "Almost Like It's Going to Break in Half"

Q: One month ago, a 17 y/o soccer player suffered a left knee injury from a tackle during a match. Not long after incurring the injury, swelling arose in the lateral (Du Bi (ST35)) and medial depression (Xi Yan (EX17)), and the popliteal fossa (Wei Zhong (UB40)) was slightly red and swollen. The patient can walk up and down stairs without any problem, but at greater degrees of knee flexion the knee feels extremely tight and painful "almost like it's going to break in half," as he described. A CT scan was performed, but only revealed swelling of the cartilage along the lateral aspect of the knee. He has not had an MRI done yet. What type of injury do you think this is?

A: With only a CT scan and *no* MRI, you cannot definitively diagnose the type of joint cavity damage or severity of sprain (i.e., stretched, partial tear, complete tear), but you could perform manual tests (i.e., anterior and posterior drawer, Lachman, McMurray) to get a better idea of the joint stability and the presence of ligament laxity or tear. Typically, if ligaments are damaged the patient will have discomfort and pain walking up and down stairs. Regardless of the specific type of injury, we know the patient suffered trauma to the knee joint and now greater degrees of flexion induce severe pain. This indicates joint malalignment (subluxation).

For best overall efficacy, you should first perform the traction-manipulation realignment ("leg-pull") maneuver to realign the joint. After realignment, bleed locally around the patella, the joint space (including Du Bi (ST35) and Xi Yan (EX17)), and anywhere else heat and swelling present; and also distally at the well points of the affected leg. Then, needle the two anatomical acupoints diagonal from the upper lateral edges of the patella (where the vastus lateralis and vastus medialis taper into tendinous tissue), Yang Ling Quan (GB34), and Yin Ling Quan (SP9).

As for TCM medicinals, I would prescribe a heat-clearing toxin-resolving formula such as Huang Lian Jie Du Tang adding The Four Lings (disinhibit water and dampness by bland percolation) and Huo Luo Dan (dispels wind and eliminates dampness, transforms phlegm and frees the network vessels, and quickens the blood and relieves pain) (starting out at 3 pills/day and gradually increasing the dose up to 6 pills/day). Once the swelling resolves in about 3–7 days, then you can begin adding in The Three Great Yang-Supplementers (starting out at small doses of 1 qian each and gradually increasing up to 5 qian each).

Typically, unless the patient has incurred a severe partial tear or complete tear (ligament or tendon), there will be noticeable improvement with pain-free range of motion after administering this formula for 2–3 weeks. Naturally, depending on the severity, you may need to refer patients with traumatic musculoskeletal injuries such as this to an orthopedic specialist for further examination. In severe cases, short-term immobilization, bracing or surgical repair accompanied by concomitant TCM treatment may offer the best outcome.

Case Study #11: Popliteal Fossa Swelling

Q: A 65 y/o male patient developed swelling of the popliteal fossa after going hiking in the mountains. I have had a similar case before, prescribing (Yu Sheng) Wu Ling San (Nephritis Formula) variant at the onset, but this treatment was not very effective. How would you treat this injury?

A: This popliteal fossa swelling sounds like a classic case of popliteal cyst (Baker's cyst))! First, you must determine if the pathocondition is still in the acute stage, indicated by the presentation of *pronounced* heat on palpation along with swelling. If so, then this can be identified as heat stasis with water-damp collecting pattern and requires administration of an yin-enriching fire-downbearing formula such as (Yu Sheng) Zhi Bo Di Huang Tang (including a large dose of Huang Bo) adding Xu Duan and Gu Sui Bu.

If there is swelling (fluid-filled cyst) in the *absence* of heat, then this can be identified as either qi or yang vacuity with water-damp collecting pattern, requiring the administration of an essence-replenishing blood-supplementing formula such as You Gui Yin or a qi- and blood-supplementing and kidney yang-supplementing formula such as Gui Qi Jian Zhong Tang. Just make sure to include The Three Great Yang-Supplementers, Niu Xi (lower extremity channel conductor), The Four Lings (disinhibit water and dampness by bland percolation), and Huo Luo Dan (dispels wind and eliminates dampness, transforms phlegm and frees the network vessels, and quickens the blood and relieves pain). And if the swelling still doesn't resolve, then that's when I would change to a kidney yang-warming qi transformation-promoting and bland-percolating dampness- and water-disinhibiting formula such as (Yu Sheng) Wu Ling San

(Nephritis Formula) variant.

As for acupuncture, in the acute stage, you should needle distal acupoints until the heat (inflammation) abates. For the post-acute and chronic stages (presenting with swelling (fluid-filled cyst) in the *absence* of heat), you should warm needle, inserting the needles in a radial pattern directly into the fluid-filled cyst and applying moxa cones on the needle handles (at least 3 cones/needle each session). At the start of treatment, you may feel a lot of resistance when needling into the taut bulbous fluid-filled sac, but after about 1 week of administering medicinals and performing warm needling, this trapped joint fluid will begin to soften up, and by 2 weeks, it will have shrunk considerably. Continue administering this approach until the cyst completely resolves. Remember! Advise the patient to avoid strenuous exercise that puts too much pressure on the affected limb, because it might irritate the synovium and prolong the healing process. Light exercise such as walking should be fine as long as there isn't excessive pain or discomfort.

Other pathoconditions such as ganglion cyst, chronic stage hematocele, hydrocele, trigger finger (stenosing tenosynovitis), compromised lymphatic return following trauma that causes swelling of the distal extremities, acute edema following trauma, and swelling of the eyelid (palpebral edema) like a ball can also be identified and treated by applying similar approaches. However, you should modify your formula to focus on the specific location and presentation of each pathocondition.

Case Study #12: If It's Gout, Don't Prescribe The Four Lings!

Q: Seven years ago, a 33 y/o male suffered trauma to his left knee, resulting in severe swelling and pain and inability to bear weight. Hospital examination revealed a torn medial collateral ligament prompting doctors to perform surgical repair. He experienced mild swelling and pain following surgery, but it was nothing that really bothered him too much.

Recently, he visited me and presented with mild swelling (bulging at Xi Yan (EX17) and Du Bi (ST35)), pronounced heat upon palpation, and pain when walking. I prescribed (Yu Sheng) Huang Lian Jie Du Tang adding The Four Lings and Huo Luo Dan, but the treatment has not been effective. What do you think about changing the formula to Zhi Bo Di Huang Tang adding Huo Luo Dan?

A: Surgical repair of a ligament tear 7 years ago, and now, swelling and pain. Hmm…sounds like inflammation to me and thus can be identified as stasis heat with water-damp collecting pattern. But remember! You must also rule out the possibility of gout. The heat-clearing toxin-resolving formula you prescribed is fine; just make sure to include large doses of Huang Bo and Huang Qin. Also, bleed the affected site and needle proximal and distal acupoints along with Xi Yan (EX17) and Du Bi (ST35).

If the patient does turn out to have increased serum uric acid (SUA) levels ($\geq$ 8.5 mg/dL), which would strongly suggest gout, then add Long Dan Cao and Shan Zha. In this case, it is *not* advisable to prescribe The Four Lings, because these bland-percolating water- and dampness-disinhibiting medicinals may increase blood viscosity and thus inhibit the elimination of SUA.

Case Study #13: Runner's Knee and Jumper's Knee

Q: Many patients have been coming to me complaining of tightness and pain in the knee joint upon walking and climbing stairs. After examination, most of them turn out to have petellofemoral pain syndrome (PFPS) or chondromalacia patella (CMP) caused by trauma or overuse. Surgery tends to be effective at remedying their condition for a while, but the symptoms commonly recur. Do you think Huang Lian Jie Du Tang variant would be effective for these types of pathoconditions?

A: PFPS is a pathocondition in which the patella rubs against the femur, becomes inflamed, and over time may progress into softening, erosion, or fragmentation of the cartilage on the posterior surface of the patella, a condition called CMP. These pathoconditions are commonly referred to as runner's knee or jumper's knee, and are common in people who participate in sports involving repetitive squatting, running, jumping, and a lot of quick braking movements (e.g., tennis, badminton, basketball). In my clinical practice, I have also treated many middle-aged hikers, who carry heavy backpacks, with these types of knee damage, as well as degenerative meniscus tears.

The first thing to do is carefully examine the patient and identify the pattern. If there is only tightness or a feeling of *"something not right"* upon bending the knee, in the *absence* of heat or swelling, then that is often a good sign, simply requiring some rest and the condition will resolve. The presence of more pronounced patellofemoral *pain*, along *with* heat and swelling, suggests inflammation (and possibly deterioration) of the cartilage, which can be identified as heat with water-damp collecting pattern. For this pattern type, you can prescribe a heat-clearing toxin-resolving formula such as Huang Lian Jie Du Tang adding The Four Lings (disinhibit water and dampness by bland percolation) and Huo Luo Dan (dispels wind and eliminates dampness, transforms phlegm and frees the network vessels, and quickens the blood and relieves pain); bleed at the affected site around the knee; and needle acupoints that are sensitive along the path of the affected site, both proximally and distally.

Established chondromalacia with softening, erosion, or complete deterioration of the cartilage, and *no* overt heat or swelling, can be identified as kidney yang vacuity pattern. In this case, you can consider prescribing a kidney yang-supplementing, qi- and blood-supplementing, and dampness-eliminating pain-relieving formula such as You Gui Yin (or Shen Qi Wan), Shi Quan Da Bu Tang, Du Huo Ji Sheng Tang, San Bi Tang, or Dang Gui Si Ni Jia Wu Zhu Yu Sheng Jiang Tang adding Huo Luo Dan. As for acupuncture, needle (using 2 or 2.5 cun needles) the proximal and/or distal grooves, both medially and laterally, formed by the protuberance of the medial and lateral facets of the patella (joining the needles on the posterior aspect of the patella), and warm needle He Ding (EX-LE2). You should see positive results after administering treatment for 2–3 months. It is also important to advise the patient to keep the body warm (specifically the legs) by wearing thick pants and thermal underwear, up to as much as 2–4 layers depending on the climate and season.

Case Study #14: Lingering Ankle Sprain with Cyst-Like Swelling

Q: Three months ago, a 42 y/o female incurred a right inversion (lateral) ankle sprain, and after going to a hospital for treatment, her condition gradually resolved. One month later swelling presented below the lateral malleolus. Her orthopedic specialist determined this was edematous fluid and thus performed aspiration on 5 separate occasions and administered a corticosteroid injection at the affected site. This treatment resolved the condition for a period of time, but eventually the cyst-like swelling returned though it felt less taut than before and there was *no* pronounced heat or pain. Do you think this is synovial fluid? If the joint capsule has been ruptured, is it necessary to undergo surgery?

A: Hmm...ankle sprain followed by repeated fluid aspiration of a cyst-like swelling with *no* pronounced heat or pain sounds like the synovial fluid accumulation of a ganglion cyst. This pathocondition can be identified as yang vacuity pattern. You should administer acupuncture treatment, needling both proximally and distally to the affected site, and also inserting needles in a radial pattern directly into the fluid-filled cyst, applying moxa cones on the needle handles (at least 3 cones/needle each session). As for TCM medicinals, you can prescribe a kidney yang-supplementing formula such as You Gui Yin or a qi- and blood-supplementing and kidney yang-supplementing formula such as Gui Qi Jian Zhong Tang, making sure to include Niu Xi, The Three Great Yang-Supplementers, and The Four Lings. This cyst-like swelling will gradually soften and completely resolve.

If the administration of this therapeutic regimen does not provide effective results, then you must also consider the possibility of joint malalignment (subluxation) due to lax or torn supporting ligaments and connective tissues. To remedy joint malalignment (subluxation), first apply the ankle compression realignment maneuver, warm needle Di Wu Hui (GB42) and Xuan Zhong (GB39), and prescribe the same formula as above. If the cyst-like swelling is not located on the site of the Ankle Joint Acupoints (Qiu Xu (GB40) proper and an extra acupoint along the inferior border of the lateral malleolus in a depression anterior to the calcaneofibular ligament and Shen Mai (UB62)), then you can warm needle there as well. This approach will provide effective treatment without recurrence of symptoms.

Case Study #15: Traumatic Rupture of Articular Cartilage

Q: I have a 33 y/o male patient who loves playing recreational soccer. Two weeks ago, he suffered a right inversion (lateral) ankle sprain with swelling, bruising, and pain. An MRI revealed ruptured cartilage between the talus and calcaneus (talocalcaneal joint). Surgical repair is not possible and the only option from Western medicine's perspective is to fuse the articular space. The patient has concerns about mobility and range of motion being limited following this procedure. Do you think there is any way TCM can treat this type of injury?

A: Ruptured articular cartilage can be classified as repletion heat pattern, and in this case the fixation procedure (arthrodesis) is a viable approach. However, despite the initial MRI findings, you should have the patient get a second opinion. There *may not* be a rupture at all, but simply malalignment (subluxation) of the tibiofibular joint or torn ligaments instead.

I would go ahead and perform the ankle compression realignment maneuver; bleed the affected site and well points of the corresponding channels; needle Di Wu Hui (GB42) and Xuan Zhong (GB39); and prescribe an yin-enriching fire-downbearing steaming bone-eliminating formula such as Zhi Bo Di Huang Tang adding Huo Luo Dan (dispels wind and eliminates dampness, transforms phlegm and frees the network vessels, and quickens the blood and relieves pain). If heat presents, include large doses of Huang Bo; and if swelling presents, include large doses of Fu Ling and add large doses of Ze Xie.

Once the swelling and heat have resolved, you can consider changing to a kidney yang-warming and -supplementing and sinew- and bone-strengthening formula such as You Gui Yin or Shen Qi Wan adding Huo Luo Dan (dispels wind and eliminates dampness, transforms phlegm and frees the network vessels, and quickens the blood and relieves pain). As long as pronounced heat and swelling do *not* present, then you can also warm needle the Ankle Joint Acupoints (Qiu Xu (GB40) proper and an extra acupoint along the inferior border of the lateral malleolus in a depression anterior to the calcaneofibular ligament and Shen Mai (UB62)), Di Wu Hui (GB42), and Xuan Zhong (GB39).

Remember! As a general rule, you should *not* needle into the joint space in the *presence* of pronounced inflammation and swelling: needle proximally and distally instead, until the inflammation and swelling have resolved (an exception would be in chronic conditions with only mild swelling and minimal, to no, heat!).

Case Study #16: Malalignment – Common Complication of Ankle Sprain

Q: About two months ago, a 29 y/o female suffered an ankle sprain (inversion sprain), resulting in mild swelling and heat. She applied RICE (rest, ice, compression, and elevation) right after the injury, and the swelling subsided up until that evening when pronounced swelling, bruising (ecchymosis), and pain developed. This prompted her to see an orthopedic specialist for a thorough examination with no noticeable fractures or structural damage found.

However, she continued to experience mild swelling and pain after standing and walking for long periods of time, as well as limited range of motion at certain angles. All her orthopedic specialist could do for her is prescribe NSAIDs, which only provided temporary relief, but never resolved the problem. That's why she came to see me. Do you think prescribing You Gui Yin adding large doses of Cang Zhu and Huang Bo will provide effective treatment for this patient's condition?

A: Your patient's history and presenting symptoms strongly suggest joint malalignment, a very common complication of ankle sprain. Since she has undergone a thorough examination (x-ray, ultrasound, MRI), you can rule out more severe injuries such as fracture, tendon rupture, and ligament tear. However, these imaging studies will *not* detect minute displacements within the articular structure as a whole, which can cause lingering problems like your patient has been experiencing over the past 2 months.

First, the joint must be realigned by performing the ankle compression maneuver that I taught you. Then, bleed the affected site and distal well points along the channels corresponding with the affected site; needle Zhong Feng (LV4), Di Wu Hui (GB42), and Xuan Zhong (GB39); and prescribe an yin-enriching fire-downbearing formula such as Zhi Bo Di Huang Tang adding Huo Luo Dan (dispels wind and eliminates dampness, transforms phlegm and frees the network vessels, and quickens the blood and relieves pain). After administering this formula for 7 days (by this time any residual inflammation and swelling resulting from the ankle compression maneuver should have resolved!), you can change to a kidney yang-supplementing formula such as You Gui Yin adding Huo Luo Dan. Also, needle the Ankle Joint Acupoints (Qiu Xu (GB40) proper and an extra acupoint along the inferior border of the lateral malleolus in a depression anterior to the calcaneofibular ligament and Shen Mai (UB62)), Zhong Feng (LV4), Di Wu Hui (GB42), and Xuan Zhong (GB39). This treatment approach will provide quick and effective results.

Remember! You must advise the patient to avoid sitting cross-legged, kneeling, or walking on the side of her affected foot; otherwise, reinjury (including the complication of malalignment) is more likely to occur. Once the condition has resolved and stabilized, you can also recommend the patient regulate the constitution by taking kidney yang-supplementing medicinals such as Shen Qi Wan or You Gui Wan to strengthen the sinews and bones.

Case Study #17: Malalignment of the Hip Joint

Q: About 1 year ago, a 33 y/o female incurred a fall that resulted in inguinal pain (right side) and inability to abduct her (right) hip. Her orthopedic surgeon diagnosed her with an inguinal ligament tear, but treatment was not effective. She was treated by a renowned TCM physician for 3 months, but without positive results. Please offer your advice and suggestions for the treatment of this patient.

A: Your description of the patient's history and symptoms suggests malalignment of the femoral head and acetabulum (which forms the hip joint, a ball-and-socket joint) and not an inguinal ligament problem. To treat this condition, I would first perform a traction-manipulation maneuver to realign the femoral head inside the joint cavity; bleed the well points of the liver, spleen, and kidney channels; needle San Yin Jiao (SP6), Tai Chong (LV3), and Nei Guan (P6); and prescribe a blood-nourishing and -quickening, stasis-dispelling pain-relieving, and network vessel-freeing channel-regulating formula such as Ru Mo Si Wu Tang adding The Three Yellows, Niu Xi, and Huo Luo Dan (dispels wind and eliminates dampness, transforms phlegm and frees the network vessels, and quickens the blood and relieves pain).

Following administration of this therapeutic regimen, once pain has been mitigated, you can begin gradually adding The Three Great Yang-Supplementers (starting out at 1 qian and increasing up to as much as 5 qian each) into your formula. At this time, you should warm needle the abovementioned acupoints along with directly needling (using a 3 to 5 cun needle, depending on the size of the patient) into the hip joint in the direction of the femoral head at insertion points from the anterior, lateral, and posterior aspects. These are Ashi (ouch) acupoints that roughly correlate, but are not specific to Wei Dao (GB28), Ju Liao (GB29), and Huan Tiao (GB30).

This therapeutic regimen will put your patient on the path of gradual improvement and recovery. Continue administering this approach and evaluating the patient's condition up until the pain and discomfort have completely resolved; the great majority anyways, but there still may be some limited range of motion or discomfort at extreme degrees, then you can consider changing the formula to either You Gui Yin, Shen Qi Wan, Shi Quan Da Bu Tang, San Bi Tang, or Du Huo Ji Sheng Tang variants to strengthen the sinews and bones and regulate the constitution.

Case Study #18: Avascular Necrosis of the Talus

Q: A 36 y/o female patient sprained her right ankle 3 years ago, and 1 year ago (2 years after the initial injury) she visited me seeking consultation. I strongly advised her to have an MRI performed then, but she procrastinated up until recently, with the results showing avascular necrosis of the talus and peripheral inflammation. Do you think the administration of Zhi Bo Di Huang Tang variant can halt this necrotic process and promote restructuring of the sclerotic bone? Now, she gets an MRI performed every 3 months.

A: During the acute and post-acute stages of avascular necrosis, I would prescribe an yin-enriching fire-downbearing formula variant such as Zhi Bo Di Huang Tang or an essence-replenishing blood-supplementing formula such as Zuo Gui Yin. However, this patient has already entered the chronic stage, which can be identified as kidney yang vacuity with cold impediment pattern. Thus, I would consider prescribing a kidney yang-supplementing formula such as Shen Qi Wan or You Gui Yin adding Di Long, Wu Gong (or Qi Cao), Xu Duan, Gu Sui Bu, Huang Bo (large dose), and Huo Luo Dan (dispels wind and eliminates dampness, transforms phlegm and frees the network vessels, and quickens the blood and relieves pain).

Continue administering this formula and advise the patient to continue having periodic MRIs performed. These MRIs will help you conduct accurate pattern identification and make the necessary modifications to your therapeutic regimen, as well as providing objective proof of efficacy!

Case Study #19: Avascular Necrosis of the Midfoot

Q: A 45 y/o female sprained her ankle about two years ago and she has been receiving both TCM (myself included) and Western medicine treatment since then. During her initial clinical visit about 1 1/2 years ago, I prescribed Ru Mo Si Wu Tang variant. After taking this formula for 2 weeks, she called in and said that her pain had diminished by 50%, but for some reason she chose not to continue with my TCM treatment at that time.

Recently, she came back for a visit saying that "the pain has come back and it's even more intense than before!" Suspecting that the process of avascular necrosis was already well underway, I advised her to get an MRI performed. The results came back as I had suspected and she was in tears about it. Her Western medical doctors told her that she needed to undergo surgery involving evacuation and curettage and then fixation (arthrodesis) with application of bone allograft. This invasive intervention scares her and she is still considering other options. Can TCM provide effective treatment for this pathocondition and alleviate the need for other invasive procedures?

A: Avascular necrosis of the hindfoot and midfoot are rare. For our humid subtropical climate here in Taiwan, during the acute stage, I would likely prescribe a blood-supplementing essence-replenishing formula variant such as Zuo Gui Yin for 3–5 weeks and then change over to a kidney yang-warming and -supplementing, blood-quickening stasis-dissipating, and sinew- and bone-strengthening formula variant such as You Gui Yin variant. Since the climate in South Korea is much colder, especially now, during the dead of winter, I recommend going ahead with You Gui Yin adding Huo Luo Dan (3 pills/3x/day) (dispels wind and eliminates dampness, transforms phlegm and frees the network vessels, and quickens the blood and relieves pain) from the start. Also, warm needle the Toe Crevice Acupoints (four acupoints located on the dorsal aspect of the foot at the proximal V-shaped bases between the 1st, 2nd, 3rd, 4th, and 5th metatarsal bones) of the affected foot.

Your treatment objective should be to first relieve pain and allow the medicinals to promote the regeneration of articular cartilage with strong and durable surface margins. Once the patient regains compressive resilience and the ability to withstand sheer and tensile forces, advise the patient to have an x-ray and/or MRI performed. These images will show visible improvement in the regeneration of healthy bone and articular cartilage.

Remember! Even after the pain resolves, the patient must continue taking TCM medicinals for at least 6 months up to 1 year (or possibly even longer) in order to ensure the complete regeneration of bone and articular cartilage. That's when you can feel confident this pathocondition has been cured!

Case Study #20: Frozen Elbow

Q: Do you think Gui Qi Jian Zhong Tang variant offers effective treatment for forty-year-old's elbow (四十肘 sì shí zhǒu)?

A: Forty-year-old's elbow (osteoarthritis), tennis elbow (lateral epicondylitis), and golfer's elbow (medial epicondylitis) typically present with arthritic stiffness and aching. They can all be classified as types of frozen elbow and identified as cold impediment pattern. Elbow injuries caused by throwing (e.g., pitchers, bowlers) tend to present with pronounced redness, heat, swelling, and pain (inflammation), especially in the acute stage and/or if the patient continues to throw despite the injury, and thus can be identified as heat pattern.

For both frozen shoulder and throwing injuries (post acute and chronic stage), I would prescribe a qi- and blood-supplementing and kidney yang-supplementing formula such as Gui Qi Jian Zhong Tang or a flesh-resolving yang-upbearing channel-coursing formula such as Ge Gen Tang adding Gan Jiang and Fu Zi. If irritation or reinjury occurs, presenting with heat and swelling, you can prescribe a heat-clearing toxin-resolving formula such as Huang Lian Jie Du Tang variant, and bleed locally at the affected site and the distal well points on the hand of the affected elbow.

Elbow injuries caused by throwing typically present with pain at the medial epicondyle of the humerus (the insertion site of the flexor/pronator tendons) near Shao Hai (HT3). This pathocondition is called flexor tendinitis, and in the acute stage can be identified as heat pattern. Again, for treatment, first bleed as mentioned above and then needle distally on acupoints corresponding to the channels of the affected site. In cases where *heat* (inflammation) is more pronounced, then prescribe Huang Lian Jie Du Tang variant, and if *cold* is more pronounced, then prescribe Gui Qi Jian Zhong Tang variant adding only small amounts of Gan Jiang and Fu Zi and relatively larger doses of The Three Yellows.

Remember! Competitive athletes (e.g., baseball pitchers) may present with a more complex clinical picture because in order to compete they may have to "grind through it" by receiving steroid injections and high doses of NSAIDS or other painkillers. These patients may present with *only* swelling and *no* heat, due to the potent "suppressant" effects of the anti-inflammatory and painkiller medication, and can be identified as true cold and false heat or cold-heat complex pattern. In these cases, if the patient had to perform, I might go ahead and prescribe Si Ni Tang to boost their metabolism and strength for competition. After the competition, I would strongly recommend the patient "treat the root" of the condition, in this case the inflammation, and then continue moving on with a comprehensive therapeutic regimen.

In cases of malalignment, subluxation, or dislocation (luxation), a traction-manipulation maneuver must be performed for elbow joint reduction, and 3–5 days after this procedure iatrogenic pronounced heat and swelling will present, which can be identified as heat pattern. Prescribe heat-clearing toxin-resolving medicinals (e.g., Huang Lian Jie Du Tang) at the onset and continue carefully evaluating the patient, modifying the formula accordingly as the heat and swelling resolve.

Remember! As a general rule, for the treatment of cold impediment pattern pathoconditions in cold climates, you should prescribe larger doses of The Three Great Yang-Supplementers and consider adding Wu Zhu Yu (warms the liver, dissipates cold, and relieves pain). The liver governs the sinews; liver cold causes spasm and contracture, and thus pain. For acupuncture, you should warm needle during the winter months, but during the summer months an infrared heat lamp will suffice.

Case Study #21: Fibrodysplasia Ossificans Progressiva (FOP)

Q: A 25 y/o female patient was diagnosed with dermatomyositis (DM) by a rheumatologist about 6 years ago. At that time, the patient felt like a common cold had set in with generalized malaise, fatigue, and soreness throughout her whole body. She was still a high school student back then and didn't think too much about it, just taking some over-the-counter medicine as a remedy. When she began university these symptoms worsened and she developed a high, unremitting fever and muscle weakness (myasthenia). One doctor diagnosed her with systemic lupus erythematous (SLE) and then following more extensive evaluation and tests, she was diagnosed with fibrodysplasia ossificans progressiva (FOP).

Her current symptoms are as follows: generalized muscle tightness; extremely sensitive skin where the slightest touch or rub incites a scream (allodynia); progressive calcification in the sinews (muscle, tendons, ligaments, fascia) around the elbow and knee; fibrosis of the lung for which a section has already been resected; and progressive fibrotic change in the chest, back, and thighs. This really is a strange and complicated pathocondition. Can the administration of TCM medicinals offer any significant results in relieving symptoms, slowing down the rate of progression, or even curing this disease?

A: FOP (aka myositis ossificans progressive (MOP)) correlates with the pathoconditions of impediment of the flesh, spasm, and congealing cold described in TCM classical texts. As for virtually all pathoconditions, TCM treatment has the capacity to provide effective relief of symptoms, slow down the rate of progression, and yes, even cure the disease. You just need to clearly evaluate the patient's history and presenting signs, symptoms, lab tests, and imaging studies in order to accurately identify the pattern as the basis for determining the optimal treatment.

This genetically acquired disease can be treated as a neurological disorder arising spontaneously or caused by trauma. Remember! Regardless of the cause, identify the pattern as the basis for determining treatment. If exterior wind-cold pattern presents, then prescribe formula variants such as Ma Huang Tang, Gui Zhi Tang, or Ge Gen Tang; and if heat (fever) presents, then add The Three Yellows and Shi Gao in your formula selection. If exterior pattern presents in the *absence* of heat in the flesh (myofascial inflammation) and there is *no* fever, or if there *is* a fever and the administration of heat-clearing toxin-resolving and vacuous heat-clearing steaming bone-eliminating medicinals (e.g., Huang Qin, Huang Lian, Qing Hao, Zhi Mu, Di Gu Pi, Xuan Shen) have failed in abating it, then consider adding The Three Great Yang-Supplementers to boost the metabolism and bolster right qi. For trauma-induced cases, stasis heat pattern will present and resolve within a few days and then manifest in cold stasis, cold stasis with dual blood and qi vacuity, cold stasis with defense yang insecurity, or cold stasis with kidney yang vacuity pattern.

For stasis heat pattern, you can prescribe a blood-quickening stasis-dispelling and network vessel- and channel-freeing formula such as Ru Mo Si Wu Tang, Tong Jing Fang, Fu Yuan Huo Xue Tang, Gui Zhi Fu Ling Wan, Dang Gui Shao Yao San, or Da Huang Zhe Chong Wan adding The Three Great Yang-Supplementers and The Three Yellows. For dual qi and blood vacuity pattern, prescribe formulas such as Bu Zhong Yi Qi Tang, Gui Qi Jian Zhong Tang, Shi Quan Da Bu Tang, and Ren Shen Yang Rong Tang adding The Three Great Yang-Supplementers, Huang Qin, and Ren Shen/Chuan Qi Powder. You could even consider kidney yang-supplementing, blood-supplementing essence-replenishing, and wind-damp dispelling formula variants like Shen Qi Wan, You Gui Yin, or Du Huo Ji Sheng Tang.

As for acupuncture, you should warm needle (burn at least 3 cones/needle for each session) acupoints that manifest as tight or spastic muscles surrounding the affected joint as well as distal acupoints and A-shi (ouch) points that respond to pressure. At first, the patient will feel distention with slightly less tension after receiving acupuncture, and as treatment continues the patient's muscles and joints will gradually loosen and become more flexible, eventually regaining mobility and range of motion.

Even after the muscle tissue and sinews dramatically improve, you must continue prescribing this regimen for 3–5 more months. If the condition remains stabilized, at that time, you can consider reducing the dosage (e.g., instead of administering a dosage of 1 packet (600 cc) of decocted medicinals 3x (200 cc each)/day, administer 1 packet over a 2 or 3 day period instead) as a means of regulating the constitution.

Case Study #22: Fibrous Dysplasia

Q: A female high school student was diagnosed with fibrous dysplasia in her femur. A thorough hospital examination ruled out osteosarcoma, determining the condition was benign (with only a minimal risk of becoming malignant). What role can TCM play in treating this pathocondition?

A: Regardless if the condition is diagnosed as fibrous dysplasia or myositis ossificans (traumatic heterotopic ossification or neurogenic heterotopic ossification), the TCM treatment approach is basically the same. First, assess whether there is heat at the affected site (femur). If so, this indicates inflammation and can be identified as stasis heat pattern, requiring administration of blood-quickening stasis-transforming formulas such as Tong Jing Fang or Ru Mo Si Wu Tang adding Zhi Mu, Huang Bo, Fu Ling, and Ze Xie. If the affected site feels cold on palpation, then this indicates cold stasis with kidney yang vacuity pattern, requiring administration of a kidney yang-supplementing formula such as You Gui Yin or Shen Qi Wan adding large doses of Gan Jiang and Fu Zi. Typically, these great yang-supplementing medicinals will provide noticeable improvements, strengthening fibrous bone and making ossified bone more pliable. These osseous changes may also be evident on follow-up scans (bone scans, MRI).

But remember! You must continue administering treatment for 3–5 months up until the lesion completely resolves. In some cases of fibrous dysplasia, the patient may opt for surgical intervention, entailing curettage and bone grafting (fixation in severe cases).

Case Study #23: Lumbar Pain in the Elderly

Q: Recently, I have been treating several elderly patients with lumbar pain upon flexion. Do you treat this common ailment any differently when it occurs in the elderly?

A: In elderly patients, both hunchback (kyphosis) and lumbar pain can be identified as kidney yang vacuity pattern. First, make sure the patient has a good appetite and well-balanced diet, and check to see if there is any lower leg edema. Lower leg edema may simply arise from poor nutritional intake, but it may also suggest chronic venous insufficiency (poor venous return) or cardiovascular and pulmonary pathologies. In fact, cardiovascular and pulmonary disease may inhibit blood flow to the lumbus and spine, which can also cause lower back pain.

Remember! You must take all of these factors into consideration when prescribing a formula. In addition to kidney yang-supplementing formulas such as You Gui Yin and Shen Qi Wan, I might also prescribe a formula variant such as Ban Xia Tian Ma Bai Zhu San (supplements the spleen and stomach, transforms damp-wind, and stabilizes wind), Xiang Sha Liu Jun Zi Tang (boosts qi and fortifies the spleen and moves qi and transforms phlegm), Bu Zhong Yi Qi Tang (fortifies the spleen and supplements qi and upbears yang), Bu Yang Huan Wu Tang (quickens the blood and supplements qi), Gui Qi Jian Zhong Tang (supplements qi, blood and kidney yang and fortifies the center), or Shi Quan Da Bu Tang (quickens the blood and supplements the blood, boosts qi and fortifies the spleen, and supplements kidney yang). As always, the choice of formula is ultimately determined by the patient's signs, symptoms, and specific pattern presentation.

Case Study #24: Ganglion Cyst

Q: I have been treating a patient with a ganglion cyst at the base of her wrist (near Shen Men (HT7)) using warm needling, but the results have been poor. It's really frustrating! Do you have any advice on treating this minor ailment?

A: You should insert the needles in a radial pattern inside the fluid-filled cyst cavity (approximately 3–5 needles depending on the cyst size) and apply the moxa cone on the needle handle (burn at least 3 cones/needle each session) as close to the skin as possible without burning (actually, mildly burning the skin would provide even faster results, but in most cases, patients will not accept this approach). When removing the needles, it's best to allow the synovial fluid to exude from the site of insertion, wiping away with a cotton swab or tissue. You can prescribe qi- and yang-supplementing medicinals, and advise the patient not to stay up late, get plenty of sleep, dress warm, don't overwork, and exercise regularly.

Remember! During this therapeutic regimen, at first the ganglion cyst will become harder, and then it will gradually soften, eventually resolving and disappearing altogether. Don't worry! Just administer this therapeutic approach and you will have no problem effectively treating this minor ailment.

VI. NEUROLOGICAL DISORDERS

Dr. Lee has been actively engaged in the research of neurological disorders in coordination with the Tri-Service General Hospital, National Defense Medical Center for the greater part of his medical career. Through these ongoing pursuits, he has gained extensive experience in the effective clinical treatment of paresis, paralysis, and other neuropathies. This section introduces some of the most common pathoconditions presenting in the TCM clinical setting.

Section 1: Facial Palsy and Trigeminal Neuralgia

Case #1: Hemifacial Spasm vs. Motor Neuron Disease

Q: What are the differences in prognosis for hemifacial spasm (HFS) and motor neuron disease (MND)?

A: There is an enormous difference in prognosis between these two conditions.

HFS is caused by involuntary muscle contractions that are controlled by the 7th cranial nerve (CN7) originating in the brainstem. This condition can be associated with facial palsy (aka Bell's palsy), which is caused by a lower motor neuron lesion, and the prognosis is very good.

MND, on the other hand, is a neurodegenerative disorder that affects motor neurons of the voluntary muscles and is typically associated with these five pathoconditions: amyotrophic lateral sclerosis (ALS), primary lateral sclerosis (PLS), progressive muscular atrophy (PMA), progressive bulbar palsy (PBP), and pseudobulbar palsy. The prognosis for MND is much less optimistic with the therapeutic goals focused on controlling the condition, preventing deterioration, extending lifespan, and preserving quality of life.

Case #2: Hemifacial Spasm, Facial Palsy, and Bell's Palsy

Q: What is the best TCM approach for treating hemifacial spasm, facial palsy, and Bell's palsy?

A: As a general rule, the Western medicine treatment protocol for diseases of inflammatory and autoimmune etiology, or virtually any other recalcitrant pathology for that matter, is the administration of corticosteroids (injection or oral route). On the contrary, TCM employs a multimodality therapeutic regimen consisting of medicinals, acupuncture and moxibustion, and tuina (facial massage). This multimodal approach provides effective treatment for hemifacial spasm and facial palsy (aka Bell's palsy) without adverse effects or complications.

The formula that I most commonly prescribe for treating these neurologic pathoconditions is the blood-quickening qi-supplementing formula Bu Yang Huan Wu Tang adding The Three Great Yang-Supplementers, Huang Qin, The Three Insects, and Ren Shen/Chuan Qi Powder.

However, acupuncture and moxibustion (warm needling) are the most important modalities for the treatment of these pathoconditions. Select acupoints based on the location of the affected site and its corresponding channels, applying moxa cones on needle handles for *body* acupoints and adhesive moxa cones directly on the skin at the base of the needle entry point for *facial* acupoints.

For the *body* acupoints, I like to warm needle Feng Chi (GB20) (for patients with longer hair that might burn, use an infrared lamp instead!), He Gu (LI4), Zu San Li (ST36), and Nei Ting (ST44).

For the *facial* acupoints, I like to warm needle Si Zhu Kong (SJ23) joining Zan Zhu (UB2) transversely along the orbital arch towards Yu Yao (EX-HN4), points on the forehead (at and parallel to Yang Bai (GB14)) directed downward towards the eyebrow, the Trigeminal Nerve Acupoints corresponding with the branched pathways of the trigeminal nerve (CNV) and facial nerve (CNVII) (starting about 1 cun out from Ting Gong (SI19) below the zygomatic arch near Xia Guan (ST7), transversely insert 3 needles in a radiating pattern joining Si Zhu Kong (SJ23), Quan Liao (SI18), and Jia Che (ST6) respectively), Jia Che (ST6) joining Di Cang (ST4), and Ying Xiang (LI20) joining Qing Ming (UB1).

My experience with moxibustion for these pathoconditions has been "blistering is the best." This entails allowing the adhesive moxa cones (typically recommend 3 adhesive moxa cones/needle each session) to burn until blisters form, which will spontaneously heal within 2 weeks without leaving a scar behind. The patient can also apply Zi Yun Gao (Purple Cloud Ointment) for faster healing. If the patient is concerned about cosmetic appearance, concealer makeup is an option. Obviously, you must first explain the details of this approach to the patient and get their consent. Male patients tend to be more accepting of this method than female patients, but not always.

Case #3: Motor Neuron Disease – Crippling Wilt and Impediment

Q: A Western medicine physician colleague of mine asked me if TCM could be administered to effectively treat motor neuron disease (MND). I don't have any experience treating patients with this type of pathocondition, and really wasn't sure how to answer. Please share your experiences in administering TCM medicinals for the treatment of MND.

A: MND correlates with the TCM pathoconditions of crippling wilt (痿躄 wěi bì) and impediment (痺 bì). These pathoconditions can manifest in a broad scope of patterns such as damp-heat, phlegm-rheum, spleen qi vacuity, spleen and lung yang vacuity, kidney and liver yin (blood) vacuity, and kidney and liver yang vacuity. In rare cases, MND may present as exterior wind-cold pattern, requiring the addition of Ma Huang, Di Long, Rou Gui, and Xi Xin into the main formula.

Right now, Western medicine typically administers Riluzole (an anti-glutamatergic) as the first-line treatment along with drugs that attempt to relieve symptoms. The use of corticosteroids has been ineffective in the treatment of this condition and attempts at using interferon, immunosuppressants, and autologous and allogenic stem cell transplants have not been successful either.

As for TCM, spleen qi vacuity and kidney yang vacuity are the two most commonly identified patterns, requiring administration of formula variants such as Bu Zhong Yi Qi Tang, Gui Qi Jian Zhong Tang, Bu Yang Huan Wu Tang, Shen Qi Wan, and You Gui Yin adding The Three Great Yang-Supplementers, Ren Shen/Chuan Qi Powder, Lu Rong (powder), Huang Qi, and Huang Qin. If the patient's condition rapidly deteriorates, then add large doses of Ren Shen (powder) (5–8 qian), Lu Rong (powder) (3–5 qian), The Three Great Yang-Supplementers (up to 1 liang each), and possibly even a small dose of Liu Huang (powder) (starting out at 1 qian and gradually increasing to 3 qian). The essence blood-boosting, qi- and blood-supplementing, interior-warming yang-assisting, yang-returning counterflow-stemming, and kidney-supplementing to promote qi absorption actions of these medicinals will give the patient a chance to rebound and continue battling.

The scary thing about this disease is how rapidly deterioration occurs. Weakness, fasciculation, spasticity, and decreases in muscle tone typically begins in the limbs and then progresses to affect swallowing, speech, breathing, and cognitive function, leading to systemic and progressive atrophy with the patient likely dying from respiratory failure. Over the years, I have devoted a considerable amount of time and energy into the research and clinical application of integrative TCM and Western medicine treatment of MND. But to date, I have only been able to slow down the rate of deterioration with the best results helping to extend the patient's life by 3–5 years. After the onset of MND, patients typically live 3 years and rarely as long as 5 years. This is a really a "tough pill to swallow" for the medical community and we all feel a sense of powerlessness as we try to confront this intractable pathocondition.

Case Study #4: Common Cold Sequelae – Facial Paralysis and Deviated Eyes and Mouth

Q: A 28 y/o male patient caught a common cold, resulting in a high fever. Two weeks later, he felt numbness on the left side of his face, pain at the back of his ear, and impaired sense of taste (dysguesia) saying, "everything tastes bitter." I diagnosed this condition as facial paralysis. Do you think Ge Gen Qin Lian Tang variant is a good formula for this condition?

A: Facial paralysis (臉癱 liǎn tān) presenting with deviated eyes and mouth (口眼歪斜 kǒu yǎn wāi xié) correlates with the modern biomedicine pathocondition facial palsy (aka Bell's palsy). In classical TCM pathophysiology, facial paralysis is caused by network strike (中絡 zhōng luò) and in this case is a sequela of external contraction (common cold), meaning that the nerves innervating the face and front and back of the ear have been affected by the pathogenic microorganism (i.e., virus) that caused the common cold.

In classical texts prior to the Jin and Yuan dynasties (1115 to 1368 AD), the etiology of *network strike* and *wind strike (stroke)* (中風 zhòng fēng) are similar in that any external contraction or internal evil may result in damage to the peripheral nervous system (PNS), peripheral vasculature, central nervous system (CNS), and cerebrovasculature. *Wind strike (stroke)* damages the channels, bowels, and viscera, which consists of the larger vessels (i.e., cerebrovasculature) and nerves (i.e., CNS), and may result in the sequelae of speech, visual, and cognitive impairment, or even hemiparesis and hemiplegia. *Network strike* damages the network vessels, which consist of the smaller vessels and nerves (e.g., CNV, CNVII), and may result in facial palsy (Bell's palsy) and deviated eyes and mouth. *Network strike* is a lower motor neuron disorder, while *wind strike (stroke)* is an upper motor neuron disorder that may result in derivative damage to the lower motor neurons (e.g., CNV, CNVII) via nuclei in the brainstem.

Prescribing a heat-clearing exterior-interior resolution and exterior-resolving channel-coursing formula such as Ge Gen Qin Lian Tang or Ge Gen Tang adding Huang Qin, Huang Lian, and Bai Zhi will be effective for exterior wind pattern *with* heat. In the *absence* of heat, I would prescribe a qi- and blood-supplementing and kidney yang-supplementing formula such as Bu Yang Huan Wu Tang or Gui Qi Jian Zhong Tang adding Gan Jiang, Fu Zi, The Three Insects, Huang Qin, Ren Shen/Chuan Qi Powder, and possibly Bai Zhi and Fang Feng (if signs or symptoms of exterior wind pattern still present).

Acupuncture should also be administered, applying the warm needling method on the affected side. Remember! The *affected* side will appear "un-deviated" and the *unaffected* side will appear "deviated"! For the *body* points, warm needle Feng Chi (GB20) (for patients with longer hair that might burn, use an infrared lamp instead!), He Gu (LI4), Zu San Li (ST36), and Nei Ting (ST44). For the *facial* acupoints, I like to warm needle Si Zhu Kong (SJ23) joining Zan Zhu (UB2) transversely along the orbital arch towards Yu Yao (EX-HN4), the Trigeminal Nerve Acupoints corresponding with the branched pathways of the trigeminal nerve (CNV) and facial nerve (CNVII) (starting at a point about 1 cun out from Ting Gong (SI19) below the zygomatic arch near Xia Guan (ST7), transversely insert 3 needles in a radiating pattern joining Si Zhu Kong (SJ23), Quan Liao (SI18), and Jia Che (ST6) respectively), Jia Che (ST6) joining Di Cang (ST4), and Ying Xiang (LI20) joining Qing Ming (UB1).

My experience with moxibustion for this type of pathocondition has been "blistering is the best." This entails allowing the adhesive moxa cones (typically recommend 3 adhesive moxa cones/needle each session) to burn until blisters form, which will spontaneously heal within 2 weeks without leaving a scar behind. The patient can also apply Zi Yun Gao (Purple Cloud Ointment) for faster healing. If the patient is concerned about cosmetic appearance, concealer makeup is an option. Obviously, you must first explain the details of this approach to the patient and get their consent. Male patients tend to be more accepting of this method than female patients. If the patient does not give consent, then simply monitor the skin after reapplying each moxa cone up until the skin appears yellowish-brown—that's when you know the burn is limited to the upper layers of the epidermis and it will *not* blister! Once the skin appears dark brownish or blackish in color, then you know it *will* likely blister and leave transient scarring, because the burn has entered deeper into the epidermis and possibly the dermis.

Case Study #5: Blepharoptosis (Ptosis)

Q: A 50 y/o female patient presented with left-sided drooping of the upper eyelid (blepharoptosis (ptosis)), and complained of numbness and mild pain (paresthesia) on the left side of her face and occasional pain in her left shoulder. An MRI (a magnetic resonance angiography (MRA) was not performed) revealed *no* abnormal findings. Do you think this could involve occlusion of a brainstem artery?

A: Left-sided drooping of the upper eyelid with mild pain suggests levator palpebrae superioris muscle palsy or an acquired demyelinating neuropathy involving the trigeminal nerve (CN5) or facial nerve (CN7). Based on your description there does *not* appear to be any noticeable signs of heat pattern, and thus I recommend administering the following therapeutic regimen:

1) Prescribe a qi- and blood-supplementing and spleen-fortifying yang-upbearing formula such as Bu Yang Huang Wu Tang, Bu Zhong Yi Qi Tang, or Gui Qi Jian Zhong Tang adding The Three Great Yang-Supplementers, The Three Insects (or Qi Cao), Ren Shen/Chuan Qi Powder, and Yu Sheng Wan.
2) Perform acupuncture (warm needling) on the *body* acupoints Feng Chi (GB20), Tian Zhu (UB10), Feng Fu (GV16), He Gu (LI4), Zu San Li (ST36), and Nei Ting (ST44); and the *facial* acupoints Ting Gong (SI19), Jia Che (ST6) joining Di Cang (ST4), and Ying Xiang (LI20) (needling transversely upwards along the septum in the direction of Qing Ming (UB1)). Remember! Apply

moxa cones on needle handles for *body* acupoints and adhesive moxa cones directly on the skin at the base of the needle entry point for *facial* acupoints.

This therapeutic approach will effectively remedy the paresthesia, and over time, resolve the ptosis.

Case Study #6: Trigeminal Neuralgia – "Sudden Jolts of Excruciating Pain"

Q: About 2 years ago, a 65 y/o female began feeling pain in the right side of her face (most pronounced in upper gums). Following a thorough examination, her doctors diagnosed her with trigeminal neuralgia and performed a nerve block procedure. Even after the procedure the patient has continued to experience 2–3 episodes of what she describes as "sudden jolts of excruciating pain" every day. The anticonvulsant and antispasmodic drugs she is currently taking don't seem to be relieving the pain much either. I prescribed Xian Fang Huo Ming Yin adding Huang Qi and The Three Insects. Do you think this is the right approach?

A: "Sudden jolts of excruciating pain" sounds like trigeminal neuralgia to me. This type of shooting or stabbing (like an electric shock!) hemifacial pain followed by a burning ache is the hallmark of trigeminal neuralgia.

You must first determine if there is any inflammation, which can be identified as *heat* pattern, and whether or not corticosteroids (anti-inflammatory and immunosuppressant effects) have been administered, which can be identified as *cold* pattern. For patients presenting with the stereotypical paroxysmal shooting or stabbing pain, you can prescribe a blood-quickening qi-supplementing formula such as Bu Yang Huan Wu Tang adding The Three Insects. If *heat* pattern presents, then add Sheng Shi Gao and Bai Zhi and Ge Gen (both enter the Yang Ming channel, resolve the exterior and dissipate wind, and free the orifices and relieve pain); and if *cold* pattern (administration of corticosteroids) presents, then add The Three Great Yang-Supplementers, Huang Qin (counterbalances the heat), and The Three Insects.

Remember! For severe cases, it is important to prescribe these

TCM medicinals in large doses (e.g., Bai Zhi and Ge Gen (at least 8 qian)). If exterior wind pattern presents, then you should consider prescribing Ge Gen Tang adding Huang Qin, Sheng Shi Gao, Bai Zhi, and The Three Insects; and if phantom pain (幻痛 huàn tòng) presents (especially for cases involving phantom pain from herpes zoster (shingles)!), then prescribe Xian Fang Huo Ming Yin variant. If signs of heat present, then bleed both locally at the site of pain, and distally at Da Zhui (GV14), Tai Yuan (LU9), and the well points of the stomach and large intestine channels.

As for acupuncture, you can needle (do *not* warm needle!) body acupoints such as Feng Chi (GB20), Tian Zhu (UB10), Ting Gong (SI19), Di Wu Hui (GB GB42), He Gu (LI4), Zu San Li (ST36), and Yang Ling Quan (GB34). For generalized facial pain, you can needle the Trigeminal Nerve Acupoints corresponding with the pathways of the 3 trigeminal nerve (CNV) branches (starting at a point about 1 cun out from Ting Gong (SI19) below the zygomatic arch near Xia Guan (ST7), transversely insert 3 needles in a radiating pattern joining Si Zhu Kong (SJ23), Quan Liao (SI18), and Jia Che (ST6) respectively). For pain around the ear and eye, you can needle facial acupoints along the gallbladder channel above and behind the ear, and Si Zhu Kong (SJ23) and Zan Zhu (UB2) transversely along the orbital arch towards Yu Yao (EX-HN4). And for pain in the lower and upper jaw, you can insert 3 needles in a radial pattern starting from Jia Che (ST6) along the pathway of the facial nerve (CN7) (and lower pathway of CN5) joining Di Cang (ST4), Xia Guan (ST7), and Quan Liao (SI18) respectively.

Case Study #7: Facial Palsy vs. Trigeminal Neuralgia – Differential Diagnosis

Q: What's a simple way to differentiate between facial palsy (aka Bell's palsy) and trigeminal neuralgia?

A: The easiest way to differentiate is to always remember this: the main symptom of trigeminal neuralgia is *pain*, whereas facial palsy is a type of impediment pattern resulting in facial paralysis with the main symptom of *deviated eyes and mouth* (口眼歪斜 kǒu yǎn wāi xié).

Case Study #8: Hemifacial Spasm

Q: A 45 y/o female has been having hemifacial spasm (HFS) for over 10 years. Following thorough examination, Western medical doctors determined that the cause was from a blood vessel compressing the facial nerve (CN7), and recommended that she undergo microvascular decompression. The patient was worried that if something happened to go wrong with the procedure her condition would become even worse. That's why she decided to seek TCM treatment. Can TCM effectively treat this pathocondition? What are your insights and experiences into the treatment of HFS?

A: A blood vessel compressing a nerve and causing HSF correlates with tremor, hypertonicity, spasm, and jerking in classical TCM pathologic terminology. Somewhere along the CN7 pathway a blood vessel (most commonly the anterior inferior cerebellar artery near where the nerve exits the brainstem) is pressing down on the nerve and disrupting conductance. Taking into consideration how long the patient has been afflicted with this condition, I would classify this as obstruction of channels and network vessels, requiring administration of the following therapeutic regimen:

1) Acupuncture (warm needle) Feng Chi (GB20), Tian Zhu (UB10), He Gu (LI4), Zu San Li (ST36), Yang Ling Quan (GB34), Ting Gong (SI19), Tai Yang (EX-HN5), Si Zhu Kong (SJ23), and Jia Che (ST6). For the facial acupoints, needle on the affected side only, but for the body acupoints you may consider selecting an acupoint or two on the channel(s) that correspond contralaterally with the spasm distribution on the affected side. Again, I use adhesive moxa cones for warm needling the facial points, applying directly on the skin at the base of the needle entry point.

2) Prescribe a qi-supplementing blood-nourishing, stasis-dispelling pain-relieving, and network vessel-freeing channel-regulating formula such as Bu Yang Huan Wu Tang, Ru Mo Si Wu Tang, or Xue Fu Zhu Yu Tang. Make sure to include Huang Qi (starting out at 1 liang and gradually increasing the dose), The Three Insects, Ma Huang, and Di Long. Based on careful assessment of signs, symptoms, and pattern identification, you can determine if it is necessary to add Gan Jiang, Fu Zi, and Huang Qin, and if so, how much.

Typically, this therapeutic regimen will provide noticeable results within 3 months, but for complete resolution, you may need to administer TCM medicinals from 6 months to 1 year.

Case Study #9: Trigeminal Neuralgia – Discontinue Drugs…Pain Rebounds!

Q: Two weeks ago, a 63 y/o female began experiencing periodic episodes of stabbing pain in her right cheek and upper and lower gums. Following thorough examination by a neurologist, she was diagnosed with trigeminal neuralgia (TN). She wanted to get a second opinion from a TCM doctor, so she came to see me. I explained to her my treatment regimen involving acupuncture and medicinals, performed acupuncture and prescribed Shi Quan Da Bu Tang adding Ge Gen and Chuan Qi.

However, the patient did not take the medicinals I prescribed; instead, she checked into a hospital where she was administered drug (unspecified) treatment and a few days later the pain disappeared. Right after being released from the hospital, she incurred nausea and vomiting and developed a severe headache. It appears that the drugs the neurologist prescribed were able to provide fast relief, but not lasting results.

She went through this treatment routine experiencing brief remission and sudden recurrence for about 1 1/2 months before she finally decided to come back and see me again. I prescribed Ban Xia Tian Ma Bai Zhu San Tang variant aimed at remedying the pain and checking vomiting. Can you offer any advice for treating this patient?

A: Right now, the Western medicine first-line treatment for neuropathic pain such as TN is anticonvulsants (e.g., carbamazepine (Tegretol), phenytoin), antispasmodics, and botulinum toxin (botox) injections. If these are ineffective, then some patients choose surgical options such as microvascular decompression and ablative therapy (e.g., Gamma knife radiosurgery), the latter involving the destruction of nerve fibers for therapeutic effect. Drugs may provide relief, but once these drugs are discontinued, the pain typically recurs. Also, long-term administration of anticonvulsants can cause harmful side effects, the most serious being Stevens-Johnson syndrome (SJS), which can be life-threatening. Similarly, surgical procedures can provide relief for a period of time, but the pain usually recurs, along with the side effects of numbness and tingling.

As for TCM medicinals, I have gotten the best results prescribing the blood-quickening qi-supplementing formula Bu Yang Huan Wu Tang adding The Three Insects, Mu Li (calms the liver and subdues yang), Long Gu (settles fright and quiets the spirit), Huang Qin, Chuan Qi (powder), and Yu Sheng Wan. In cases where exterior wind-heat or exterior-interior heat pattern presents, I would prescribe a formula such as Ge Gen Tang, Ge Gen Qin Lian Tang, Xian Fang Huo Ming Yin, or Wen Dan Tang adding The Three Insects and Yu Sheng Wan. Regardless of the pattern type and formula selection, I always make sure to include The Three Insects and Yu Sheng Wan for their brain electrical activity-regulating, network vessel-freeing, and pain-relieving actions.

As for acupuncture, needle (do *not* warm needle!) the following acupoints both ipsilateral and contralateral to the affected side: Feng Chi (GB20), Tian Zhu (UB10), He Gu (LI4), and Zu San Li (ST36). On the affected side, transversely insert needle(s) just above the root of the helix at the crease of the ear (corresponding with the semilunar ganglion of CN5) directed towards Yu Wei (EX-HN37) and Tai Yang (EX-HN5); transversely needle Si Zhu Kong (SJ23) joining Zan Zhu (UB2) along the orbital arch towards Yu Yao (EX-HN4); and starting about 1 cun out from Ting Gong (SI19) directly below the zygomatic arch just above Xia Guan (ST7), transversely insert three radiating needles corresponding with the 3 main trigeminal nerve (CN5) pathways. In cases where heat pattern presents, prior to performing acupuncture, bleed Da Zhui (GV14), Ting Gong (SI19), and the well points of channels corresponding with the distribution of facial pain.

As for the formula you have chosen, rarely would I prescribe the spleen- and stomach-supplementing, phlegm-damp transforming, and wind-stabilizing formula variant Ban Xia Tian Ma Bai Zhu San variant for trigeminal neuralgia, but you can give it a try. Remember! Regardless of the formula, at the onset of treatment your primary objective is to relieve the painful symptoms!

Case Study #10: Post-Stroke Periodontal Phantom Pain

Q: This patient has a history of incurring three cerebrovascular accidents (CVAs)—cerebral infarction (once) and cerebral hemorrhage (twice). After his first cerebral hemorrhage 8 years ago, he began experiencing periodontal pain that he said "feels like someone is stabbing my gums." The way he describes it sounds a lot like trigeminal neuralgia (TN). He has tried all types of drugs and therapies without success. Now, the only thing he can do is resort to monthly botulinum toxin (botox) injections, blocking the nerve and temporarily mitigating the pain. As far as other physical and cognitive sequelae from stroke, he is actually quite fortunate: he is able to walk on his own with a steady gait, can speak and communicate normally, and has full control of his bladder and stool. What do you think the best approach is for treating this patient?

A: Post-stroke periodontal pain is suggestive of phantom pain. If the patient remains free of neurological deficits and cognitive impairment despite multiple CVAs as you explained, then the key here is to focus on relieving the pain. You can prescribe the heat-clearing toxin-resolving, swelling-dispersing hardness-breaking, and blood-quickening pain-relieving formula Xian Fang Huo Ming Yin adding The Three Insects and Yu Sheng Wan; and needle the acupoints Feng Chi (GB20), Tian Zhu (UB10), He Gu (LI4), Zu San Li (ST36), Nei Ting (ST44), Ting Gong (SI19), Xia Guan (ST7), Jia Che (ST6), Da Ying (ST5), and Di Cang (ST4). Administration of this therapeutic regimen will provide pain relief, and in time, remedy this pathocondition.

Another possibility would be to prescribe the blood-quickening qi-supplementing formula Bu Yang Huan Wu Tang adding The Three Insects and Yu Sheng Wan, along with needling the acupoints just mentioned above. This approach will serve the dual function of remedying the post-stroke sequelae of phantom pain now and preventing another CVA from occurring in the future.

Section 2: Postherpetic Neurological Complications

Case Study #1: Herpes Zoster (Shingles) – Girdling Snake Cinnabar, Fire-Girdle Sore, and Snake Cinnabar

Q: I am in the process of compiling background information and case reports to substantiate the clinical efficacy of TCM treatment of postherpetic neurological complications. Eventually, I'd like to publish a paper entitled *TCM Treatment of Postherpetic Neurological Complications*. It would appear that the stress of modern life may be part of the reason for the increasing incidence of herpes zoster (shingles) (i.e., reactivation of the varicella-zoster virus (VZV) following initial infection presenting as chickenpox (varicella) earlier on in life). Postherpetic complications typically manifest as severe pain, heat pain, cold pain, residual heat, qi vacuity, palsy, cold impediment, and wilting pattern.

Detailed differentiation and pattern identification of these clinical features and complications are documented in classical TCM texts. For instance, the complication of paralysis (麻痺 má bì) (an umbrella term to describe neuropathies that may manifest as palsy, paresthesia, paresis, and plegia) can be further differentiated into the anatomical site (e.g., eyes, ears, face) affected and its manifestations. Classical TCM texts abound with both specific and non-specific pathologic term correlations, explanations, and therapeutic approaches. Plying through the canons of TCM classical literature to find these correlations is a laborious process. I was wondering if you could give me any suggestions or ideas about how I could best go about this process.

A: The documentation and description of classical TCM pathologic terms and pathoconditions, such as girdling snake cinnabar (蛇丹 shé dān), fire-girdle sore (缠腰火丹 chán yāo huǒ dān), and snake cinnabar (蛇纏腰 shé chán yāo), directly correlate with the initial phase of herpes zoster (shingles). As for the complications, modern biomedicine describes these manifestations with terms such as facial tics, trigeminal neuralgia, ptosis, facial spasm, and facial palsy. In classical TCM texts, the manifestation of these complications correlate with terms such as impediment (痺 bì), pain (痛 tong), wilting (痿

wěi), disablement (廢 fèi), twitching (振跳 zhèn tiào), convulsion (抽搐 chōu chù), headache, and hemilateral headache (偏頭疼 piān tóu téng) among others. There are ample descriptions of pathoconditions that correlate with herpes zoster complications in numerous classical TCM external medicine texts. You can analyze them for yourself, make distinctions, and differentiate the various clinical manifestations.

Remember! The process of learning is the root of discovery, so don't be hesitant about putting in the extra time and effort; in the end, you will realize it was worth it! One contemporary book I would recommend is *Practical Integrative Traditional Chinese Medicine and Western Medicine Neurology* (實用中西結合神經病學). This book will give you some ideas to start on as you reference other TCM texts from China, Japan, and Korea. You can also include your own clinical cases to support your material. This will provide a valuable contribution to the entire medical community. Get to work and good luck!

Case Study #2: Postherpetic Peripheral Neuropathy

Q: A 79 y/o female patient (looks like she is about 60 y/o) developed herpes zoster skin eruptions on her lower left leg and stayed in the hospital for 10 days receiving drug treatment. The medication resolved the rash, but after returning home she couldn't dorsiflex (raise upward) her left foot or her third and fourth toes. She thought it might have been a side effect of the medication, prompting her to seek TCM treatment.

Though I have quite a bit of experience treating herpes zoster (prescribing Long Dan Xie Gan Tang variant) and have even successfully treated several cases of the postherpetic complication of ptosis (prescribing Xian Fang Huo Min Yin variant), but I have never treated a case like this before. What signs and symptoms do you use to differentiate and determine pattern identification? What's the best approach for treating this patient?

A: Phantom pain (postherpetic neuralgia), phantom heat (paresthesia), phantom cold (paresthesia), and phantom noise (auditory hallucination) are the most common complications of herpes zoster. However, encephalitis, myelitis, cranial and peripheral nerve palsies (e.g., myoclonus, ataxia, spasticity, flaccid paralysis), and a syndrome of delayed contralateral hemiparesis may also occur. In some patients, skin lesions are deep and extensive, with scarring and myofascial adhesions manifesting after the eruptions have healed.

For this patient with foot drop, you can still administer Xian Fang Huo Ming Yin adding Huang Qi (2 liang), Di Long (5–8 qian), Ma Huang (2–3 qian), and Niu Xi (5 qian); and if phantom pain (postherpetic neuralgia) presents, then add The Three Insects. You can perform acupuncture as well as needling acupoints corresponding to the channels of the affected site.

One thing is for sure, I have never come across a herpes zoster case that has presented as cold pattern. All of my patients have presented as heat pattern, with the most common being ascendant hyperactivity of liver yang (肝陽上亢 gān yáng shàng kàng), liver channel depressed heat (肝經鬱熱 gān jīng yù rè), stasis obstruction, qi vacuity, and innominate toxin swelling (無名腫毒 wú míng zhǒng dú). You should also consider including Long Dan Cao (drains fire in the liver and gallbladder), The Three Yellows (clear heat and resolve toxin), Qing Hao, Zhi Mu, and Di Gu Pi (enrich yin and downbear fire and clear vacuity heat and eliminate steaming bone), and Sheng Shi Gao and Sheng Mu Li (clear heat and drain fire). Naturally, your medicinal selections should be based on the presentation of specific signs and symptoms and detailed pattern identification.

Case Study #3: Postherpetic Peroneal Nerve Palsy

Q: A 69 y/o female patient suffered from a bout of shingles last year. Everything seemed to be healing up just fine until she began noticing muscle weakness, and eventually, the inability to raise her right foot. This postherpetic peroneal nerve palsy (foot drop) has lingered on since then, prompting her to visit me for treatment. I prescribed Bu Zhong Yi Qi Tang (including Huang Qi (2 liang)) adding Di Long (8 qian), Niu Xi (8 qian), and The Three Great Yang-Supplementers (3 qian each), but it's already been 2 weeks now without any improvement in her muscle weakness and foot drop. What do you think I should do?

A: This is a good formula for postherpetic peroneal nerve palsy, but I would include larger doses of Gan Jiang and Fu Zi, a smaller dose of Niu Xi, and add Ma Huang and Ren Shen/Chuan Qi Powder. Also, perform acupuncture (warm needle), manipulating the needles with strong supplementing techniques (e.g., swirling and rotating) prior to changing the moxa cones (burn at least 3 cones/needle each session). The patient will have noticeable improvement within 3 months of administering this therapeutic regimen, but it will likely take about 6 months for the patient to fully recover.

Case Study #4: Postherpetic Deviated Eyes and Mouth

Q: This is a 59 y/o female patient who is among the large population of Chinese people of Korean descent living in Jilin Province, China. About 1 month ago, she developed herpes zoster skin eruptions on the right side of her face near her ear. For the past 3 weeks, her TCM physician in China has been treating her with local injections, topical medicinal paste (not sure what type), and acupuncture. Her condition has not shown any improvement, and that's why one of her relatives here in South Korea contacted me for assistance.

A: For the herpes zoster complication of facial palsy, as long as the skin eruptions have already healed, you can treat this condition just as you would for deviated eyes and mouth (口眼歪斜 kǒu yǎn wāi xié). There are many types of folk medicine therapies with antispasmodic actions for the treatment of facial palsy, such as Ba Dou (Croton Seed, Fructus Crotonis) and Qian Zheng San topical umbilical therapy and the orally administered decoction Yu Zhen San, but they aren't very effective. The problem with these therapies is that they don't *treat the root* (治本 zhì běn) of the pathocondition.

The root of postherpetic deviated eyes and mouth can be identified as qi and blood vacuity with blood impediment (血痹 xuè bì) pattern, and the focus of treatment is on enhancing cerebrovascular circulation, innervating the central nervous system (CNS), and rectifying the aberrant electrical conductance of the myelin sheath to restore normal innervation of the affected peripheral nerve(s). This requires the administration of qi- and blood-supplementing medicinals adding The Three Insects.

The treatment of blood impediment with qi- and

blood-supplementing medicinals is described in the TCM classic *On Cold Damage and Miscellaneous Diseases* (傷寒雜病論 shāng hán zá bìng lùn), which classifies wind strike (stroke) (中風 zhòng fēng) as blood impediment. Remember! Make sure to include The Three Insects for these types of peripheral nerve disorders (cranial nerves are peripheral nerves!). However, for pathologies of the central nervous system resulting in neurologic deficits, such as cerebrovascular accident (CVA), paralysis (癱 tān), and disablement (廢 fèi), The Three Insects will *not* provide therapeutic efficacy.

As for medicinals, I would prescribe Bu Yang Huan Wu Tang adding The Three Great Yang-Supplementers, The Three Insects, Huang Qin, and Ren Shen/Chuan Qi Powder. If residual heat pattern presents, then consider adding Qing Hao, Yu Sheng Wan, and a small dose of Long Dan Cao; and if hemilateral headache presents, then add Tian Ma (or Wu Zhu Yu).

Also, perform acupuncture (warm needling) on the following acupoints: Feng Chi (GB20), Tian Zhu (UB10), He Gu (LI4), and Zu San Li (ST36); transversely needle towards the back of the head at the crease of the ear along the zygomatic arch (corresponding with the semilunar ganglion of CN5); transversely needle Si Zhu Kong (SJ23) joining Zan Zhu (UB2) along the orbital arch towards Yu Yao (EX-HN4); and starting at a point directly below the zygomatic arch near Xia Guan (ST7), transversely needle three radiating points joining Si Zhu Kong (SJ23), Quan Liao (SI18), and Jia Che (ST6) respectively (corresponding with the three main pathways of the facial nerve (CN7) and trigeminal nerve (CN5)).

Remember! Warm needling will give you quicker results than just needling. For *body* acupoints, you can directly apply moxa on the skin (or moxibustion on ginger) at the location of acupoints or fit moxa cones on the needle handles; and for *facial* acupoints you can apply adhesive moxa cones directly on the skin at the base of needle entry points. My experience for *facial* acupoints has been that "blistering is the best," which entails burning the adhesive moxa cones until the skin turns a dark brownish or blackish color. A blister will subsequently appear where the moxa cones had been placed: within 3 days a scab will form and within 10–14 days the scab will fall off, leaving no sign of discoloration or scarring. Obviously, you must explain the details of this approach to the patient and get their consent first.

Also, during this therapeutic regimen, the eyelid and cheek may feel swollen and distended and paroxysmal drooling may occur. This is nothing to be concerned about! You can assure the patient that these are just temporary therapeutic responses and a part of the healing process. The results from administration of this therapeutic regimen will make both the patient and doctor very happy!

Case Study #5: Postherpetic Neuralgia – It's Just "Phantom Pain"

Q: A 30 y/o male patient came down with a bout of herpes zoster about 1 1/2 years ago. At the time, he was administered Zovirax (acyclovir) cream, which he applied topically for 1 1/2 months until the skin eruptions completely resolved. The rash healed, but he felt pain in the right shoulder and upper back, which got worse over time, with severe pain now occasionally radiating along the pathway of the triple burner channel of his right arm. Symptoms arise both in the day and at night. What's the best way to treat this condition?

A: For postherpetic neuralgia (aka phantom pain) you can prescribe a heat-clearing toxin-resolving and blood-quickening pain-relieving formula such as Xian Fang Huo Ming Yin adding The Three Insects (Quan Xie, Wu Gong, and Bai Jiang Can) and Yu Sheng Wan. But remember! You must also advise the patient to *relax*, and by all means, *don't get stressed out* about this condition, because stress will only make it worse! Assure the patient that this TCM therapeutic regimen will provide rapid relief of "phantom pain."

Section 3: Olfactory and Gustatory Nerve Palsy

Case Study #1: Olfactory Nerve Palsy – "I Still Can't Smell!"

Q: A 34 y/o overweight female patient became ill with a high fever and an upper respiratory tract infection earlier this spring. And about 1 month later, she noticed bilateral loss of her sense of smell (anosmia). It's already been 2 months now and she said emphatically, "I still can't smell!" What's the best approach for treating anosmia resulting from olfactory nerve palsy? How long will it take before treatment shows results? How long before complete recovery?

A: There are many causes of anosmia including external contraction (common cold) affecting the cranial nerves, iatrogenic origin (e.g., a complication of anesthetics, chemotherapy, or radiotherapy), trauma, polyps, and tumors. It sounds like your patient's condition results from a complication of microbial infection (likely a virus!), in which the virus (邪氣 xié qì) may have not been completely resolved and/or the metabolic waste from the immune response fighting the virus has impaired olfactory nerve (CNI) function.

Thus, I would consider prescribing a heat-clearing phlegm-transforming formula such as Wen Dan Tang adding Lai Fu Zi, Ma Huang, Fu Zi, Xi Xin, and Sang Bai Pi. For Ma Huang, incrementally increase the dose up until it affects the patient's sleep, and then bring it down a bit, to where sleep is unaffected (that's the maximum optimal dose!). The patient will begin regaining her sense of smell within 3–5 weeks.

If your patient had begun taking this formula immediately after incurring loss of smell, then results would appear as quickly as 1–2 weeks. As for other types (patterns) of anosmia, I have also prescribed formulas such as Bu Yang Huan Wu Tang and Ma Huang Fu Zi Xi Xin Tang combining Bu Yang Huan Wu Tang to effectively treat this condition.

Case Study #2: Anosmia Following a Bout of the Common Cold

Q: A 43 y/o male patient complained of anosmia starting 5 years ago following a common cold. I *confidently* prescribed a 2-week dosage of Wen Dan Tang combining Ma Huang Fu Zi Xi Xin Tang adding Bai Jie Zi and Lai Fu Zi. The patient returned after 2 weeks without any noticeable improvement whatsoever. I am very disappointed and a bit embarrassed for being overly confident! Can you give me some advice on this case?

A: Loss of sense of smell (anosmia) for the past 5 years following external contraction (外感 wài gǎn) (common cold) clearly indicates olfactory nerve palsy. Continue prescribing your original formula, but include large doses of Ma Huang, Gan Jiang, Fu Zi, and Sang Bai Pi; Xi Xin (up to 3 qian) and Xin Yi and Cang Er Zi (8 qian or more). Remember! For Ma Huang, you should incrementally increase the dose up until it affects the patient's sleep, and then bring it down a bit, to where sleep is unaffected. Administering this approach will provide effective results.

Case Study #3: Chronic Nasal Congestion – Hyposmia and Hypogeusia

Q: A 16 y/o male patient has had chronic nasal congestion since childhood. Three years ago, he began noticing the inability to sense bitter and salty flavors; and then as time passed, even the sweet taste of his favorite chocolate candy bar had no flavor, and he began losing some sense of smell as well. I believe chronic nasal congestion is the cause of the patient's gustatory and olfactory nerve palsy, presenting as hyposmia (partial loss of the ability to smell) and hypogeusia (partial loss of the ability to taste). Based on this diagnosis, I prescribed Wen Dan Tang variant. Do you think this is a good approach?

A: For this patient presenting with chronic nasal congestion, hyposmia, and hypogeusia, it would be fine to prescribe a heat-clearing phlegm-transforming formula such as Wen Dan Tang adding Ma Huang, Xin Yi, Bai Zhi, Sheng Pu Huang, Mu Dan Pi, and Zhi Zi. This formula variant is appropriate for wind-cold or wind-heat exterior (external contraction) pattern that evolves into repletion heat pattern with gustatory and olfactory nerve palsy sequelae.

However, you must remember that the etiology and pathomechanisms of gustatory and olfactory dysfunction may be identified as different patterns for each specific case. For instance, if heart heat pattern presents, then consider prescribing Tian Wang Bu Xin Dan variant; if heart blood vacuity presents, then consider Bu Yang Huan Wu Tang variant; and if qi and blood vacuity presents, then consider a formula such as Bu Zhong Yi Qi Tang, Gui Qi Jian Zhong Tang, Shi Quan Da Bu Tang, or Ren Shen Yang Rong Tang adding Ma Huang, Di Long, Chuan Qi, Xi Xin, Xin Yi, and Sang Bai Pi.

Remember! You must identify the pattern as the basis for determining treatment. As you know, different pattern types require the administration of corresponding formulas.

Case Study #4: Gustatory Nerve Palsy – Longstanding Anosmia

Q: I have a 65 y/o female patient who explained that 34 years ago (about 6 months after giving birth to her oldest daughter) she suddenly, in the absence of any apparent causative factors, incurred a complete loss her sense of taste (ageusia). She has tried both TCM and Western medicine treatment over the years, but nothing has been effective. Do you think it's still possible to treat this condition after so many years have elapsed?

A: This case of anosmia can be classified as gustatory nerve palsy, with the root of the dysfunction likely in the brainstem. The principle cranial nerves that innervate the tongue are the facial nerve (CNVII), glossopharyngeal nerve (CNIX), and vagus nerve (CNX): the nuclei of these nerves are bunched together in the brainstem. Damage to the brainstem, ganglia, and nerves proper anywhere along their respective courses may lead to gustatory nerve palsy. This damage may be caused by a viral infection, iatrogenic origin (e.g., side effects from drugs, radiotherapy), neurological and endocrine disorders, tumors, and even anxiety.

You will have to carefully examine your patient's medical history and make a definitive determination yourself, but it sounds to me like it very well could be a case of visceral agitation (臟躁 zàng zào). For this pathocondition, I would prescribe a blood-quickening qi-supplementing formula such as Bu Yang Huan Wu Tang along with the center-harmonizing agitation-calming and stagnation-dissipating phlegm-transforming formula Gan Mai Da Zao Tang Combining Ban Xia Hou Po Tang adding Ma Huang, Di Long, Chuan Qi (powder), and Yu Sheng Wan.

At this stage, after so many years have passed, you shouldn't approach this pathocondition from the perspective of residual heat or Shao Yang heat pattern (e.g., Wen Dan Tang, Xiao Chai Hu Tang). Remember! The tongue belongs to the heart, the heart connects to the brain-marrow, and the heart holds the office of monarch, whence the spirit light emanates. This is the reason why I would try prescribing the formula above. Indeed, it has been a long time, but you can give it a try!

Section 4: Post-Traumatic Neuropathies

Case Study #1: Broken Wrist Results in Numb Fingers

Q: A 22 y/o female pianist got into a car accident and fractured her left wrist. After the fracture healed, she felt cutaneous numbness on the back of her hand and first, second, and third fingers. Her range of motion is good, but when she raises her arm it trembles. How would you treat this patient?

A: Distal radius fracture resulting in numbness of the fingers and back of hand (peripheral neuropathy) can be identified as qi vacuity pattern.

As for treatment, I would prescribe the qi- and blood-supplementing and kidney yang-supplementing formula Gui Qi Jian Zhong Tang (including large doses of Huang Qi) adding small doses of Fu Ling and Ze Xie, and Yu Sheng Wan. But there are many other dual qi- and blood-supplementing formula variants that will also be effective, such as Bu Zhong Yi Qi Tang, Bu Yang Huan Wu Tang, Shi Quan Da Bu Tang, and Hui Yang Sheng Xian Tang. Just make sure to include some yang-supplementing medicinals in your formula.

Naturally, you should perform acupuncture as well. I would warm needle (fitting moxa cones on the needle handle and burning at least 3 cones/needle each session) the Finger Crevice Acupoints (four acupoints located on the dorsal aspect of the hand at the proximal V-shaped bases between the 1st, 2nd, 3rd, 4th, and 5th metacarpal bones), Wai Guan (TB5), and Shou San Li (LI10). Plus, moxatherapy can be administered by applying adhesive moxa cones on the well points of the corresponding channels of the affected hand.

Actually, any of a variety of dual qi- and blood-supplementing formula variants, such as Bu Zhong Yi Qi Tang, Bu Yang Huan Wu Tang, Shi Quan Da Bu Tang, and Hui Yang Sheng Xian Tang, will provide effective treatment. Just make sure to add yang-supplementing medicinals and perform acupuncture (warm needling).

Remember! You must advise your patient to actively mobilize her affected hand, do stretching exercises to keep it loose, and soak it in hot water and/or apply a heating pad. Encouraging your patient to stay positive and avoid the mental traps of becoming mired in frustration and depression by this physical setback is another important aspect of your therapeutic regimen. Make her aware that if she dwells on the injury too much, her anxiety might very well lead to *psychogenic* numbness. This is why I would also prescribe Yu Sheng Wan, because it functions as a mild sedative that relieves anxiety.

Case Study #2: Progressive Muscular Atrophy Following Car Accident

Q: I have a male patient who got into a serious car accident 7 years ago and fractured his skull. For a period of time right after the accident, he was still able to walk. After the skull was sutured, he incurred a sudden increase in intracranial pressure (ICP), resulting in left-sided hemiparesis, but his condition improved following treatment.

This summer he incurred paroxysmal severe lumbar pain and weakness in his left leg that has continued worsening. After receiving treatment with acupuncture and TCM medicinals from other physicians without noticeable results, he decided to see what I could do for him. How would you treat this patient with progressive paresis in his left leg?

A: This patient's history and clinical presentation suggests CNS compression resulting in progressive muscular atrophy (PMA). You should advise your patient to have an MRI performed to see if there are any CNS obstructions or compressions within the brain, spine, or lumbar region. I would start out by prescribing either Paralysis Formula #2 (Shi Quan Da Bu Tang Variant) or Paralysis Formula #3 (You Gui Yin Variant) including large doses of Ma Huang (incrementally increasing the dose up until it affects the patient's sleep, and then bring it down a bit, to where sleep is unaffected—that's the maximum optimal dose!), Di Long, Gan Jiang, Fu Zi, Lu Rong (powder), Ren Shen/Chuan Qi Powder. If constipation presents, then incrementally increase the dose of Da Huang, while also increasing the doses of Rou Gui and Ren Shen/Chuan Qi Powder to maintain a balanced draining to supplementation ratio.

Section 5: Cold Impediment

Case Study #1: UB Channel and SI Channel Cold Impediment

Q: A 64 y/o male patient with a history of fifty-year-old's shoulder (五十肩 wǔ shí jiān) has recently felt soreness and pain in the left scapular region when he gets up every morning. He feels particularly sharp pain near Gao Huang (UB43) and Tian Zong (SI11), but still has normal strength and function. Results of MRI and cardiology tests were all normal. I prescribed Gui Qi Jian Zhong Tang adding Ma Huang, Ge Gen, and Di Long without noticeable effects. What would you do for this type of patient?

A: That's right! For pain in the Gao Huang region, you can administer the qi- and blood-supplementing and kidney yang-supplementing formula Gui Qi Jian Zhong Tang. Ma Huang and Ge Gen are good additions, but you don't need to add Di Long.

You should also perform Tui Na (Chinese massage therapy) techniques to search for and "untangle" (loosen up) those muscle knots (myofascial trigger points) along the pathways of the urinary bladder (UB) channel (e.g., Gao Huang (UB43), Tian Zhu (UB10)), small intestine (SI) channel (e.g., Tian Zong (SI11), Jian Zhen (SI9)), and gallbladder channel (e.g., Feng Chi (GB20), Wan Gu (GB12)).

After "untangling" the muscle knots, needle (or warm needle) the acupoints Feng Chi (GB20), Tian Zhu (UB10), Jian Zhen (SI9), Hou Xi (SI3), and Wei Zhong (UB40); and apply heat therapy to the affected area with an infrared lamp. Also, encourage the patient to regularly stretch the neck, arm, shoulder, and upper back muscles; and focus on good posture. This approach will produce effective results.

Case Study #2: Cold Impediment in the Gao Huang (UB43) Region

Q: I have a 56 y/o male patient with a history of type 2 diabetes mellitus, hyperlipidemia, and proteinuria. About 2 months ago, he began feeling the sensation of heat and pain along the lower border of his left scapula in the Gao Huang (UB43) region, and lying down exacerbated the pain. He underwent a thorough medical examination, but results failed to identify any potential causes of this pain (e.g., fractured rib, herpes zoster, and neuropathy). Do you think this is a type of myopathy?

A: It sounds like a typical case of cold impediment (寒痹 hán bì). All you need to do is perform Tui Na (Chinese message therapy); needle (or warm needle) the acupoints Feng Chi (GB20), Tian Zhu (UB10), Hou Xi (SI3), Wai Guan (TB5), and Wei Zhong (UB40); and apply heat therapy to the affected area with an infrared lamp. Heat therapy, warm needling, and moxatherapy are especially important during the cold weather seasons!

As for TCM medicinals, you can prescribe the spleen- and stomach-supplementing and phlegm-damp transforming formula Ban Xia Tian Ma Bai Zhu San adding Sang Bai Pi (8 qian), Huang Qi (2 liang), and Sheng Du Zhong (4 qian). Administering this approach will completely resolve this condition in a short period of time, as well as provide preventive therapy for the patient's type 2 diabetes mellitus, hyperlipidemia, and proteinuria.

Case Study #3: Cold Impediment – Skewed Handwriting

Q: A 52 y/o male patient had been under heavy stress about 3 years ago and incurred a sudden episode of reversal cold (厥冷 jué lěng) over the right half of his body. Ever since this incident his handwriting has been skewed (can't write clearly on a straight line); and at night, he feels heat in the heart of the palms and soles and has stabbing pain in his right shoulder. However, he does *not* have any cognitive impairment resulting from this incident, and follow-up MRIs have shown *no* structural abnormalities or lesions. Please offer your opinions and guidance on this case.

A: Your description of this patient's history and presenting symptoms suggests the possibility of Parkinson's disease (PD), frozen shoulder (fifty-year-old's shoulder), or simply cold impediment (寒痹 hán bì). You should make sure the patient has been tested for PD and conduct a frozen shoulder exam on your own.

More than likely, it is a simple case of cold impediment, for which I would proceed as follows:

1) Needle the Three Shoulder Acupoints (corresponding to Jian Yu (LI15), Jian Liao (TB14), and a point snugly wedged between the coracoid process and the humeral head), He Gu (LI4), Shou San Li (LI10), Zhong Zhu (TB3), Wai Guan (TB5), Bei Lao Gong (located in opposition to Lao Gong (PC8) on the dorsal aspect of the hand at the proximal V-shaped base between the 3rd and 4th metacarpal bones), and Zu San Li (ST36).

2) Prescribe Gui Qi Jian Zhong Tang variant. After the pain has been effectively remedied, then the patient will gradually regain normal handwriting function.

If the condition is diagnosed as fifty-year-old's shoulder (frozen shoulder), then also perform the overhead traction-compression maneuver to disband the adhesion; bleed the well points of the hand channels of the affected side; and needle He Gu (LI4), Shou San Li (LI10), and Wai Guan (TB5).

Case Study #4: Reversal Cold of the Extremities – Psychogenic Etiology

Q: A 48 y/o male patient presented with the following history: About 20 years ago, he began experiencing coldness in his hands and feet that lasts pretty much all year round, except for summertime, when the symptoms subside for a while. Occasionally, his face and torso *feel* "hot," but his extremities are "cold." Soaking in hot springs or a heated spa provides relief, but it only lasts for a few hours and then the coldness returns. He even avoids shaking hands with people because he feels embarrassed by how cold his hands are.

I prescribed Dang Gui Si Ni Tang Jia Wu Zhu Yu Sheng Jiang Tang variant for 1 month without noticeable effect. He has a lot of pent up tension and anxiety; as the eldest son, he must take care of his ailing mother. I am considering changing the formula to Jian Ling Tang variant. What do you think the best approach would be for this case?

A: If the coldness in the extremities only occurs in the hands and feet, then this may suggest that the patient simply doesn't exercise enough and/or has too much stress and anxiety. Stress and anxiety in itself can induce peripheral vascular spasm via perturbations of the autonomic nervous system.

For this type of reversal cold of the extremities (手足厥冷 shǒu zú jué lěng), you should try to conduct a detailed pattern identification and consider prescribing formulas such as Zhi Bo Di Huang Tang (enriches yin and downbears fire and eliminates steaming bone), Shen Qi Wan (supplements the kidney and assists yang), You Gui Yin (warms and supplements the kidney), or Ban Xia Tian Ma Bai Zhu San (supplements the spleen and stomach, transforms damp-wind, and stabilizes wind) adding medicinals such as Gan Cao and Da Zao (nourish the blood and calm the spirit) and, if necessary, Long Gu and Mu Li (calm the liver and subdue yang).

Case Study #5: Elbow Weakness and Pain Upon Flexion

Q: A 46 y/o female patient was lifting weights at a fitness center 2 months ago when she felt a sensation "like an electrical shock" in her left arm; and since then, she has experienced weakness and pain upon flexion of her left elbow. How would you treat this patient?

A: This case of elbow pain and weakness upon flexion can be identified as cold impediment pattern, resulting from a muscle strain, pull, or tear that occurred 2 months ago while lifting weights.

I would prescribe a qi- and blood-supplementing and kidney yang-supplementing formula such as Gui Qi Jian Zhong Tang (including large doses of The Three Great Yang-Supplementers and Huang Qi) adding Huo Luo Dan and Yu Sheng Wan. You should also perform acupuncture (warm needling) on Nei Guan (P6), He Gu (LI4), and Hou Xi (SI3). Remember! Remind the patient to keep her joints warm, whether it's wearing extra layers of clothing or an elbow sleeve.

Section 6: Sciatica and Lumbar Pain

Case Study #1: Gluteal Intramuscular Injection – UB Channel Cold Impediment

Q: A female patient explained that she had received an intramuscular (IM) injection in the gluteal region (right side) while in the hospital undergoing treatment for enteritis. After the injection, she incurred right-sided urinary bladder channel neuropathy—numbness and pain extending from the buttocks (near Huan Tiao (GB30)) to the 4th and 5th toes along the urinary bladder and gallbladder channels.

A: Typically, an iatrogenic complication resulting from IM injection such as this can be identified as cold impediment (寒痹 hán bì) pattern and treated like a case of cold impediment presenting in sciatica. Generally, for this pathocondition, I would prescribe a kidney yang-supplementing formula variant such as You Gui Yin and warm needle acupoints such as Guan Yuan Shu (UB26), Huan Tiao (GB30), Yang Ling Quan (GB34), and Wei Zhong (UB40).

However, there are some factors that I would take into consideration first in order to accurately identify the pattern as the basis for determining treatment.

1) For young and/or nulliparous women of reproductive age, you must also consider endometriosis compressing on the lumbosacral plexus. This pathocondition can be identified as stasis heat, stasis heat entering the network vessels (瘀熱入絡 yū rè rù luò), or heat entering the blood chamber (熱入血室 rè rù xuè shì) pattern, requiring the administration of medicinals such as Ru Mo Si Wu Tang adding Huang Qin, Mu Dan Pi, Zhi Zi, Sheng Mu Li, Niu Xi, and Sheng Du Zhong. Also, needle these acupoints: Guan Yuan Shu (UB26), Huan Tiao (GB30), Wei Zhong (UB40), Zu San Li (ST36), Tai Chong (LV3), and Gong Sun (SP4).
2) If the patient is parous, then the condition can be identified as cold impediment pattern, requiring the administration of medicinals and warm needling as mentioned above.
3) For women going through menopausal transition who present with yin vacuity heat or Shao Yang heat symptoms, you

might consider prescribing an essence-replenishing blood-supplementing formula variant such as Zuo Gui Yin or an yin-enriching fire-downbearing formula variant such as Zhi Bo Di Huang Tang. Also, needle (or warm needle) acupoints such as Guan Yuan Shu (UB26), Huan Tiao (GB30), Yang Ling Quan (GB34), Wei Zhong (UB40), Nei Guan (P6), Shen Men (HT7), San Yin Jiao (SP6), Feng Chi (GB20), and Tai Chong (LV3).

Case Study #2: Cold Impediment – Soak and Decoct Medicinals in Rice Wine

Q: Three months ago, a 45 y/o male bus driver began feeling numbness and pain near his right Huan Tiao (GB30) region. X-ray images showed no abnormalities, but an MRI revealed mild swelling of the right femoral head, prompting his orthopedician to suspect osteomyelitis. His doctor repeatedly administered antibiotic injections to treat this condition over the course of 2 months with unremarkable results.

Right now, at rest he has no pain, but when he moves around, he still has pain and describes the feeling of walking as "stiff" and "awkward." I suspect that his condition may be occupational in nature, caused by poor posture while working. Thus, I advised him to take some time off and prescribed Zhi Bo Di Huang Tang variant. Do you think there is a more effective approach?

A: This description of your patient's history and symptoms suggests that he has cold impediment (or fixed impediment (著痺 zhuó bì)) of the hip (acetobulofemoral) joint resulting in sciatica. It doesn't sound like osteomyelitis to me, because Western medicine treatment of osteomyelitis administering antibiotics and corticosteroid injections is very effective at quickly resolving inflammation and remedying the condition. I think the patient likely suffers from qi and blood deficiency (lack of perfusion) to the tissues surrounding the acetobulofemoral joint, a pathocondition that can be identified as kidney vacuity cold-damp with qi and blood vacuity pattern.

As for TCM medicinals, I would prescribe a kidney yang-supplementing, qi- and blood-supplementing, and dampness-eliminating pain-relieving formula such as You Gui Yin or

(Yu Sheng) Du Huo Ji Sheng Tang (including large doses of Gan Jiang and Fu Zi) adding Ma Huang and Di Long (add in towards the end of the decocting process), Huo Luo Dan, and Yu Sheng Wan. Alternatively, you could prescribe the yin-enriching fire-downbearing and steaming bone-eliminating formula Zhi Bo Di Huang Tang, but make sure to add The Three Great Yang-Supplementers, Du Zhong, Ma Huang, and Di Long to ensure efficacy.

You should also perform acupuncture (warm needling) on Guan Yuan Shu (UB26), Huan Tiao (GB30), Yang Ling Quan (GB34), Zu San Li (ST36), Wei Zhong (UB40), and Ba Liao (UB31–34). Note: My Huan Tiao (GB30) is actually located about half the distance between the standard Huan Tiao (GB30) and Huan Zhong (EX-LE10), and depending on the thickness of the patient's buttocks, you should use anywhere from a 3 cun to a 6 cun needle, making sure that the needle sensation is felt in the pelvis or inguinal area. This strong needle sensation will ensure optimal efficacy.

Remember! Don't presume that all Western medicine diagnoses are unequivocally correct; in fact, up to 30–40% of diagnoses based on MRI images are "false positive." This is especially true for cold climates in northern regions, such as South Korea, where cold impediment is a widely prevalent condition. You must have confidence in your examination, pattern identification, and diagnostic skills!

One last thing! For cold impediment pathoconditions, it's best to first steep the raw medicinals in a mixture of 1 1/2 bowls (approx. 300 ml) rice wine and 4 1/2 bowls (approx. 900 ml) water for 30 min. up to 2 hours prior to decocting. Soaking the medicinals in the mixture of rice wine and water will enhance the liver and kidney-warming supplementing, blood-quickening network vessel-freeing, and wind-dispelling cold-dissipating actions of these medicinals.

Case Study #3: Sciatica – Gallbladder and Urinary Bladder Channel Cold Impediment

Q: I have a 61 y/o female patient with the following history: For over 1 year now, the patient has experienced lumbar pain that radiates down along the back and side of the left leg, swelling and pain at the anterior medial aspect of the left knee along the joint space, and varicose veins at the left popliteal fossa. What's the best approach for encompassing all three of these pathoconditions into a single, comprehensive treatment regimen?

A: The history you described suggests either gallbladder channel and/or urinary bladder channel cold impediment, both of which directly correlate with sciatica. Varicose veins may cause aching and heaviness in the calves, and unless it's a severe case, you can simply advise the patient to regularly exercise (going on walks is easiest and the best!), get up out of a seated position at least once every hour to stimulate circulation, and elevate the legs when resting. For the knee pain, you should verify whether there is a history of trauma (possibly a ligament sprain or tear), assess if there is heat and swelling, and determine what types of movement or activities induce the pain prior to administering treatment (e.g., bleeding, acupuncture, medicinals).

Since sciatica is the chief complaint, I would administer the following therapeutic regimen:

1) Needle the acupoints Guan Yuan Shu (UB26), Yao Yang Guan (DU3), Huan Tiao (GB30), Feng Shi (GB31), Xi Yang Guan (GB33), Wei Zhong (UB40), Yang Ling Quan (GB34), Yin Ling Quan (SP9), and Du Bi (ST35) and Xi Yan (EX17).

2) Prescribe the kidney yang-warming and -supplementing formula You Gui Yin adding Huo Luo Dan (dispels wind and eliminates dampness, transforms phlegm and frees the network vessels, and quickens the blood and relieves pain).

3) Advise the patient to make sure she keeps warm, especially from the waist down, by wearing extra clothing and thermal underwear.

Case Study #4: Sciatica – TCM Pattern Identification and Treatment

Q: I recently treated a patient suffering from sciatica with a 4-year history of lumbago and radiating pain and numbness in the left leg. After administering 3 sessions of acupuncture (warm needling) over a 2-week period, she said that her pain was completely gone. I didn't even prescribe medicinals! The patient was so happy with the results that she has recommended me to her family and friends. Is sciatica always this easy to treat?

A: Sciatica (lumbar radiculopathy) is typically *not* a difficult pathocondition to treat (*unless* disc protrusion, prolapse, or herniation is severe!), and indeed, acupuncture offers very effective treatment.

The majority (about 95%) of patients present with wind-cold-damp impediment pattern, which can be further differentiated into cold impediment (aka painful impediment (痛痺 tòng bì)), fixed (damp) impediment (著痺 zhuó bì), and moving (wind) impediment (行痺 xíng bì) patterns, while the remaining patients present with heat impediment (熱痺 rè bì) pattern. Common causes of wind-cold-damp type are muscle strain (e.g., wrenched lumbus (閃腰 shǎn yāo), poor posture), fatigue, exposure to the elements, radiculopathy (e.g., bulging disc, herniated disc), and vertebral compression fractures; and common causes of heat type are external contraction (e.g., microbial infection) and autoimmune disease.

Since the body and its pathologies are a living, fluid process, there is bound to be some overlap and ambiguity when attempting to rigidly define them into static categories. For instance, in the acute stage of virtually every wind-cold-damp type injury, there will be an inflammatory response (i.e., heat) and likely local swelling; and once this heat and swelling subside, then the pathocondition enters the post-acute and chronic stages. Naturally, each stage of the pathocondition will require administration of the optimal treatment (e.g., medicinal, acupuncture, moxibustion, bleeding, medicinal paste applications, traction-manipulation maneuvers) based on pattern identification as the basis for determining treatment.

In the acute stage of wind-cold-damp type injury, treatment may require the administration of heat-clearing toxin resolving, bland-percolating dampness- and water-disinhibiting, blood-quickening stasis-resolving, and yin-enriching fire-downbearing medicinals; whereas in the post-acute and chronic stages, administration of kidney yang warm-supplementing and blood-quickening stasis-resolving medicinals should be administered.

For wind-cold-damp impediment (i.e., cold impediment (aka painful impediment), fixed impediment, and moving impediment) patterns, I typically prescribe (Yu Sheng) You Gui Yin variant, modifying the formula based on the presentation of specific signs and symptoms. Remember! For herniated disc (aka ruptured disc or slipped disc) cases—caused by the degeneration and cracking of the fibrocartilaginous cushions (intervertebral discs) between the vertebrae and resulting in the compression of spinal nerves, I would first perform the back-to-back traction maneuver that I taught you.

For vertebral compression fractures, you can prescribe the blood-nourishing blood-quickening and network vessel-freeing pain-relieving formula Ru Mo Si Wu Tang adding Huang Qin, Sheng Du Zhong, Niu Xi, Di Long, and Ma Huang. For heat impediment pattern resulting from autoimmune disease, I recommend formula variants such as (Yu Sheng) Hyperactive Immune Formula, Er Miao San, San Miao San, Si Miao San, or (Yu Sheng) Zhi Bo Di Huang Tang (which contains Er Miao San). For external contraction pattern, I recommend formulas such as Di Long San, Da Qing Long Tang, Ma Huang Tang, or Ge Gen Tang adding The Three Yellows, Di Long, Sheng Du Zhong, and Niu Xi. For any of the above patterns, if yang vacuity pattern concomitantly presents, then add The Three Great Yang-Supplementers; and if steaming bone pattern concomitantly presents, then add Qing Hao, Zhi Mu, and Di Gu Pi.

As for cases of spinal stenosis, cauda equina syndrome (CES), spinal tumors, and spinal epidural abscess, though there may be sciatica-like symptoms of impediment pattern, these pathoconditions typically present with more debilitating symptoms and a more complex overall clinical picture. Thus, these pathoconditions can be classified as paralysis and should be treated accordingly.

Case Study #5: Herniated Disc – Foot Numbness and Diminished Sensation

Q: Two years ago, a 51 y/o female patient began feeling diminished sensation (hypoesthesia) and numbness on the dorsal aspect of her right foot, and over time these symptoms have spread up her leg and into the lumbar region. I have had many patients presenting with a similar clinical picture. She underwent a thorough neurological examination and was diagnosed with herniated (prolapsed) disc. Based on your clinical experience, about how long does it usually take for the patient to begin showing improvement and ultimately have a complete recovery.

A: For diminished sensation and numbness of the foot caused by compression on the spinal nerves (radiculopathy) from herniated disc, I recommend the following therapeutic regimen:

1) Perform the back-to-back traction maneuver.

2) Administer acupuncture (warm needling) on acupoints along the urinary bladder, gallbladder, and stomach channels.

3) Prescribe the kidney yang-warming and -supplementing formula You Gui Yin adding Huang Qi, Ma Huang, and Di Long. Herniated disc will take some time to treat, usually a minimum of 1–2 months for the improvement of symptoms, and at least 3–5 months for complete recovery.

Remember! You must advise these types of patients to have an MRI and CT scan performed to rule out the possibility of a spinal tumor or stenosis.

Case Study #6: Compression Fracture – Lumbar Pain and Lower Extremity Neuropathy

Q: A 67 y/o female patient suffers from longstanding lumbar pain and severe neuropathy in her lower extremity (left side). She refuses to undergo surgery as her neurologist has advised. What do you think the best approach for this patient would be?

A: The lumbar pain is likely the result of a recent vertebral compression fracture. The severe neuropathy in her lower extremity should gradually improve, or completely resolve over time, once the anatomical structures (i.e., muscles, tendons, ligaments) restabilize from the "fallout" of the compression fracture. If your patient happens to have a longstanding lumbar compression fracture that continues to be symptomatic, then you should warm needle, use an infrared lamp, and advise the patient to wear extra clothing (e.g., thermal underwear) to maintain warmth and promote circulation.

In both scenarios (recent and longstanding), I would prescribe a kidney yang-supplementing, qi- and blood-supplementing, and dampness-eliminating pain-relieving formula variant such as You Gui Yin, Du Huo Ji Sheng Tang, San Bi Tang, or Paralysis Formula #3 (You Gui Yin Variant). Also, I would needle the acupoints Shen Shu (UB23), Pi Shu (UB20), Guan Yuan Shu (UB26), Wei Zhong (UB40), Huan Tiao (GB30), Kun Lun (UB62), Tai Chong (LV3), Di Wu Hui (GB42), Zu San Li (ST36), and Yang Ling Quan (GB34). If the weakness and numbness persist, then add large doses of Ma Huang, Di Long, Huang Qi, Gan Jiang, and Fu Zi; and apply strong supplementing needle manipulation techniques during your acupuncture sessions.

Remember! For cases of longstanding lumbar compression fracture (over 1 year up to decades), I would also perform the back-to-back traction maneuver, make sure to warm needle (burning at least 3 cones/needle each session), and recommend hot compress therapy and warm water therapy.

Case Study #7: Sciatica – Three Years After Femur Fracture

Q: Three years ago, a 72 y/o female slipped and fell, fracturing her femur. An open reduction and internal fixation (ORIF) surgical procedure was performed, and since then she has incurred pain that radiates down from Huan Tiao (GB30) to Yang Ling Quan (GB34). Why would gallbladder channel impediment persist so long after surgery and healing? Could there still be nerve edema? Her Western medical doctors told her that it's possible the internal fixation plate has come loose. Do you think this could be the cause?

A: You should conduct a careful examination of the patient. Is there any heat and swelling (edema) of the lower leg? If there *is*, then prescribe a heat-clearing toxin-resolving formula such as Huang Lian Jie Du Tang combining Wu Ling San (disinhibits water and dampness by bland percolation) adding Niu Xi and Sheng Du Zhong. If there is *not*, then prescribe a kidney yang-supplementing, sinew- and bone-strengthening, blood-supplementing essence-replenishing, and dampness-eliminating pain-relieving formula variant such as You Gui Yin, Gui Zhi Ren Shen Tang, Zuo Gui Yin, Shen Qi Wan, San Bi Tang, or Du Huo Ji Sheng Tang.

Yes, internal fixation brace loosening and osteomyelitis are potential complications. And so is reduction malalignment which would require reoperating to remove and correct the reduction and fixation, or possibly even undergoing a hip replacement prosthetic implant procedure. Fractures can be a pain!

Section 7: Cervical Radiculopathy and Myelopathy

Case Study #1: Numbness in Arms and Legs – It Could Be Radiculopathy, Myelopathy or Basilar Artery Stenosis

Q: A 72 y/o female patient visited me with numbness in both hands and feet, which presents both at rest and during activity, and she occasionally feels dizziness. I prescribed Ban Xia Tian Ma Bai Zhu San variant. Do you think this is a good approach?

A: These symptoms suggest either cervical radiculopathy (irritation and/or compression of the spinal nerve root) or cervical myelopathy (compression of the spinal cord), which may result from a variety of causes including degenerative changes of the spine (spondylosis), spondylolisthesis, blunt trauma, infection, spinal stenosis, tumors or cysts, and autoimmune disorders (e.g., rheumatoid arthritis (RA), ankylosing spondylitis (AS)). However, you must also make sure to rule out the possibility of basilar artery stenosis (BAS).

Remember! Carefully examine the patient and request Western medicine diagnostic scans and tests as tools to help you conduct accurate differential diagnosis and pattern identification. For radiculopathy and myelopathy, it would be better to prescribe a dual qi- and blood-supplementing and channel-freeing network vessel-quickening formula such as Paralysis Formula #2 (Shi Quan Da Bu Tang Variant) (including large doses of Huang Qi) adding Tian Ma and Ren Shen/Chuan Powder. If it turns out to be BAS, then prescribing a blood-quickening qi-supplementing formula such as (Yu Sheng) Bu Yang Huan Wu Tang to promote and maintain vasculature patency would be best.

Case Study #2: Paroxysmal Numbness and Weakness in Both Hands – (Yu Sheng) Gui Qi Jian Zhong Tang Variant

Q: A 45 y/o male patient explained that 3 weeks ago he began experiencing paroxysmal numbness and weakness in both hands, headache and painful stiff nape (頭項強疼 tóu xiàng qiáng téng), and intermittent numbness and weakness in both feet. These symptoms exacerbated upon bending his neck forward (neck flexion).

When he came for a clinic visit yesterday, the lower body symptoms had completely resolved and the upper body symptoms only present in certain postural positions, with no pain whatsoever lying flat or standing erect. Stool and urine are normal and there are no exterior pattern symptoms. Taking these factors into consideration, the first week I prescribed (Yu Sheng) Gui Qi Jian Zhong Tang adding Ge Gen (8 qian) and small doses of The Three Insects; and the second week, I increased the dose of Huang Qi. Do you think this is a good approach?

A: Yes, this prescription should effectively treat this patient's condition. Western medicine really has no effective treatment for this type of ailment, but TCM formulas like Gui Qi Jian Zhong Tang that have qi- and blood-supplementing, spleen- and kidney yang-warming, and channel-freeing network vessel-quickening actions can effectively remedy these types of neuropathies. You can count on excellent success rates for the majority of these types of cases. This is an example of another therapeutic niche for TCM, because up to now Western medicine just hasn't come up with an effective treatment protocol. TCM has been doing this for thousands of years!

Case Study #3: Postsurgical Shoulder Immobility – Gui Qi Jian Zhong Tang Variant

Q1: A patient of mine incurred shoulder immobility (could not raise his arm at all) following a surgical procedure for cervical myelopathy. My first prescription was (Yu Sheng) Gui Qi Jian Zhong Tang adding Ge Gen, which produced marginal results. And then I tried adding Gan Jiang, Fu Zi, Gui Zhi, Ma Huang, Huang Qin, Chuan Qi, and Di Long. Amazing! Three days later, the patient was able to raise his arm to shoulder level, and 1 week later, he could raise his arm above his head. Thanks for your clinical advice and guidance!

A: Yes, Gui Qi Jian Zhong Tang variant works great—a perfect example of the therapeutic efficacy of TCM in the treatment of neurological pathoconditions. Postsurgical complications of this nature can be classified as the classical TCM pathologic term paralysis (麻痺 má bì). Signs, symptoms, patterns, pathoconditions, diagnoses, therapeutic regimens, and prognoses for the gamut of human disease are chronicled throughout the timeless pages of TCM classics. For instance, passages on headache and painful stiff nape (頭項強疼 tóu xiàng qiáng téng) presented in *Treatise on Cold Damage and Miscellaneous Diseases* directly correlate with cervical spine disorders.

Remember! The more you delve into the classical texts, the more clinical success you will have!

Q2: This is a follow up to the patient with postsurgical shoulder immobility. During the patient interview on his first clinical visit, he gave a detailed history of his condition. At the onset, prior to surgery, he incurred numbness in the fingers of his right hand. He went in for an examination, which revealed adhesions along C2-C6 vertebrae, so his doctors decided to go ahead with surgery. Following surgery, the patient didn't have any numbness in his fingers; however, 6 days later, he woke up that morning unable to raise his arm at all. Further nerve conduction studies and an MRI revealed *no* abnormalities. Why would this complication present 6 days later and not right after surgery? Does the etiology and pathomechanism involve qi vacuity with blood stasis pattern?

A: Inadvertent (iatrogenic) damage to the spinal nerves may have occurred during the debridement procedure with subsequent inflammation and swelling. Corticosteroid injections are typically administered to suppress the initial inflammation and swelling, but once the effects wear off in about 3 to 5 days, the immune system springs back into action, resulting in nerve swelling and compression. It's also possible that scarring and arachnoid adhesions have formed which would disrupt nerve conduction. This would account for the delayed presentation of symptoms.

I would identify this condition as qi vacuity with kidney yang vacuity pattern, but (Yu Sheng) Gui Qi Jian Zhong also includes Dang Gui in it so it does have blood-supplementing actions as well. In addition to prescribing Gui Qi Jian Zhong Tang variant, I would also acupuncture (warm needle) combinations of the following acupoints on the affected side: He Ge (LI4), Hou Xi (SI3), Zhong Zhu (TB3), Shou San Li (LI10), Chi Ze (LU5), Jian Zhen (SI9), Ju Gu (LI16), Tian Zong (SI11), Qu Yuan (SI13), Feng Chi (GB20), and Tian Zhu (UB10).

Case Study #4: Postsurgical Complications in Lower Extremities

Q: One year ago, this patient underwent surgery (anterior cervical discectomy and fusion (ACDF)) in hopes of providing relief for the symptoms of numbness and weakness in both hands and feet. Following surgery, these original symptoms subsided, but other symptoms presented: numbness in the 2nd, 4th, and 5th toes, and paresthesia (aching and tingling) in both ankles. What's the best approach for treating this condition?

A: It is common in this type of surgical procedure to damage the myelin sheath of the nerves and spinal meninges (dura mater, arachnoid mater, and pia mater), inducing swelling and adhesions that may result in nerve compression and lead to numbness and paresthesia of the hands and feet. For this condition, I would prescribe a dual qi- and blood-supplementing, kidney yang-supplementing, and channel-freeing network vessel-quickening formula such as Paralysis Formula #2 (Shi Quan Da Bu Tang Variant) (including large doses of Huang Qi and Di Long) adding Ren Shen/Chuan Qi/Rou Gui Powder (at a ratio of 3:3:1).

Remember! You must clearly explain, and reiterate time and again, the following unavoidable fact to your patient: "Pain is part of the pathway to recovery!" Meaning that during the TCM therapeutic regimen, which includes oral administration of medicinal formulas, acupuncture (warm needling), and physical therapy, patients will incur *intensified* aching, numbness, distention, and pain (some patients would say *excruciating!*). This is a positive sign, indicating that the nerves remain active with the potential to regenerate, and that the TCM treatment is indeed showing efficacy.

I have seen this occur time and again during my clinical treatment of neuropathies. You must reassure the patient that this is a part of the process towards recovery. If they are able to overcome (*endure!*) the initial discomfort, then gradually, over time, their symptoms will improve. It's not easy, but to date, this is the only alternative the patient has for regaining functional capacity. Regenerative medicine (cell-based therapies), including targeted gene therapy using CRISPR/Cas9, still has a long way to go for clinical application in human patients.

Case Study #5: Cervical Herniated Disc – Acupuncture Is Effective!

Q: A 58 y/o female patient suffered from paroxysmal cervical herniated disc. After 1 week in the hospital, she returned home and didn't experience any symptoms while sitting or lying down. However, when she stood up, she felt severe pain in the 1st and 2nd fingers and upper back (Gao Huang (UB43) region) on her right side. She explained that the pain was so bad she couldn't carry out daily activities. Do you think this can be identified as a blood stasis pattern, requiring administration of Ru Mo Si Wu Tang variant?

A: In the acute stage of cervical herniated disc (aka prolapsed or extrusion), blood stasis pattern does typically present, but in the subacute and chronic stages, I would identify this pathocondition as qi vacuity with kidney yang vacuity pattern. Prescribing Ru Mo Si Wu Tang variant is still a viable option as long as you make sure to add The Three Great Yang-Supplementers, Huang Qin, Huang Qi (at least 2 liang), Di Long, and Ma Huang.

And regardless of the formula you choose, you should also acupuncture (warm needle) the following points: Feng Chi (GB20), Tian Zhu (UB10), Jian Jing (GB21), Jian Zhen (SI9), Gao Huang (UB43), Tian Zong (SI11), Qu Yuan (SI13), Ju Gu (LI16), Hou Xi (SI3), and He Ge (LI4). Acupuncture is effective! It will give you faster and more effective results.

Case Study #6: Cervical Herniated Disc – Postsurgical Finger Numbness

Q: Two years ago, an 80 y/o female patient experienced paroxysmal numbness in the fingers of her right hand and weakness in her left foot. Her neurologist suspected cerebrovascular accident (CVA), but after further evaluation, an MRI revealed a cervical herniated disc for which surgery was performed. Unfortunately, surgery did not resolve her symptoms, so she decided to make a special 300 km trip from another city seeking my assistance. This elderly lady is really counting on me! How would you treat this case?

A: Postsurgical neuropathy is not at all uncommon. Iatrogenic damage to nerve tissue may result from the surgical procedure proper (i.e., compression, stretch, contusion, transection) or from the administration of anesthesia (i.e., mechanical trauma, local anesthetic toxicity, ischemia). Despite the advent of microsurgery and computer-assisted surgery, which helps minimize the potential for error, it is still difficult to perform surgery without complications.

In my opinion, the "ideal" approach would have been to begin administering a TCM formula decoction through the patient's nasogastric (NG) tube immediately following surgery. I would have prescribed Ru Mo Si Wu Tang adding large doses of Ze Xie, Fu Ling, and Huang Qin (or Huang Lian), Ma Huang, Di Long, and Ren Shen/Chuan Qi Powder. This blood-nourishing blood-quickening, stasis-dispelling pain-relieving, network vessel-freeing channel-regulating, and swelling-dispersing flesh-engendering formula effectively resolves inflammation and swelling and promotes the patency of damaged nerves.

For cases in which *not that much time* has elapsed since surgery, I would first find out if she has recently been administered corticosteroid injections. If *not*, then prescribe Ru Mo Si Wu Tang adding Ma Huang, Di Long, Huang Qin, Niu Xi, and Ren Shen/Chuan Qi/Rou Gui Powder (at a ratio of 3:3:1). If *so*, then prescribe the dual qi- and blood-supplementing and channel-freeing network vessel-quickening formula Paralysis Formula #2 (Shi Quan Da Bu Tang Variant).

If a *long period of time* has elapsed since surgery (it sounds like this is the case for your patient!), then the pathocondition can be identified as qi vacuity with kidney yang vacuity pattern, requiring administration of (Yu Sheng) Gui Qi Jian Zhong Tang (including large doses of Huang Qi) adding Ma Huang, Di Long, and Yu Sheng Wan. And as is typical for almost all types of neuropathy, acupuncture (warm needling in cases of qi or yang vacuity pattern) is an important part the therapeutic regimen.

Case Study #7: "Pectoral Muscle Paralysis" – It's Not That Uncommon!

Q: Three years ago, a 34 y/o male began feeling neck pain (right side) and could not internally rotate his arm at the elbow, prompting him to seek medical examination that revealed paralysis of the pectoral muscle. After undergoing neurosurgery, the neck pain symptoms improved, but motor function of the arm was still impaired and the chest muscles remain atrophied. I thought about prescribing (Yu Sheng) Gui Qi Jian Zhong Tang (containing Gan Jiang, Fu Zi, and Rou Gui) variant. Do you think this is the right approach?

A: This patient you describe as having "pectoral muscle paralysis" may have incurred damage to the recurrent laryngeal nerve, cervical nerves from C3 on down, or somewhere along the brachial plexus (i.e., brachial plexus injury (BPI), which commonly affects the lateral pectoral nerve). However, the possibility of this condition arising from compression of an artery somewhere in the neck, chest or cervical spine (i.e., anterior spinal artery syndrome) must also be ruled out. In severe cases, all of these potential etiologies may lead to varying degrees of paresthesia, paralysis, and compromised respiratory function if the patient doesn't receive adequate treatment.

As for the therapeutic regimen, I would prescribe a blood-quickening qi-supplementing formula such as (Yu Sheng) Bu Yang Huan Wu Tang (containing Yin Xing Ye) adding The Three Great Yang-Supplementers, Huang Qin, Ren Shen/Chuan Qi Powder, Di Long, and Ma Huang. Also, perform acupuncture (warm needle) on acupoints such as He Ge (LI4), Shou San Li (LI10), Wai Guan (TB5), Bei Lao Gong (located in opposition to Lao Gong (PC8) on the dorsal aspect of the hand at the V-shaped base between the 3rd and 4th metacarpal bones), Yu Men (LU2), Zhong Fu (LU1), Jian Zhen (SI9), Tian Zong (SI11), and Ju Gu (LI16). Remember! Be careful not to needle too deeply on chest and upper back points, you don't want to have a mishap that leads to pneumothorax!

There is the potential that the patient's condition could deteriorate and lead to complete paralysis on the affected side (hemiplegia). Thus, you must advise the patient to continue follow-up examinations with a neurologist; and if necessary, have the patient undergo further surgery to correct the problem. If for some reason the patient doesn't want to undergo surgery or surgery is deemed inappropriate, then you can still "fight the battle alone." With accurate pattern identification and the right therapeutic regimen, you can achieve positive results!

The formula you prescribed—(Yu Sheng) Gui Qi Jian Zhong Tang—may also be effective, but you would definitely need to add Ma

Huang, Di Long, and Xing Ren to open up the orifices and free the channels and quicken the network vessels. These additional medicinals will both promote healing of the affected nerve and serve as a preventive measure against acute respiratory distress syndrome (ARDS).

Section 8: Lumbar Radiculopathy and Myelopathy

Case Study #1: Lumbar Stenosis

Q: About 1 month ago, this patient began having back pain upon walking and felt weakness in both legs. Following examination at several hospitals, he was diagnosed with lumbar stenosis. His doctors opted for a conservative approach, holding off on surgery for now and waiting to see how the patient's condition progressed.

Dr. Lee, I distinctly remember you telling me one time that this pathocondition could not be completely cured. If that's the situation, then what is the best way for me to handle this case?

A: Surgery will only provide a brief respite in the great majority of cases, with the symptoms recurring and sometimes even worsening. Typically, the only option from a Western medicine standpoint is long-term administration of pain killers and corticosteroids. In nearly all cases, TCM treatment can effectively relieve the patient's symptoms and greatly improve quality of life; and in some cases, complete resolution of symptoms can be achieved.

Typically, the TCM therapeutic regimen will take a minimum of 1 month and a maximum of 8 months before noticeable results appear. The patient must maintain a healthy diet and lifestyle and may need to be administered follow-up TCM treatment (medicinals and acupuncture (warm needling)) to regulate the constitution if they feel overfatigued or incur pain.

For medicinals, I would prescribe a kidney yang-supplementing (or dual qi- and blood-supplementing) and channel-freeing network vessel-quickening formula such as You Gui Yin, Shi Quan Da Bu Tang, Paralysis Formula #2 (Shi Quan Da Bu Tang Variant), or Paralysis Formula #3 (You Gui Yin Variant) adding Da Huang (adjust the dose of Da Huang up until the patient maintains 2–3 stools/day), Ze Xie (large doses up to 1.5 liang), and The Three Great Yang-Supplementers (gradually adding up to 5–7 qian each). For acupuncture (warm needling), I like to needle Hua Tuo's paravertebral points, as well as urinary bladder channel distal points. By implementing this regimen, you will achieve progressively positive results.

Case Study #2: Sciatica – "It *Feels* Like Somebody Else's Skin"

Q: A 45 y/o male patient presented with paresthesia (numbness and tingling) along the lateral aspect of his right thigh with no pain or itchiness. He said that "it *feels* like somebody else's skin" and explained the affected area continues expanding. How would you approach this case?

A: Numbness along the lateral aspect of the thigh is a stereotypical symptom of L2 spinal nerve root compression (lumbar radiculopathy). As for treatment, I would first perform the back-to-back traction maneuver; administer acupuncture (warm needle) on the acupoints Guan Yuan Shu (UB26), Ba Liao (UB31–34), Huan Tiao (GB30), local A-shi (ouch) points, Yang Ling Quan (GB34), and Xi Yang Guan (GB33); and prescribe a kidney yang-supplementing, blood-quickening stasis-dissipating, and sinew- and bone-strengthening formula such as You Gui Yin or Shen Qi Wan or a dual qi- and blood-supplementing formula such as Shi Quan Da Bu Tang adding Huang Qi, Du Zhong, Ma Huang, and Di Long. If this approach does not offer satisfactory results, then consider changing the formula to either Wu Zhu Yu Tang or Dang Gui Si Ni Tang Jia Wu Zhu Yu Sheng Jiang Tang adding Du Zhong, Niu Xi, Huang Qi, Ma Huang, and Di Long.

If you put in some extra effort to perform the back-to-back traction maneuver, stimulate the acupoints with supplementing needle manipulation techniques, and apply at least 3 moxa cones during each acupuncture session, in most patients symptoms will completely resolve within 3–5 months. In cases where symptoms have been present for a long duration, you could also consider referring the patient to a neurologist for the possibility of surgery. Following surgery, TCM medicinal decoctions should be administered as soon as the patient is able to ingest fluids. This will promote rapid healing of the surgical site and greatly reduce the possibility of complications.

Section 9: Paralysis

Case Study #1: Transverse Myelitis of the Thoracic Spinal Cord Paralysis Formula #2

Q: Six months ago, a 41 y/o male patient began experiencing back pain and spasms in both legs. Under the care of a neurosurgeon, an MRI was performed revealing transverse myelitis involving the second thoracic vertebra (T2). He has been administered corticosteroids since the diagnosis to control the inflammation. The patient still has problems independently regulating urination and stool, weakness in both legs, and abdominal tightness and pain; but *no* fever. What's the best approach for treating this condition?

A: After 6 months, transverse myelitis has already entered the chronic stage, meaning that the ongoing administration of steroids will likely not provide substantive effects. I would immediately prescribe a dual qi- and yang-supplementing and channel-freeing network vessel-quickening formula such as Paralysis Formula #2 (Shi Quan Da Bu Tang Variant) adding Da Huang (incremental doses up until the patient maintains 3 stools/day) and Ren Shen/Chuan Qi/Rou Gui Powder (at a ratio of 3:3:1). This is the best approach I have found for treating paralysis of infectious origin.

Case Study #2: Spinal Compression Fracture – Partial Paralysis

Q: This morning a Mr. Ge called and asked: "Can you prescribe me the same medicinals as Dr. Lee?" I wasn't aware of this patient's case, but he said he would come to my clinic late this evening seeking treatment. This must be a patient of yours from Taiwan. Can you please send me details about his case? Thank you!

A: Mr. Ge is a Korean citizen of Taiwanese descent. The last time he returned to Taiwan for a visit he suffered a spinal compression fracture of the L4 vertebra, resulting in partial paralysis (weakness in both legs and urinary and fecal incontinence). It sounds like he felt the formula I prescribed was effective, so he wants to continue taking it. Below is a basic outline of formula variations and modifications:

1) First, I administered the kidney yang-supplementing and channel-freeing network vessel-quickening formula (Yu Sheng) Paralysis Formula #3 (You Gui Yin Variant) (including Ma Huang (2 qian)) adding Ren Shen/Chuan Qi/Rou Gui Powder (at a ratio of 3:3:1 qian), and Yu Sheng Wan (1 pill/1x/day).

2) Then, a bit later on in the therapeutic regimen I *added* Gan Jiang (4 qian), Di Long (5 qian), Rou Gui (4 qian), Fu Zi (2 qian), and Ma Huang (3 qian) into the main formula composition.

3) Later on, I *changed* over to the dual qi- and blood-supplementing and channel-freeing network vessel-quickening formula (Yu Sheng) Paralysis Formula #2 (Shi Quan Da Bu Tang Variant), which the patient has been continually administered for a long duration (about 8 months). The relatively large dose of Ma Huang (*no* difficulties falling asleep) was in part aimed at the patient's chronic tearing on exposure to wind (迎風落淚 yíng fēng luò lèi) condition.

4) Recently, his blood glucose levels have been mildly high, so I *changed* the formula to Zhi Bo Di Huang Tang (subtracting Gan Cao) adding Sang Bai Pi (1 liang), Di Long (8 qian), and Mu Dan Pi (4 qian) (30 packets/1 packet/day/3x/day).

5) Next, I *added* Lu Rong (1 g) and Dai Zhe Shi (5 g) to the main formula (30 packets/1 packet/day/3x/day).

Case Study #3: Cervical Spine Fracture – Paralysis Formula #2 (Shi Quan Da Bu Tang Variant)

Q: A 58 y/o female patient suffered a cervical spine fracture (C5-C7) in an automobile accident, requiring internal fixation. After this surgical procedure, the patient regained sensation in her thumb and index finger, but with pronounced weakness; and had mobility in her shoulder, but complete paralysis below the shoulder.

Unsatisfied with these results, she decided to give TCM a try. I prescribed Paralysis Formula #2 (Shi Quan Da Bu Tang Variant) adding The Three Great Yang-Supplementers (5 qian each), Da Huang (1.5 qian), Ren Shen (powder)/Chuan Qi (powder) (1.5 qian each), and Han Lian Cao (5 fen each). Right now, PLT is only 70,000 (normal range 150,000–400,000 μL), and it was even lower prior to surgery. Do you think this is the right approach for treating this condition?

A: That's a great formula. You will be able to effectively treat paralysis patients with this approach!

Case Study #4: Cervical Spinal Cord Injury (Paralysis) – Therapeutic Responses Indicating TCM Treatment Efficacy

Q: In the treatment of paralysis resulting from cervical spinal injury, I still have some uncertainties. For instance, how do I know if the TCM medicinals are having a positive effect? Below are some of the questions I have come across during the clinical treatment of paralysis. I hope you can help put me on the right path!

1) Stabbing pain: After 2 weeks of administering TCM medicinals to a patient with paralysis resulting from cervical spinal cord injury, there is no improvement in motor function, but the patient does begin to feel a heightened sense of intense pain. Is this a sign of efficacy?

A: That's right! Paralysis patients will progress from a complete absence of sensory perception to a heightened sense of pain (hyperesthesia, allodynia and hyperalgesia). This indicates that the nerves are innervating and the process of regeneration is underway. You indeed prescribed the correct medicinals, so keep administering this formula!

Remember! You must clearly *explain* and *reiterate*, time and again, the "therapeutic responses (瞑眩反應 míng xuàn fǎn yìng)" involved throughout the course of the TCM therapeutic regimen. That way the patient knows what to expect along the path towards recovery. The path may indeed be rough at times, but if the patient knows what to expect, he/she will gain confidence in your ability and be more likely to continue treatment.

I once successfully treated a cervical spinal cord paralysis patient whom had been paralyzed in a wheelchair for 9 years—it was obvious that he didn't have a lot of faith in TCM from the beginning. After taking my prescription for a while, he came back for a consultation telling me: "All of the sudden, I started to feel this pain," and I responded by congratulating him, saying "Your nerves are innervating!" as a way of encouraging him to stay the course with treatment. As I had hoped, the patient was emboldened with confidence—taking the TCM medicinal decoction everyday and actively engaging in motor skill rehab exercises. In about 5 years, he was standing independently and learning how to walk again, feeling absolutely jubilant. So you can see that even after 9 years of paralysis, it is still possible to promote nerve regeneration. Pain is a sign that the nerves are innervating and beginning to regenerate!

2) Excessive urine output (polyuria): A 60 y/o female patient visited me with a history of cervical spinal cord injury (C8 on down), a classic case of paralysis. I prescribed Paralysis Formula #2 (Shi Quan Da Bu Tang Variant) adding Gan Jiang, Fu Zi, and Rou Gui (7 qian each), Da Huang (2 qian), and Di Long (5 qian). One week later she came back for a follow-up visit and said her urine volume had dramatically increased (900 cc/4 hours). The patient felt this was an inconvenience and worried she might not be able to get to the toilet in time. Thus, she wasn't compliant with my treatment (only taking 1 dosage (200 ml) of decocted medicinals/day, instead of 3 (600 ml)/day). Eventually, she developed a bladder infection (cystitis) and urinary catheterization was performed. Is increased urine output a sign of efficacy?

A: Yes! Increased urine output indicates heightened nerve conductance below the cervical lesion. The heart is pumping larger volumes of blood to the kidneys via the celiac artery and the kidneys are autonomously regulating filtration volume. This is a very positive sign! Keep encouraging your patient to stay the course with your therapeutic regimen. In 3–5 days urine output regulation should be back to normal, and at that time, the edema in the abdomen, chest, and lower extremities will also resolve. This is definitely a sign that the condition is improving!

The fact that your patient feels distention in her bladder indicates that nerve conductance is already occurring down to L1, and if your patient can feel urine being passed, then that means conductance is open down to S5. You must try your best to clearly *explain* and *reiterate* the beneficial actions of TCM medicinals on the central nervous system, and how these actions have already jumpstarted the patient's self-repair and regeneration mechanisms. Encourage the patient to continue staying the course with the TCM therapeutic regimen, because based on these initial signs, the odds of achieving significant improvement and recovery are very good!

3) Sensory perception in the buttocks: A patient with paralysis resulting from cervical spinal cord injury recently complained of feeling sensations of heat and pain in the buttocks region. Is this a positive sign as well?

A: Yes! Paralysis patients typically spend long periods of time either lying on their back or sitting. This factor combined with a dulled sensory perception (hypoesthesia) make these patients susceptible to developing bedsores and ulcerations. If the patient has sensory perception, that indicates the nerve is innervating, which is a positive sign! You should explain the significance of this "good news" to the patient and their family, and encourage them to continue with the TCM therapeutic regimen. Staying the course will gradually lead to significant improvement and recovery!

Case Study #5: Therapeutic Responses – Soreness, Numbness, Distention, and Pain

Q: I have been treating a myelitis patient, who happens to be a pastor. Recently, he told me that the therapeutic responses he has been experiencing from taking TCM medicinals was "just too much to handle, so I want to stop taking them." I tried explaining repeatedly to him that this was just a process on the path towards improvement and recovery, but he wouldn't accept my reasoning. I feel so frustrated knowing that I can help this patient!

A: You must continue trying to get through. There's no doubt about it, the manifestation of these *positive* therapeutic responses (瞑眩反應 míng xuàn fǎn yìng) can be difficult to tolerate and accept, but the patient must have the patience and courage to make it through. That's the only way they will see improvement.

Recently, I have been treating a woman who suffered a cervical herniated disc from an automobile accident 3 years ago. Two weeks after taking my TCM prescription, she felt aches throughout her entire body, but after a few days these symptoms had already diminished by 30%. The patient was really happy about these results, explaining that it was her first time to experience this type of "innervating" sensation, despite receiving all types of TCM and Western medicine therapies, including laser surgery. I recommend prescribing a qi- and blood-supplementing and kidney yang-supplementing formula such as (Yu Sheng) Gui Qi Jian Zhong Tang adding Ge Gen and Ren Shen/Chuan Qi Powder. Your patient's condition will improve over time.

Case Study #6: Spinal Cord Injury – Paralysis

Q: A 50 y/o male got into a traffic accident and suffered fractured vertebrae (T8-T9). Following a vertebral fixation procedure, the patient remained paralyzed in both legs (diplegia) and he is still in the hospital after 1 1/2 months following surgery. The patient's wife and children came to visit me right after the patient's surgery, and we arranged for a trip to see the patient in the hospital. The pinprick test on his toes generated no response at all, and he also has neurogenic bladder and neurogenic bowel.

I prescribed Shi Quan Da Bu Tang adding Fu Ling, Ze Xie, Ren Shen, and Chuan Qi, which the patient has been taking now for 5 weeks. Recently, the pinprick test on his toes revealed slight sensory perception. The patient (and family members) thought that his condition had indeed improved. However, I really don't think his pace of progression is occurring fast enough. I am just curious. Do you think his condition would have improved to this level even without the administration of TCM medicinals?

A: Based on my 40 years of clinical experience, I know that the administration of TCM medicinals *can* and *does* promote repair and regeneration of the central nervous system. Patients have a much greater chance of recovery when a TCM therapeutic regimen is administered. The sooner accurate pattern identification and treatment is administered, the better chances of positive results. So get moving!

You should immediately prescribe Paralysis Formula #2 (Shi Quan Da Bu Tang Variant). If atrophy sets in for too long, it is that much more difficult to initiate recovery. The patient's nervous system can still be repaired and regenerated, but there will be extremely trying neurologic "therapeutic responses" along the path to recovery that includes spasticity, rigidity, clonus, myoclonus, spontaneous pain, hyperalgesia, allodynia, and numbness. Remember! Paralysis of the sphincter muscles will take relatively longer to recover.

Case Study #7: Aversion to Cold Following Spinal Tumor Surgery

Q: A 62 y/o male patient underwent surgery for a spinal cord tumor (neoplasm). Following surgery he experienced an aversion to cold from the chest (Tan Zhong (Ren17)) on down, and the patient is still being administered corticosteroids. My initial idea was to treat this condition as paralysis resulting from spinal cord injury. Then I had second thoughts, wondering whether the administration of the great yang-supplementing medicinals (e.g., Gan Jiang, Fu Zi, Rou Gui) included in the paralysis treatment regimen would have the deleterious effect of tumor proliferation. How would you approach this case?

A: Well, I would first need to determine the nature of the neoplasm. Is it a primary tumor (e.g., ependymoma, astrocytoma, meningioma, neurinoma) or secondary (i.e., metastatic)? What type of surgical procedure was performed: spinal decompression (e.g., laminectomy) or tumor resection? And if tumor resection was performed, then how much of the tumor was successfully removed? Did the patient receive adjuvant radiotherapy and/or chemotherapy?

If only spinal decompression was performed and/or it was only possible to achieve partial resection of the tumor, then I would first focus on treating the "root" (i.e., cancer); and once the cancer has been managed, then treat the "tip" (i.e., spinal cord and nerve compression symptoms).

For treating the "root," I would prescribe the blood-nourishing blood-quickening, stasis-dispelling pain-relieving, and network vessel-freeing channel-regulating formula Ru Mo Si Wu Tang adding large doses of Fu Ling, Ze Xie, Huang Qin (or Huang Lian), Huang Bo, Di Long, Ma Huang, Niu Xi, Sheng Du Zhong, and Wan Ling Dan.

After the tumor shrinks and eventually resolves, that's when you can consider treating the "tip." If complete resection was achieved and it appears that the tumor has been completely resolved, then you can treat this condition as "paralysis," by prescribing one of formulas in the (Yu Sheng) Paralysis Formula Series.

Obviously, if the tumor is of metastatic origin, then you will need to conduct a comprehensive evaluation, including complete blood count, tumor marker levels, and imaging studies, to determine if carcinogenesis has occurred in other organs or tissues. This adds another dynamic that you will have to take into consideration. You are definitely starting to see the big picture now, clearly recognizing the subtle nuances and multivariable complexities at the heart of TCM clinical applications. Let's go!

Case Study #8: Paralysis, TCM Treatment, and Corticosteroids

Q: Last October, this male patient suddenly incurred an episode of severe weakness in both legs, which continued worsening over time to the point where he couldn't walk and had to get around in a wheelchair. His neurologist administered corticosteroid injections, and since then, the severity of symptoms has worsened to complete immobility of both legs, not even a twitch!

After administering TCM medicinals (Paralysis Formula #2 (Shi Quan Da Bu Variant)) for 1 week, the patient noticed a slight improvement in strength; after 2 weeks of treatment, the patient regained some motor function in both legs, but also began feeling mild distention and pain; after 3 weeks of treatment, the distention and pain in both legs intensified; and after 1 month of treatment, the patient regained strength in both legs, but also recorded a mild fever fluctuating from 37–39 C° along with intensified pain and distention. The patient was concerned about these therapeutic responses and decided to discontinue TCM treatment. Finally, I convinced him to start taking the TCM medicinals again.

Two weeks later, he could walk 20 to 30 m and 3 weeks later 50 to 80 m, and the distention and pain upon micturition had disappeared. Then, 1 month later, he suddenly experienced another episode of weakness in both legs. I explained to the patient that this was a normal manifestation during the treatment regimen, and that the weakness would resolve within 1 week. However, he said that he had had enough and went back to the hospital where he received large-dose steroid injections. While in the hospital, spinal cord atrophy spread up into the brainstem and he was admitted into ICU where he is in a coma receiving continuous hydrocortisone infusions. This has been such a frustrating case. Do you have any advice?

A: A paralysis patient in a coma admitted into ICU, who is receiving continuous corticosteroid infusions and still remains unconscious. There must be some other complication involved. I would consider these possibilities:

1) Progressive spinal cord atrophy.

2) Large doses of continuous corticosteriod infusions make the cerebral vasculature susceptible to atherosclerosis, which may lead to cerebral infarction, atrophy, and hydrocephalus.

3) Long-term administration of corticosteroid infusions makes the walls of the cerebral vascular thin and brittle and susceptible to rupture, which may lead to cerebral hemorrhage and intracerebral hemorrhage.

I don't think this is an exacerbation of the original condition. If the family is willing and you have the consent of the ICU attending physician, you can see the patient and get a clearer understanding of the situation. Most likely, you will want to prescribe a blood-quickening stasis-transforming formula adding qi- and yang-supplementing, bland-percolating water-disinhibiting, and stool-freeing medicinals. It should be possible to revive the patient back to consciousness; otherwise, it won't be long before he passes away.

Case Study #9: Traumatic Brain Injury – Hemiparesis, Diplopia, and Strabismus

Q: Seven years ago, a 34 y/o female suffered traumatic brain injury (TBI) on the right side of her brain from an automobile accident, resulting in left-sided hemiparesis and apraxia of speech. Now, she still participates in speech rehabilitation, gets along well on her own, and leads a relatively normal life.

However, recently she has been having problems with incomitant (paralytic) strabismus and diplopia (sees 3 or 4 images), particularly troubling since she is studying hard right now in preparation for a professional certification exam. Her ophthalmologist said he couldn't do anything for her. Right now she is not taking any medication, has normal blood pressure, and normal stool and urine. I want to prescribe Bu Yang Huan Wu Tang adding The Three Insects and Ren Shen/Chuan Qi Powder. What do you think about this approach?

A: Left-sided hemiparesis obviously resulted from head trauma and intracerebral hemorrhage caused by the automobile accident, but I don't think your patient's current problems with diplopia are related to that injury. If these vision problems were caused by TBI, then they would have presented along with the other symptoms following the accident, not 7 years later.

The likely etiologies of these visual disorders are as follows: a newly arising compression or infection involving the preoptic chiasma; a newly arising hemorrhage, tumor, or embolism near the thalamus; or ocular muscle or orbicularis oculi muscle spasm or nerve compression resulting in one side being normal and the other affected, resulting in an abnormal accommodation response. Most likely the third scenario is involved and caused by overuse (e.g., focusing on the computer screen too long!) and insufficient sleep (e.g., staying up too late studying!) that results in hyperperfusion, angiogenesis, or hemangioma and leads to diplopia.

You can advise her to have an MRI performed and consider prescribing the following TCM therapeutic regimen:

1) If blood stasis and heat (inflammation) present, then prescribe a blood-quickening stasis-transforming formula such as Ru Mo Si Wu Tang, Sheng Yu Tang, or Bu Yang Huan Wu Tang adding combinations of these medicinals: Huang Qin, Huang Lian, Mu Dan Pi, and Zhi Zi (clear heat and cool the blood), Bai Zhu, Fu Ling, and Ze Xie (disinhibit water by bland percolation), Long Gu, Mu Li, and Dai Zhe Shi (calm the liver and subdue yang), Niu Xi (quickens the blood and conducts fire downward), Chuan Qi (powder) (transforms stasis and stanches bleeding), and Da Huang (clears heat and drains fire and quickens the blood and dispels stasis). Remember! Chuan Qi is an essential medicinal here, so it must be included. At this time, you shouldn't prescribe The Three Great Yang-Supplementers, and if you do, only in very small doses.

2) If headache, nausea and vomiting, and dizziness present, then this suggests increased intracranial pressure (ICP), requiring the addition of Tian Ma, Bai Zhu, Fu Ling, Ze Xie, Da Huang, and Ban Xia into the main formula.

3) If the patient has been administered corticosteroids, then you can consider prescribing a qi- and blood-supplementing formula such as Gui Qi Jian Zhong Tang or Bu Yang Huan Wu Tang adding The Three Great Yang-Supplementers, Ren Shen/Chuan Qi (powder), and Huang Qin, or possibly Tian Ma, Ru Xiang, Mo Yao, and Di Long as well.

Case Study #10: Cutaneous Numbness – Lateral Aspect of Thigh

Q: A 56 y/o female patient visited me with a chief complaint of lateral femoral cutaneous neuropathy (right side). Originally, I was considering prescribing Paralysis Formula #2 (Shi Quan Da Bu Variant) or Paralysis Formula #3 (You Gui Yin Variant), but the patient also explained that she has chronic active hepatitis B (CAH-B). How would you approach this case?

A: Indeed, Paralysis Formula #2 and #3 would be effective in the treatment of lateral femoral cutaneous neuropathy, and despite her CAH-B, you could still prescribe one of those formulas if you wanted. But remember! If AST and ALT levels are increased, then add large doses of The Three Yellows (up to 8 qian each) into your formula. This will serve the dual function of treating both the neuropathy and lowering AST and ALT.

However, if it were my patient, I would likely go ahead with Ru Mo Si Wu Tang adding Huang Qin, Huang Lian, Huang Qi (large dose), Du Zhong, Ma Huang, and Di Long. Chronic hepatitis of viral etiology can be identified as exterior heat pattern, which is the logic behind the use of Ma Huang Lian Qiao Chi Xiao Dou Tang for jaundice with exterior pattern as described in *Treatise on Cold Damage and Miscellaneous Diseases*. Just remember to add a large dose of Huang Qi into the formula for the neuropathy and also needle acupoints along the urinary bladder and gallbladder channels. This approach should bring you positive results. One other thing, you must take into consideration South Korean dietary and alcohol consumption habits, which predisposes patients to a mild secondary heat pattern amidst the primary cold pattern (more cold than heat (熱少寒多 rè shǎo hán duō))!

Section 10: Neuropathy of the Upper and Lower Extremities

Case Study #1: Mother's Wrist and Radial Neuropathy

Q: Recently, I have been treating a number of patients with mother's wrist, but with mixed results. How do you treat this pathocondition? How about other upper extremity neuropathies?

A: De Quervain's tenosynovitis (mother's wrist) is a common malady involving the wrist. Mother's wrist can be identified as lung channel residual heat pattern spreading to the wrist. It can be treated by first bleeding the affected site and then needling Chi Ze (LU5), He Gu (LI4), and Ah Shi (ouch points) acupoints along the radial aspect of the wrist in between the abductor pollicis longus (APL) and extensor pollicis brevis (EPB) tendons. As for medicinals, I would typically prescribe a heat-clearing exterior-solving formula such as Huang Lian Jie Du Tang adding Gui Zhi (or Sheng Ma) or Yang Dan Tang adding Sang Bai Pi. Remember! Do *not* perform tui na (massage) directly on the affected site, because this will only exacerbate the inflammation!

Of course, you could also apply the splint-fixing therapy. This entails placing a traditional TCM wood slat splint over the palmar aspect of the first metacarpal bone (the thenar eminence of the hand near the acupoint Yu Ji (LU10)) fixed in place with string (or tape) and wrapped in bandage. This is an excellent method for ensuring the tendons get adequate rest and produces faster results, but it may present an inconvenience for many people in carrying out daily activities, so most patients won't accept this approach.

Just for future reference, brachial plexus injury (BPI) can also cause upper extremity neuropathy (radial neuropathy). For this condition, you must assess the severity of nerve compression. If there is already complete paralysis from the thumb to the forefinger, then advise the patient to have decompression surgery and prescribe a spleen-fortifying qi-supplementing yang-upbearing formula such as Bu Zhong Yi Qi Tang variant to promote healing and repair.

If the condition is milder, then this can be identified as qi vacuity pattern, for which you can acupuncture (warm needle) acupoints on the affected side, such as He Gu (LI4), Yu Ji (LU10), Bei Lao Gong (located in opposition to Lao Gong (PC8) on the dorsal aspect of the hand at the V-shaped base between the 3rd and 4th metacarpal bones), Wai Guan (TB5) joining Nei Guan (P6), Shou San Li (LI10), Qu Chi (LI11), Chi Ze (LU5), Shao Hai (HT3), and Ji Quan (HT1); and possibly even Zu San Li (ST36) contralaterally.

As for medicinals, I would prescribe a spleen-fortifying qi-supplementing yang-upbearing formula such as Bu Zhong Yi Qi Tang or a blood-quickening qi-supplementing formula such as Bu Yang Huan Wu Tang adding The Three Great Yang-Supplementers, Huang Qin, Chuan Qi (powder), Ma Huang, Di Long, and Yu Sheng Wan. Remember! Regardless of your formula selection, you need to include large doses of Huang Qi (at least 2 liang) and warm needle!

Case Study #2: Radial Neuropathy and Carpal Tunnel Syndrome – "Everything Feels Like Sandpaper"

Q: Three years ago, a 53 y/o female suddenly experienced numbness in both hands. All of the fingers in her right hand and the 1st, 2nd and 3rd fingers in the left hand are affected, and she feels pain near the acupoint Zhuo Liao (LI12) on her right arm. This condition has continued getting worse since the onset. Now, her hands feel cold all the time, numbness is more pronounced in the morning, and she says that "everything feels like sandpaper." What's the best approach for treating this condition?

A: Numbness in both hands…hmm…based on her history it sounds to me like the patient may have radial neuropathy on the left side and carpal tunnel syndrome (CTS) on the right side. In TCM, both conditions can be identified as qi vacuity pattern.

As for treatment, you can prescribe a qi- and blood-supplementing formula such as Gui Qi Jian Zhong Tang, Bu Yang Huan Wu Tang, or Sheng Yu Tang adding The Three Great Yang-Supplementers, Huang Qin, Chuan Qi (powder), and Yu Sheng Wan. Also, acupuncture (warm needle) Shou San Li (LI10), Wai Guan (TB5) joining Nei Guan (P6), He Gu (LI4), Bei Lao Gong, Zhong Zhu (TB3), and Hou Xi (SI3).

This therapeutic regimen will provide rapid results. Initially, the patient will notice a reduction in the frequency and distribution of the numbness, then a therapeutic response manifesting as a distended feeling will present, and finally the numbness with completely resolve.

Case Study #3: Arm Numbness When Hanging Down at the Sides – Qi Vacuity Pattern

Q: I have a female patient who feels numbness in the five fingers of both hands when they are hanging down at her sides. The strange thing is that when her arms are placed in other positions there is no numbness, only when hanging down. What could be the reason for this anomaly?

A: Upper extremity numbness can be identified as qi vacuity pattern. Numbness presenting when the arms are hanging down at the sides suggests either median nerve entrapment somewhere along its pathway or Raynaud phenomenon (primary or secondary).

As for treatment, I would prescribe the qi- and blood-supplementing and kidney yang-supplementing formula (Yu Sheng) Gui Qi Jian Zhong Tang (including large doses of Huang Qi (at least 2 liang)) adding Fu Ling and Ze Xie. Additionally, I would acupuncture (warm needle) Shou San Li (LI10), Wai Guan (TB5) joining Nei Guan (P6), He Gu (LI4), Zhong Zhu (TB3), Bei Lao Gong (located in opposition to Lao Gong (PC8) on the dorsal aspect of the hand at the V-shaped base between the 3rd and 4th metacarpal bones), and Hou Xi (SI3).

Case Study #4: Numb Fingers – Only During the Summertime!

Q: A 60 y/o male patient has been incurring numbness (no tremor) in the fingers of both hands every year for more than 10 years now, but only during the summertime! He has undergone thorough examinations, including MRIs and electrocardiography, which have *not* revealed any abnormalities. Please offer your advice and guidance on this case?

A: Finger numbness only during the summertime suggests yang vacuity along with qi vacuity pattern. However, you must also take into consideration the possibility of excessive perspiration during the summertime, resulting in liquid and qi depletion (津氣虧虛 jīn qì kuī xū) and yin and essence depletion (陰精虧損 yīn jīng kuī sǔn) that may lead to detriment to yin affects yang pattern (陰損及陽症 yīn sǔn jí yáng zhèng). Thus, preserving fluid, liquid, yin and essence is also an essential aspect of treatment.

I would consider prescribing a heat-clearing phlegm-transforming formula such as Xiao Chai Hu Tang or Wen Dan Tang; a blood-quickening blood-cooling formula such as Di Gu Pi Yin adding Huang Qi (2 liang), Gan Cao and Hong Zao (or Long Yan Gan) (large doses), and Fu Ling and Ze Xie (small doses); or a dual qi- and blood-supplementing formula such as Bu Zhong Yi Qi Tang, Bu Yang Huan Wu Tang, or Gui Qi Jian Zhong Tang adding Qing Hao, Zhi Mu, Di Gu Pi, Fu Ling, and Ze Xie.

Case Study #5: Lower Leg Cutaneous Paresthesia – Gallbladder Channel Cold Impediment

Q: A 50 y/o male patient explained he felt the sensation of tingling and soreness along the lateral aspect of the right lower leg (calf) whenever cool or cold air blew on his legs. He went to see a neurologist for an examination, and eventually, followed the advice of his neurosurgeon to undergo surgery on his L4 and L5 vertebrae.

Ever since the surgery 2 months ago, he has had the feeling of "pins and needles" (soreness, numbness, prickling, and tingling) in the skin of his right lower leg. I prescribed Paralysis Formula #3 (You Gui Yin Variant) (including Gan Jiang and Fu Zi, and large doses of Rou Gui and Di Long) and administered acupuncture (warm needling). Do you think this is a good approach?

A: Regardless if the etiology is lumbar radiculopathy or peroneal mononeuropathy, the distribution of the paresthesia (feeling of "pins and needles") corresponds with the path of the gallbladder channel, and thus can be classified as gallbladder channel cold impediment. Yes, I would prescribe Paralysis Formula #3 (You Gui Yin Variant) adding Huang Qi, Chuan Xiong, and Wu Zhu Yu. Remember! Advise the patient to wear warm clothing (e.g., multiple layers, thermal underwear) and exercise regularly (e.g., go for walks).

Case Study #6: Restless Leg Syndrome

Q: A 66 y/o female patient has a 10-year history of pronounced pricking, tingling, and aching in both lower legs and heat in the heart of the soles. The discomfort gets so bad that it affects her sleep at night and has resulted in chronic insomnia. It started out with just a tingling feeling in both lower legs and then spread throughout the muscles of her entire body (*not* the skin, but the muscle tissue), and sometimes there is even cramping in the lower legs.

She has been taking Western medicine drugs as treatment over the past 6 years, which initially provided some relief, but has not proven effective in the long run. Originally, I identified this as lower burner damp-heat pattern and prescribed San Miao San variant. This was not effective, so I added The Three Great Yang-Supplementers, which resolved the cramping, but the other symptoms remain. Do you have any suggestions for treating this patient?

A: This sounds more like a case of cold-damp pattern restless leg syndrome (RLS) to me, and that's why her condition improved once you added The Three Great Yang-Supplementers to your formula. Typically, as in this case, patients will only seek TCM treatment after long-term administration of Western medicine drugs have proven ineffective and/or side effects manifest. Drugs prescribed for neurological and psychiatric disorders (e.g., antidepressants, dopamine agonists, benzodiazepines, anticonvulsants, opioid analgesics, hypnotics, sedatives) function as "suppressants," effectively dampening and subduing physiological mechanisms. For this reason, if these types of drugs are being administered, then the pathocondition can be identified as either cold-damp or cold stasis pattern.

In the absence of Western medicine drug intervention, I would typically identify this pathocondition as ascendant hyperactivity of liver yang pattern (肝陽上亢 gān yáng shàng kàng) and prescribe a liver-settling wind-extinguishing and yin-enriching yang-subduing formula such as (Yu Sheng) Jian Ling Tang (includes Niu Xi) adding Huang Bo, Cang Zhu, Long Yan Gan, Da Zao, and Yu Sheng Wan.

For this case, the first thing I would do is advise the patient to begin gradually reducing the dosage of these drugs and prescribe either a heat-clearing dampness-drying formula such as San Miao San adding The Three Great Yang-Supplementers, Long Yan Gan, and Hong Zao; or a dual qi- and blood-supplementing formula such as Gui Qi Jian Zhong Tang adding Niu Xi, Long Yan Gan, and Hong Zao.

As the patient continues reducing the dosage of these drugs and weaning away from the "suppressant" effects, then this pathocondition can be identified as damp-heat pattern. At this time, if symptoms have not fully resolved yet, then you can consider prescribing San Miao San adding The Three Yellows, Gan Cao, Long Yan Gan, Da Zao (large dose), and Yu Sheng Wan; or an yin-enriching fire-downbearing formula such as Zhi Bo Di Huang Tang adding Yu Sheng Wan. If symptoms still haven't resolved once the drugs have been completely discontinued, then the condition can be identified as having returned to the "essential state" of ascendant hyperactivity of liver yang pattern described above. The "essential state" is simply the true manifestation of the pathocondition in the absence of influence from "suppressant" drugs.

This TCM therapeutic regimen should be administered up until the neurologic symptoms completely resolve and normal sleeping patterns are restored, and then you can begin to gradually reduce the dosage and eventually discontinue treatment. Remember! You should also advise her to maintain a well-balanced diet containing essential minerals (e.g., Fe, Mg, Na, Cl, K, P, Ca) and vitamins (e.g., D, B-complex, C, A). Nutritional deficiency can also lead to generalized distention and aches throughout the entire body!

Case Study #7: Polyneuropathy – Bilateral Numbness

Q: A female patient visited me with a chief complaint of numbness and coldness in both hands and feet. She explained that it started out as just a tingling sensation and then gradually developed into numbness and coldness, with darkening of the skin and palpably lower temperature at the affected sites, similar to the symptoms of diabetic neuropathy. I diagnosed the condition as polyneuropathy. Can you offer any insights into this case?

A: Bilateral numbness of the hands and feet suggests polyneuropathy. This condition can be effectively treated with a variety of approaches based on detailed pattern identification as the basis for determining treatment.

In cases of qi- and blood-vacuity pattern and kidney yang vacuity pattern you can consider prescribing formulas such as Shi Quan Da Bu Tang or Shen Qi Wan adding Ma Huang and Di Long; Paralysis Formula #2 (Shi Quan Da Bu Tang Variant) or Paralysis Formula #3 (You Gui Yin Variant) adding Huang Qi; or Gui Qi Jian Zhong Tang or Bu Yang Huan Wu Tang adding Gan Jiang, Fu Zi, Huang Qi, Huang Qin, Ma Huang, and Di Long. And in cases of exterior wind pattern, you could prescribe Ge Gen Tang or Gui Zhi Tang adding Gan Jiang, Fu Zi, Huang Qi, Huang Qin, Ma Huang, and Di Long.

Naturally, you should also perform acupuncture (warm needle), selecting acupoints locally at the affected site and distally along the corresponding channels. The patient will notice pronounced improvement within 3–5 months of administering this therapeutic regimen.

Case Study #8: Polyneuropathy – Carpal Tunnel Syndrome and Tarsal Tunnel Syndrome

Q: One year ago, a 42 y/o male began feeling "like there was something wrong" in both legs from the ankle down to the toes, and then, numbness set in! At first, he thought it was just poor circulation, but 3 months later, numbness presented in both arms from the wrists down to the fingers. Now, he has numbness and coldness in both hands and feet, and he has developed an uncharacteristic bad temper, even getting angry and swearing at friends. He doesn't get enough sleep either, because he wakes up frequently (almost every hour) during the night. Do you think this could be multiple sclerosis or could it be simply psychosomatic?

A: The patient's history and symptoms suggest polyneuropathy affecting the median nerve of the upper extremities and the posterior tibial nerve of the lower extremities. This condition can be identified as qi vacuity with kidney yang vacuity pattern, and the treatment approach is similar to carpal tunnel syndrome (CTS) and tarsal tunnel syndrome (TTS).

You can prescribe a dual qi- and blood-supplementing and kidney yang-supplementing formula such as Bu Yang Huan Wu Tang, Bu Zhong Yi Qi Tang, Sheng Yu Tang, Hui Yang Sheng Xian Tang, Gui Qi Jian Zhong Tang, or Shi Quan Da Bu Tang. Just make sure to include Huang Qi (up to 2 liang), The Three Great Yang-Supplementers, Huang Qin, Ma Huang, Di Long, Ren Shen/Chuan Qi Powder, and Yu Sheng Wan. If the patient has constipation, then add Da Huang; and if the patient has trouble sleeping, then add Da Zao (and/or Long Yan Gan). Also, perform acupuncture (warm needle) on acupoints such as Shou San Li (LI10), Zu San Li (LI36), Wai Guan (TB5) joining Nei Guan (P6), He Gu (LI4), Bei Lao Gong (located in opposition to Lao Gong (PC8) on the dorsal aspect of the hand at the V-shaped base between the 3rd and 4th metacarpal bones), Zhong Zhu (TB3), San Yin Jiao (SP6), Di Wu Hui (GB42), Hou Xi (SI3), and Shu Gu (UB65).

If the patient is being administered corticosteroids or immunotherapy (e.g., interferons, immunoglobulins), then advise him to gradually reduce the dose once his symptoms have resolved, and eventually discontinue these drugs altogether. After the Western medicine drugs have been discontinued, you should continue administering TCM medicinals for 1–2 more months, and then gradually discontinue TCM medicinals altogether. In the future, if the patient catches the common cold (external contraction) advise him to immediately see a TCM physician to quickly resolve the condition with a heat-clearing exterior-resolving formula (regardless of the formula, make sure to add large doses of Huang Qin); bleed Da Zhui (GV14) (above, on, and below), Cun Kou (Tai Yuan (LU9)), Shang Yang (LI1), and Li Dui (ST45); and needle acupoints such as Feng Chi (GB20), Tian Zhu (UB10), He Gu (LI4), Zu San Li (ST36), San Yin Jiao (SP6), and Jing Bai Lao (EX-HN15).

Based on my clinical experience, you can be confident in proclaiming that the condition has been cured if the patient has incurred 2–3 common colds (external contractions) or after going through 1 full winter without recurrence of symptoms. Remember! You must be aware that many Western medicine drugs (e.g., chemotherapeutic agents, cobalt-60) will damage motor neurons.

Case Study #9: Left Hand Tremor

Q: A 25 y/o male injured his left upper arm moving artillery while serving his compulsory military service. Since then, he has had tremor in his left hand. I prescribed Gui Qi Jian Zhong Tang adding The Three Insects along with administering acupuncture (warm needling). After the first week, there was noticeably less tremor, but it has already been 3 weeks now and the condition has not completely resolved. What is the best approach for getting quicker results?

A: Positive results after the first week sounds pretty good to me! And you've only been providing treatment for a total of 3 weeks! Continue administering the TCM therapeutic regimen, maybe trying warm needling (burn at least 3 cones/needle each session) on some different acupoints. I am confident this approach will result in complete recovery.

Remember! During the treatment process, if the patient happens to develop transient swelling (edema) in the extremities, don't be concerned about it. This is simply a therapeutic response due to increased blood perfusion throughout the body that temporarily "overwhelms" the lymph capillaries and vessels in the extremities, compromising their capacity to absorb the influx of interstitial fluid from the tissues and propel it back to the larger collecting ducts towards the center of the body. This increased blood perfusion results from the combined actions of these principal medicinals: Dang Gui (supplements and quickens the blood), Huang Qi (supplements qi and upbears yang), Gan Jiang (warms the channels and the center and frees the channels and network vessels), Fu Zi (returns yang and stems counterflow, assists yang and supplements fire, and frees the channels and network vessels), and Rou Gui (supplements fire and assists yang and warms the channels and frees the vessels). Just add Fu Ling and Ze Xie to your formula and the swelling (edema) will readily resolve!

Case Study #10: Ulnar Nerve Entrapment – Finger Numbness

Q: I have a patient whose 3rd and 4th phalanges are numb. I diagnosed the condition as ulnar nerve entrapment at Shao Hai (HT3) of the hand Shao Yin heart channel. I plan on treating this condition with acupuncture. Do you have any suggestions for this case?

A: That may be, but typically if there is ulnar nerve entrapment at Shao Hai (HT3), then numbness would occur starting from the elbow on down. Your patient just has numbness in the fingers, suggesting that the site of entrapment is at the wrist and involves either the median or ulnar nerve. If it does turn out to be entrapment of the ulnar nerve at Shao Hai (HT3), you might want to inquire about the patient's sitting habits to determine if any adjustments can be made to avoid putting pressure on the ulnar nerve while seated.

For this condition, I would acupuncture (warm needle) Shen Men (HT7), Bei Lao Gong (located in opposition to Lao Gong (PC8) on the dorsal aspect of the hand at the V-shaped base between the 3rd and 4th metacarpal bones), Zhong Zhu (TB3), Wai Guan (TB5) joining Nei Guan (P6), Shao Hai (HT3), and Hou Xi (SI3).

Case Study #11 Head, Neck, and Upper Back Pain – It's Very Common!

Q: In my clinical practice, I frequently see female patients who present with aches and pain in the right upper extremity, upper back and shoulder (near Gao Huang (UB43)), neck (near Feng Chi (GB20)), and ocular region (near Tai Yang (EX-HN5)); and occasionally, impediment in the lower extremities. Why do you think these presentations are so prevalent?

A: There are many potential causes of upper extremity, head and neck, and upper back pain, including postural and work-related musculoskeletal disorders (i.e., occupational overuse syndrome (OOS) (aka repetitive strain injury (RSI)), cervical radiculopathy, and lumbar radiculopathy. However, for 30 to 50 y/o women in particular, you also need to consider the possibility of stress and anxiety producing psychosomatic symptoms.

Thus, I would start out prescribing a spleen- and stomach-supplementing, phlegm-damp transforming, and wind-stabilizing formula such as Ban Xia Tian Ma Bai Zhu San adding Gan Cao, Du Zhong, Long Yan Gan, and Yu Sheng Wan; and acupuncture Feng Chi (GB20), He Gu (LI4), Hou Xi (SI3), Wai Guan (TB5), Guan Yuan Shu (UB26), Huan Tiao (GB30), Yang Ling Quan (GB34), Wei Zhong (UB40), and Di Wu Hui (GB42). For pain in the ocular region (near Tai Yang (EX-HN5)), you can acupuncture Feng Fu (GV16), Wan Gu (GB12), Zan Zhu (UB2), Si Zhu Kong (TB23), Ting Gong (SI19), and Shang Xing (DU23). You can also advise your patients to dress warmly (e.g., extra layers of clothing, thermal underwear), exercise regularly (e.g., going for walks), and get 8–10 hrs of sleep every night.

Case Study #12: Heat in the Heart of the Palms and Soles

Q: Do you prescribe Zhi Bo Di Huang Tang variant for patients presenting with heat in the heart of the palms and soles? It's been my experience that this formula is only effective for patients with normal stool and urine, and not very effective at all in those with sloppy stools (溏便 táng biàn). Is this similar to your experience?

A: Heat in the heart of the palms and soles (手足心熱 shǒu zú xīn rè) is one of the symptoms that the classical TCM pathologic term vexing heat in the five hearts (五心煩熱 wǔ xīn fán rè) encompasses. This pathocondition can be identified as Shao Yang heat, heart heat, steaming bone heat, "phantom heat," or damp-heat pouring downward (濕熱下注 shī rè xià zhù) (disruption of the lumbosacral nerves) pattern. Remember! Other conditions such as paralysis and stroke sequelae can also cause these types of symptoms.

That's why it is so important to carefully interview and examine the patient, and if necessary, attain lab reports and image study results, so you can accurately identify the pattern as the basis for determining treatment.

Typically, for patients with vexing heat in the five hearts in the *absence* of a distinguishable underlying etiology, I would prescribe an yin-enriching fire-downbearing steaming bone-eliminating formula variant such as Jia Wei Xiao Chai Hu Tang, Zhi Bo Di Huang Tang, or Di Gu Pi Yin.

For patients identified with heart heat pattern, I would prescribe Zhi Zi Bo Pi Tang, Tian Wang Bu Xin Dan, Qing Yan Li Ge San, Qing Shang Fang Feng Tang, or Liang Ge San variants.

For damp-heat pouring downward pattern, I would prescribe Er Miao San, San Miao Wan, Jia Wei Er Miao San, Si Wei Wan, or Long Dan Xie Gan Tang.

Typically, the most difficult type to treat is "phantom heat" in the elderly, for which I would prescribe either Zhi Bo Di Huang Tang adding Long Gu and Mu Li; Xiao Chai Hu Tang adding Long Gu and Mu Li; or Jian Ling Tang adding Da Zao, Long Yan Gan, Qing Hao, Zhi Mu, Di Gu, Huang Bo, The Three Insects, and Di Long. It takes a long time for effects to appear. Sometimes it's best to refer the patient to a neurologist or psychiatrist who will likely administer antidepressants, while also concomitantly administering TCM medicinals. If this turns out to be an enduring and incalcitrant neurological problem, then it may be necessary for the patient to undergo nerve block, cauterization, or other surgical procedure performed by a neurosurgeon.

For patients with vexing heat in the five hearts in the *presence* of sloppy or thin stool, you can consider prescribing either Wu Ling San (Zhang Zhong-jing's original formula containing Gui Zhi!), Chai Ling Tang, or Chai Ping Tang adding medicinals such as Qing Hao, Zhi Mu, Huang Bo, Di Gu Pi, Long Gu, and Mu Li

Case Study #13: Bilateral Big Toe Coldness

Q: A 56 y/o female patient frequently feels coldness in both of her big toes. At first, it was on the tips of her toes and later it spread throughout the entire toe up to Tai Chong (LV3). I prescribed Paralysis Formula #3 (You Gui Yin Variant) including large doses of Gan Jiang, Fu Zi, and Rou Gui. Do you think this is a good approach?

A: Coldness in both big toes suggests involvement of the L5 spinal nerve caused by either wind-cold, viral infection, or compression (radiculopathy). So, yes, I think Paralysis Formula #3 (You Gui Yin Variant) is the right approach, because of its kidney yang-warming and -supplementing, channel-freeing network vessel-quickening, and sinew- and bone-strengthening actions. However, it would be best for the patient to have an MRI performed to help make a definitive diagnosis and rule out the possibility of other pathologies. This will save everyone a lot of time and energy in the long run.

If the condition is longstanding or it only manifests during the winter months, then you can consider prescribing a qi- and blood-supplementing and kidney yang-supplementing formula such as

Gui Qi Jian Zhong Tang, Shi Quan Da Bu Tang, You Gui Yin, San Bi Tang, or Dang Gui Si Ni Tang adding Wu Zhu Yu and Gan Jiang. You can also apply adhesive moxa cones at local acupoints or apply Ai Cao Gao (Mugwort Ointment) on the affected site along with heat therapy using an infrared lamp. Remember! You must remind your patient to dress warmly (e.g., extra layers, thermal underwear) and exercise regularly (e.g., going for walks).

Section 11: Other Neurological Disorders

Case Study #1: Multiple Sclerosis or "Fatigue from Overworking"?

Q: A 39 y/o male patient visited me explaining that he has been experiencing aching and stiffness of the extremities, headache, and grogginess over the past 1 month. When he gets out of bed in the mornings his arms and legs ache and feel stiff. At rest, this impediment subsides, and when active, it worsens again. He told me that the cause of his recent symptoms is probably "fatigue from overworking." Do you think these symptoms could indicate multiple sclerosis?

A: I would advise the patient to have a neurological exam performed as well as a thorough lab workup including electrolyte levels (e.g., K, Ca, Mg), enzymes (e.g., creatine kinase (CK)), antinuclear antibodies (ANA), and thyroid function (e.g., T3, T4, TSH) to rule out other potential causes. If the symptoms are immediately relieved once the patient takes a rest, then you should also consider the possibility of periodic paralysis (PP) triggered by stress or physical activity.

Typically, multiple sclerosis (MS) can be identified as either wilting (痿 wěi) with qi vacuity and phlegm-rheum pattern or kidney yang vacuity pattern. By accurately conducting pattern identification as the basis for treatment, TCM can provide effective relief of symptoms, promote remission, and improve the overall quality of life for MS patients.

Case Study #2: Periodic Paralysis

Q: A 30 y/o female patient incurred paroxysmal aversion to cold, weakness of the extremities, and generalized aches with symptoms more pronounced at nighttime. At night when lying in bed she is unable to lift her limbs, but in the daytime the condition improves. She doesn't have a fever, but in some aspects her symptoms resemble those of a common cold (external contraction). Please offer your advice and suggestions.

A: Your description suggests that the patient may have periodic paralysis (PP). Most of the patients who I have treated with PP present with signs and symptoms that can be identified as wind-cold exterior pattern along the Shao Yang channel. For this condition I would consider using one of these three formulas: 1) Ge Gen Tang combining Si Ni Tang, 2) Dang Gui Si Ni Tang adding Wu Zhu Yu, Gan Jiang, Fu Zi, and Huang Qin, or 3) Ban Xia Tian Ma Bai Zhu San adding Ma Huang and Wu Zhu Yu. Also, perform acupuncture (warm needle, burning at least 3 cones/needle each session) at local and distal acupoints along the corresponding channels.

Case Study #3: Amyotrophic Lateral Sclerosis

Q: Three days from now an amyotrophic lateral sclerosis (ALS) patient will visit me. I have never attempted to treat this type of patient. Can TCM offer effective treatment for ALS?

A: ALS is a □ progressive disease that affects people differently. Typically, this disease will manifest in the following three ways: 1) gradually progressive decline; 2) the patient improves and their condition stabilizes for a period of time, and then once again, the symptoms recur and the disease continues exacerbating (the precipitating factors for this recurrence could be external contraction (microbial infection), childbirth, pregnancy, use of anticancer agents, or possibly even exposure to pesticides); and 3) once the condition has stabilized, the patient can expect an extended life expectancy (as long as 15–20 years from the time of onset!).

This pathocondition can be identified as a type of wilting pattern (痿證 wěi zhèng), and specifically, thymus gland wilting and myofascial wilting pattern. Treatment of this pathocondition requires administration of a qi-, blood-, and yang-supplementing formula such as Bu Zhong Yi Qi Tang, Gui Qi Jian Zhong Tang, Bu Yang Huan Wu Tang, Shi Quan Da Bu Tang, or Sheng Yu Tang adding The Three Great Yang-Supplementers, Huang Qin, Ren Shen (powder), and possibly Lu Rong. If residual damp-heat presents, then add Er Miao San, San Miao Wan, or Si Miao Wan to your main formula; and since enduring illness enters the brain (i.e., enduring illness affects the kidney, kidney governs the bones and engenders marrow, and the brain is the sea of marrow) you may also consider adding Ma Huang (opens the nine orifices) and Di Long (frees the channels and network vessels).

Remember! For most types of wilting pattern pathoconditions, it is essential to add large doses of Huang Qi, The Three Great Yang-Supplementers, and Ren Shen (powder).

VII. THYROID DISEASE

There is more to thyroid disorders than just simple enlarged thyroid (goiter). Conditions of hypothyroidism and hyperthyroidism have varying etiologies including autoimmune disorders such as Hashimoto's thyroiditis and Grave's disease.

Case Study #1: Hypothyroidism – Phlegm-Heat Pattern

Q: A 38 y/o female was diagnosed with hypothyroidism 3 months ago and has been taking thyroid hormone replacement since then to control her condition. Subsequent lab tests now show normal thyroid hormone levels, but she still feels generalized weakness, heaviness, and has an enlarged thyroid. How should I treat this patient?

A: Right now Western medicine still doesn't offer definitive treatment for thyroid disorders (e.g., hyperthyroidism, goiter, thyroid nodules, thyroid cancer, and Hashimoto's thyroiditis) except for surgical resection (thyroidectomy). For hypothyroidism, unfortunately, in many patients oral administration of levothyroxine (L-thyroxine) causes side effects such as mental sluggishness, dulled reactions, edema, palpitations, and lack of sexual desire.

The underlying pathological mechanism causing these symptoms of fatigue and heaviness may involve congestion or obstruction of the synaptic receptors, which inhibits the transfer of chemical signals across synaptic clefts. Regardless of the precise mechanism, I would simply identify this pathocondition as phlegm-heat pattern and prescribe the heat-clearing phlegm-rheum transforming formula (Yu Sheng) Wen Dan Tang adding Bai Jie Zi, Lai Fu Zi, Ge Gen, and Mai Men Dong. This therapeutic approach will provide effective relief for your patient's condition.

Case Study #2: Enlarged Thyroid (Goiter)

Q: Recently, I have had a number of patients seeking treatment for enlarged thyroid (goiter). Some have had *decreased* thyroid hormone levels (hypothyroidism), some have had *increased* thyroid hormone levels (hyperthyroidism), and others have had *normal* thyroid hormone levels (euthyroidism). Please share your clinical insights into the treatment of this pathocondition?

A: Thyroid hormone (FT3 and FT4) levels, both *increased* and *decreased*, are not the only cause of an enlarged thyroid gland (goiter); patients with *normal* thyroid hormone levels (euthyroid) also present with goiter. The most common causes of enlarged thyroid (goiter) are iodine deficiency, hyp*o*thyroidism (e.g., Hashimoto's thyroiditis, certain drugs, iatrogenic), and hyp*er*thyroidism (e.g., Graves' disease, toxic nodular goiter).

In TCM, an enlarged thyroid (goiter) can typically be identified as either repletion heat swelling pattern (i.e., hyp*er*thyroidism) or vacuity swelling (or possibly true cold and false heat) pattern (i.e., hyp*o*thyroidism). You can look at it like a company with a surplus of funds that indiscriminately expands (i.e., hyp*er*thyroidism); or a company with insufficient funds that has to borrow money to maintain a façade of buoyancy (i.e., hyp*o*thyroidism).

For enlarged thyroid (goiter) in patients with *increased* thyroid hormone levels (hyp*er*thyroidism), you can consider prescribing a formula such as Jian Ling Tang, Chai Hu Long Gu Mu Li Tang, Hyperactive Immune Formula, Huang Lian Jie Du Tang, Gua Lou Niu Bang Zi Tang, Liang Ge San, or Xian Fang Huo Ming Yin adding Xia Ku Cao (channel conductor for the thyroid) and Yuan Hu.

For enlarged thyroid in patients with *decreased* thyroid hormone levels (hyp*o*rthyroidism), you can consider prescribing a formula such as Gui Zhi Jia Long Gu Mu Li Tang, Shen Fu Tang, Shi Quan Da Bu Tang, You Gui Yin, Shen Qi Wan, or Li Zhong Tang. Just make sure to include The Three Great Yang-Supplementers, Huang Qin, Sheng Long Gu, and Sheng Mu Li.

If the goiter is surgically removed, regardless of whether it develops again, the patient will likely be left with *underactive* thyroid hormone production (depending on the extent of resection); and if it does grow back again, then the thyroid levels could "rebound," producing *excessive* thyroid hormone (hyp*er*thyroidism). If aspiration of fluid is performed, the swelling typically only goes down for a few days before it fills back up again. And in surgery, there is always the risk of either directly damaging or causing swelling of the recurrent laryngeal nerve, which may result in dysphonia, hoarseness, and in severe cases, aphonia; or even cause thyroid storm (an acute exacerbation of hyp*er*thyroidism), a rare, life-threatening postoperative complication.

Another rare, life-threatening condition is myxedema coma, occurring late in the progression of uncontrolled hyp*o*thyroidism. In severe cases where longstanding hyp*o*thyroidism is not appropriately treated, myxedema crisis (myxedema coma) may evolve, which can depress respiratory function and cause death. At the onset of myxedema crisis, the patient will have a dark complexion, dry skin, and weight gain (regardless of how much they eat, they don't feel full!).

Case Study #3: Gui Qi Jian Zhong Tang – Shrinks Goiter!

Q: I have a patient whose chief complaint is right shoulder pain, but she also has a history of *decreased* thyroid hormone levels (hyp*o*thyroidism) and an enlarged thyroid. My treatment was focused on the shoulder pain, so I prescribed (Yu Sheng) Gui Qi Jian Zhong Tang (including Huang Qi (2 liang)). To everyone's surprise, 3 days later her enlarged thyroid (goiter) had begun to noticeably shrink down to about 2/3 its original size. Is this a normal reaction?

A: Regardless if the enlarged thyroid results from *increased*, *decreased* or *normal* thyroid hormone levels, administering a qi- and blood-supplementing and kidney yang-supplementing formula such as (Yu Sheng) Gui Qi Jian Zhong Tang (including Huang Qi (2 liang)) may produce this type of "surprise" for some goiter (瘿 yǐng) patients. I have seen a similar type of rapid resolution of swelling in patients with generalized edema who have taken this formula. Your patient's case provides yet another testimonial!

I attribute this effect to two possible physiological processes: 1) directly stimulates the production of hormones and 2) restores the homeostatic balance between the brain (i.e., hypothalamus and pituitary gland) and the feedback mechanism of hormone and endocrine regulation throughout the body.

Case Study #4: Thyroid Carcinoma Resection – May Induce Thyroid Storm

Q: A 48 y/o female patient presented with a history of uterine fibroids (leiomyomas), which were resected; and on another occasion, a thyroid tumor (carcinoma), which was resected and followed up by a regimen of chemotherapy (she did *not* receive radiotherapy). After the surgery and adjuvant chemotherapy, she incurred weakness in her extremities, finger tremor "on an empty stomach" (low blood sugar levels I presume), poor memory, mental sluggishness, poor appetite, tidal heat, and heat flashes in the face. Recently, she has begun to feel pain in her left eye. What is the best approach for treating this patient?

A: Your thyroid carcinoma patient's history suggests she may be incurring thyroid storm (thyrotoxic crisis). I would identify this condition as dual qi and blood vacuity along with yang vacuity pattern and prescribe a formula variant such as Shi Quan Da Bu Tang or Bu Yang Huan Wu Tang. Remember! This is a life-threatening condition that can lead to nausea, vomiting, hypertension, atrial fibrillation, congestive heart failure, delirium, seizures, coma and death.

Case Study #5: Subclinical Hyperthyroidism – Menstrual Irregularities

Q: A 15 y/o female patient with a history of subclinical hyperthyroidism (SCH) and liver disease explained that it's been over 3 months since her last period, and that she has been losing weight (unintentionally). Her most recent lab tests showed TSH 0.0131 (normal range 0.5–6 uU/ml), and T3 and T4 normal. What are your impressions of this case?

A: *Low* TSH levels with normal T3 and T4 suggests yang vacuity pattern. However, I would also advise the patient to get lab tests done for FSH and LH (low levels may cause oligomenorrhea and amenorrhea) to determine if there is a problem involving the pituitary gland. If all of these hormone levels are *low*, then I would definitely prescribe a yang-supplementing or neutral supplementation formula such as Gui Zhi Jia Long Gu Mu Li Tang, Shen Fu Tang, Shi Quan Da Bu Tang, You Gui Yin, Shen Qi Wan, or Li Zhong Tang adding The Three Great Yang-Supplementers and Huang Qin.

Administer this formula up until the patient's regular menstrual cycle returns. The pathocondition can be considered remedied once the patient incurs 2–3 consecutive normal periods. In TCM pathologic terms, this can be classified as delayed menstruation (經遲 jīng chí) or menstrual block (閉經 bì jīng).

In a case overt hyperthyroidism where the patient presents with *low* TSH levels and *increased* T3 and T4, this can be identified as yin vacuity with yang hyperactivity, requiring the administration of a liver-settling wind-extinguishing and yin-enriching yang-subduing formula variant such as Jian Ling Tang.

Case Study #6: Thyroid Carcinoma Postsurgical Complication – Vocal Cord Paralysis

Q: Last year, a 35 y/o female patient underwent surgery to remove a thyroid tumor (malignant), and following surgery she lost her voice (aphonia). How would you treat this patient?

A: Loss of voice (aphonia) is a common postsurgical complication of thyroid carcinoma. Recently, for a patient with the same type of condition, I prescribed the spleen-fortifying qi-supplementing yang-upbearing formula Bu Zhong Yi Qi Tang adding Huang Qi (1 liang), He Zi (5 qian), Ren Shen/Chuan Qi Powder (starting out at 2 g each and gradually increasing the dose), and Yu Sheng Wan (1 pill). After only 2 weeks, the condition resolved. You can also consider this approach.

However, you must first assess the thyroglobulin (Tg) levels (used as a tumor marker to determine the presence of any remaining thyroid gland tissue), and if Tg levels are normal or low, then add The Three Great Yang-Supplementers and Huang Qin. It's been over a year now since the onset of this complication, so she has already entered the chronic yang vacuity pattern stage. Since enduring illness enters the brain (i.e., enduring illness affects the kidney, kidney governs the bones and engenders marrow, and the brain is the sea of marrow) you may also consider adding Ma Huang (opens the nine orifices) and Di Long (frees the channels and network vessels).

Case Study #7: Hyperthyroidism – Antithyroid Drug Side Effects

Q: A male patient diagnosed with hyperthyroidism was prescribed antithyroid drugs (iodides). After taking the medication, he began having a sore throat that was worse when swallowing and speaking, and in the afternoon it felt swollen and distended. Do you think prescribing Huang Lian Jie Du Tang adding Fu Ling, Ze Xie, Bai Zhu, Jie Geng, and Lian Zhao would be effective?

A: Many types of Western medicine drugs (including antithyroids) cause side effects involving swelling and irritation of the mucus membranes that result in sore throat, a burning sensation in the throat, hoarseness, shortness of breath, and panting.

All the patient needs to do is reduce the dosage of these drugs and the side effects should resolve spontaneously. Monitor T3, T4, and TSH levels to accurately identify the pattern and determine the optimal TCM medicinals for treatment. The heat-clearing toxin-resolving formula you mentioned will treat inflammatory type hyperthyroidism and should also quickly resolve the patient's throat symptoms. However, in recent years, I have had even better success prescribing my Hyperactive Immune Formula, which is composed of The Three Yellows adding yin vacuity-heat clearing and yin-enriching medicinals. You can give it a try!

Case Study #8: Hashimoto's Thyroiditis, Graves' Disease, and Thyroid Cancer – Diagnostic Indices and TCM Pattern Identification

Q1: I have a female patient with a history of generalized weakness and heaviness, fatigue, and soft stools (3–4 stools/day). She has visited both TCM and Western medicine doctors, but neither has given her a definitive diagnosis.

During her initial consultation with me 1 month ago, I suspected hypothyroidism, and thus advised her to get a lab workup. The results showed extremely high levels of TSH 250 (0.5–6 uU/ml) and T3 and T4 slightly lower than normal, prompting me to diagnose her with Hashimoto's thyroiditis. Her endocrinologist subsequently confirmed this diagnosis, prescribing a dosage of 1 L-thyroxine pill/day, while I concomitantly prescribed Gui Qi Jian Zhong Tang variant.

Following this treatment regimen her enlarged thyroid (goiter) shrank by 2/3 the original size. Last week her lab tests showed TSH 130 and T3 and T4 normal. Her endocrinologist increased her L-thyroxine dosage to 1.5 pills/day, while I changed my formula to Gui Zhi Jia Long Gu Mu Li Tang adding Gan Jiang and Fu Zi.

I have a general understanding of the etiology, presentation, diagnosis, and treatment of thyroid disorders, but not much clinical experience at all. Please clearly explain to me the pathophysiological relationships between TSH, T3, and T4 in the thyroid and brain (hypothalamus, anterior pituitary gland) and the implications for pattern identification, diagnosis, and treatment.

A: Good work! It's not easy to make an accurate diagnosis of

Hashimoto's thyroiditis. I haven't treated all that many Hashimoto's thyroiditis patients myself, but I can share with you what I know. The key diagnostic factors you must consider are free triiodothyronine (FT3), free tetraiodothyronine (thyroxine, FT4), thyroid-stimulating hormone (TSH), thyroglobulin (Tg), and thyroid antibodies (TSH receptor antibody (TRAb), thyroid peroxidase antibody (TPOAb), thyroglobulin antibody (TgAb), and thyroid-stimulating immunoglobulin (TSI)). My understanding of these diagnostic indices and their relationships to pattern identification and treatment are as follows:

1) If T3 and T4 levels are *low* and TSH *high*, then this indicates overt hypothyroidism in the late stage of Hashimoto's thyroiditis, which can be identified as yang vacuity pattern. You just need to further differentiate between qi and blood, spleen and stomach, and kidney patterns.

2) If T3 and T4 levels are *normal* or *slightly high* and TSH *high*, then this indicates subclinical hypothyroidism in the progression of Hashimoto's thyroiditis, which can be identified as qi, blood, and yin vacuity along with yang hyperactivity pattern.

3) If T3 and T4 levels are *normal* and TSH *extremely high*, then this indicates the presentation of Hashimoto's thyroiditis, which can be identified as yang hyperactivity with yang straying outward pattern (陽亢陽越 yáng kàng yáng yuè).

4) If Tg is *high* or possibly *extremely high* (*several times higher* than normal!), then this suggests thyroid carcinoma and can be identified as yang hyperactivity with yang straying outward pattern; and if Tg is *over ten times higher* than normal, then this can be identified as yang straying outward with great heat pattern.

5) *Elevated* thyroid antibody (TRAb, TPOAb, TgAb, and TSI) levels indicate the presence of an inflammatory autoimmune response. TRAb is specific to Graves' disease, TPOAb and TgAb to Hashimoto's thyroiditis, and Tg is a key follow-up biomarker for thyroid carcinoma.

6) If TSH and Tg are *both high*, then this suggests thyroid carcinoma. Levels may also be increased following treatment of thyroid carcinoma (e.g., surgical resection, radioactive iodine ablation (RAIA), chemotherapy, radiotherapy).

7) Be aware! After the L-thyroxine replacement therapy has been completely discontinued and the TCM therapeutic regimen continues to be administered over a period of time, TSH and

> thyroid antibody levels may suddenly *"rebound."* If these levels are only *slightly increased*, then it can be identified as phlegm-rheum, yin vacuity, or liver depression pattern, requiring the addition of small doses of Sheng Long Gu and Sheng Mu Li to the main formula; and if these levels are *extremely high*, then it can be identified as yang straying outward pattern, requiring a formula such as Jian Ling Tang.

This is a great topic to compile into a case report and publish a paper on. You can present the efficacy in treating Hashimoto's thyroiditis through an integrative TCM and Western medicine therapeutic approach, and with TCM treatment alone, once the Western medicine drugs have been discontinued!

Q2: The most recent lab test results for this Hashimoto's thyroiditis patient are as follows: TSH 13.89 (0.5–6 uU/ml), TgAb 99.50 (< 20 IU/ml), and TPOAb 31.65 (< 35 IU/ml). I recently prescribed the yin and yang neutrally-supplementing and subduing and settling securing and astringing formula Gui Zhi Long Gu Mu Li Tang (adding Gan Jiang and Fu Zi), and the patient is also still receiving Western medicine treatment. Do you think I need to add heat-clearing toxin-resolving medicinals to suppress the overactive immune response? Or should I just continue prescribing yang-supplementing medicinals?

A: Congratulations! You already have achieved some clinical success at treating Hashimoto's thyroiditis: it's not easy to bring TSH levels down that quickly. In my opinion, you should go ahead and add The Three Yellows, which will effectively regulate the overactive immune response and thus continue to bring down TSH and TgAb. Adding heat-clearing toxin-resolving and welling-abscess-dispersing bind-dissipating medicinals, such as Pu Gong Ying and Lian Qiao, would be effective as well.

However, in my clinical practice, I have found that The Three Yellows provide the best clinical efficacy at quickly and effectively resolving all types of heat (inflammation) resulting from a broad spectrum of etiologies (i.e., microbial infections, autoimmune disorders). Just add a relatively large dose of Huang Qin, Huang Bo, and Huang Lian (5–8 qian each) and you are good to go!

Case Study #9: Hashimoto's Thyroiditis – Optimal Therapeutic Approach

Q1: A 31 y/o female patient whom I had previously treated for Hashimoto's thyroiditis recently came for a follow-up visit. Her most recent lab tests showed *normal* TSH, T3, FT4, TPOAb, and TgAb levels, and she is currently taking L-thyroxine. The first time I treated this patient for low thyroid hormone levels (hypothyroidism) was 4 years ago. At that time, I prescribed Gui Zhi Jia Long Gu Mu Li Tang variant, which effectively improved her symptoms of abdominal fullness, heaviness in the lower abdomen, fatigue, and poor sleep.

You mentioned before that once treatment successfully brings thyroid hormone levels back to normal and shrinks the enlarged thyroid, the patient should gradually discontinue both Western medicine and TCM medicinals. Can you explain this approach in greater detail?

A: In its "essential state," Hashimoto's thyroiditis can be identified as heat pattern. But the reality is that the majority of patients with this pathocondition will receive Western medicine drug treatment. Levothyroxine (T4) replacement therapy (L-thyroxine) is the first-line therapy for the treatment of Hashimoto's thyroiditis and other types of hypothyroidism.

L-thyroxine functions as a "suppressant." So when this synthetic hormone is being taken by the patient you can go ahead and prescribe a neutral supplementation, dual qi- and blood-supplementing, or a kidney yang-supplementing formula such as Gui Zhi Jia Long Gu Mu Li Tang, Shi Quan Da Bu Tang, Li Zhong Tang, Shen Fu Tang, You Gui Yin, or Shen Qi Wan. Just make sure to include The Three Great Yang-Supplementers, Huang Qin, Sheng Long Gu, and Sheng Mu Li.

After administering these yang-supplementing or neutrally supplementing medicinals for a period of time, once FT4 (FT3 has a much shorter half-life, so is a less significant indice) and TSH levels have stabilized for 1–2 months, then you can advise the patient to begin gradually reducing the dosage of Western medicine drugs, with the aim of eventually discontinuing administration altogether. This may take 3–5 days at the quickest, and at the slowest 1–2 weeks, before complete discontinuation. Implementing a gradual reduction in dosage will make it less likely for a "rebound" and minimize the potential risk of thyroid storm.

Remember! Once this synthetic hormone has been completely discontinued, you must change to a heat-clearing toxin-resolving and yin vacuity-heat clearing yin-enriching formula such as Hyperactive Immune Formula adding Xia Ku Cao (thyroid channel conductor, clears liver fire and dissipates binding depression) and Zi Su Zi (downbears qi and transforms phlegm).

Note: Hashimoto's thyroiditis patients who receive long-term administration of corticosteroids, undergo radioactive iodine (I-131) (aka radioactive iodine ablation (RAIA)), or partial (with too much resected) or complete thyroidectomy will typically present with low thyroid hormone (FT3, FT4) levels. Thus, for these patients, I would apply the same approach as above, prescribing Gui Zhi Jia Long Gu Mu Li Tang, Shi Quan Da Bu Tang, Li Zhong Tang, Shen Fu Tang, You Gui Yin, or Shen Qi Wan and making sure to include The Three Great Yang-Supplementers, Huang Qin, Sheng Long Gu, and Sheng Mu Li.

Q2: The most recent lab test results for this Hashimoto's thyroiditis patient showed *normal* TSH, T4, and T3 levels, and *elevated* TPOAb; and the patient complained of mild generalized aches. Thus, I prescribed Xiao Chai Hu Tang combining Huang Lian Jie Du Tang (including Huang Qin, Huang Bo, and Zhi Zi (8 qian each)) adding Sheng Long Gu and Sheng Mu Li. My treatment regimen hasn't lowered antibody levels. Do you think it would be best to change the formula?

A: Increased antithyroid antibody (TOPAb, TRAb, TgAb) levels are not the cause of the symptoms (i.e., mild generalized aches), and may simply reflect a "carrier" state in which the body remains poised in response. Thus, it's not absolutely imperative to bring antithyroid antibody levels completely back down to *normal*. Let's take rheumatoid arthritis (RA) as an example: even though RF may remain elevated, if ESR and CRP are normal, then it's not absolutely imperative to bring RF levels down to *normal*. You just need to monitor and follow-up on the patient's condition, and then once the condition has stabilized, gradually discontinue administration of medicinals.

Case Study #10: Hashimoto's Thyroiditis – Phlegm-Rheum Fatigue and Potential Complications

Q1: A 13 y/o female Hashimoto's thyroiditis patient presented with extreme fatigue, sluggishness, and generalized weakness, and virtually the only thing she feels like doing all day is sleeping. Her most recent lab test results are as follows: *normal* thyroid metabolism (TSH, Tg, FT3, and FT4), *elevated* antithyroid antibodies (TgAb 73.24 (< 20 IU/mL) and TPOAb 2170 (< 35 IU/mL)), and *normal* MCHC 29.4 (32–36). What are your thoughts on this case?

A: Monitor the patient's potassium (K) levels and pulse (discern if it is *forceful* or *fine, faint and nearly expired*) and inspect the patient's skin complexion (discern if it is *normal* or *pale*). I am thinking this patient may have periodic paralysis (PP) or an atypical Hashimoto's thyroiditis. Actually, regardless of whether the patient has been diagnosed with Hashimoto's thyroiditis or not, you can simply proceed as follows:

If the pulse is *forceful* and she has a *normal* complexion, then this pathocondition can be identified as phlegm-rheum fatigue (倦怠 juàn dài), summerheat (暑 shǔ), or damp cumbersome fatigue (困倦 kùn juàn) pattern and you can prescribe a heat-clearing phlegm-transforming formula such as Wen Dan Tang or Chai Ling Tang.

If the pulse is *fine, faint and nearly expired* along with a *pale* complexion, then you can prescribe a channel-warming exterior resolving formula such as Ma Huang Fu Zi Xi Xin Tang or a spleen- and stomach-supplementing and phlegm-damp transforming formula such as Ban Xia Tian Ma Bai Zhu San adding Ma Huang, Xi Xin, Gan Cao, Long Yan Gan, and Ren Shen (powder). Remember! This latter approach can also be applied for the treatment of chronic fatigue syndrome (CFS).

Q2: For this 13 y/o female Hashimoto's thyroiditis patient, if her TgAb and TPOAb are *elevated*, do you think Ban Xia Tian Ma Bai Zhu San variant would be a good formula to prescribe?

A: The TCM treatment of Hashimoto's thyroiditis is much more involved than simple yang supplementation alone. That's the kind of singular, rigid approach Western medicine resorts to in the treatment of complex pathoconditions, administering antithyroid drugs (thionamides and iodides), corticosteroids, and immunosuppressants simply by default.

If the thyroid gland is *not* hyperactive, but there are symptoms of fatigue, intermittent low-grade fever, and generalized weakness, then you must consider the possibility of "crisis" evolving from hyperthyroidism (thyroid storm) or hypothyroidism (myxedema coma), or the concomitant presentation of either thyrotoxic myopathy, hypothyroid myopathy, or thyrotoxic periodic paralysis (TPP). In this situation, potassium (K) is a key diagnostic reference.

Dilated cardiomyopathy (DCM) resulting from Hashimoto's thyroiditis can be identified as heat pattern. Thus, unless the patient *has* already been administered high dose pulse intravenous corticosteroid therapy, then you can consider prescribing a blood-cooling heat-clearing and blood-quickening qi-supplementing formula such as Di Gu Pi Yin, Ru Mo Si Wu Tang, Sheng Yu Tang, or Bu Yang Huan Wu Tang adding Huang Qin and Huang Lian. Generally, unless the patient *has* undergone surgical resection of the thyroid that leads to hypothyroidism, thyroid pathoconditions can be identified as heat, hyperactive yang, yang straying outward, or phlegm-heat pattern.

Remember! Patients with a longstanding history of hypothyroidism are susceptible to developing myxedema coma, a potentially life-threatening state of decompensated hypothyroidism that can lead to impaired mental status, low blood sugar (hypoglycemia), hyponatremia, hypoxia, respiratory depression (hypoventilation), hypothermia, and carbon dioxide retention (hypercapnia). You must be aware and stay vigilant!

Case Study #11: Graves' Ophthalmopathy

Q: A 36 y/o female patient presented with an enlarged thyroid (goiter) and has a longstanding history of hyperthyroidism and bulging eyes (exophthalmos). She was diagnosed with Graves' disease and has been taking Western medicine drugs (β-blockers and antithyroid drugs) to treat this pathocondition ever since. Three months ago, she gave birth to a baby boy (no complications). Right now her chief complaint is the exophthalmos and goiter. She has tried both TCM and Western medicine treatment, but none have been effective in resolving these symptoms. What's the best approach for treating this patient?

A: Treatment of Graves' ophthalmopathy takes a long time. In my experience, if you can shrink the bulging just a little bit over a 3 month period, that would be considered "good" results; and if you could completely resolve the bulging over 6 months to 1 year, then I would be "very satisfied."

As for medicinals, I would consider prescribing a Shao Yang-harmonizing phlegm-dispelling, swelling-dispersing hardness-breaking, and liver-calming yang-subduing formula such as Gui Zhi Fu Ling Wan, Chai Hu Long Gu Mu Li Tang, San Zhong Kui Jian Tang, Wen Dan Tang, Xian Fang Huo Ming Yin, or Jian Ling Tang. Just make sure to include Sheng Long Gu, Sheng Mu Li, Bai Jie Zi, Lai Fu Zi (or Zi Su Zi), Xia Ku Hua (or Xia Ku Cao), and Bie Jia (or San Leng and E Zhu).

Case Study #12: Thyroid Hematocele

Q. A 42 y/o female patient suddenly developed a lump on her left thyroid lobe. Upon hospital examination, it was diagnosed as a thyroid hematocele. She had blood aspirated twice (4 cc and 9 cc respectively), but it filled back up again. The hematocele is pliable and the fluid inside is dark. Do you think Ru Mo Si Wu Tang adding The Four Lings and Xia Ku Cao would be effective for this?

A: In my opinion, thyroid and parathyroid cysts and hematoceles should not be aspirated, because it will simply fill back up again within 3–7 days. However, for some cases, it may be necessary to perform fine-needle aspiration biopsy to rule out malignancy.

Does your patient have *elevated* thyroid hormone (FT3, FT4) levels? If *so*, then typically I would treat both the "root" (hyperthyroidism) and the "tip" (hematocele) with a formula such as Chai Hu Jia Long Gu Mu Li Tang or Xian Fang Huo Ming Yin adding Sheng Mu Li, Sheng Long Gu, Pu Gong Ying, Huang Qin, Fu Ling, and Ze Xie. If the patient has a rapid heart rate (tachycardia), I would add Gan Cao and Long Yan Gan.

Ru Mo Si Wu Tang adding The Four Lings and Xia Ku Cao should effectively resolve the hematocele. Xia Ku Cao (thyroid channel conductor that clears liver fire and dissipates binding depression) will also lower elevated thyroid hormone levels if prescribed in large doses. When thyroid hormone levels are normal or low, you should limit the dose of Xia Ku Cao to 3 qian and add Huang Qin and Huang Lian. If after a period of time the Ru Mo Si Wu Tang variation isn't providing effective results, then you can consider changing the formula to Xue Fu Zhu Yu Tang variant.

Case Study #13: Simple Nontoxic Goiter – "Something in My Throat"

Q: Three years ago, a 44 y/o female patient developed a simple nontoxic goiter on her right thyroid lobe. After waiting to see if it would resolve on its own, she decided to get it checked out, and by that time, it had already grown to 1 cm. Other than feeling like there was "something in my throat," she had no other symptoms. Her endocrinologist advised her to undergo surgical resection, but I think we should hold off on invasive intervention and take Wen Dan Tang variant instead. Do you think this formula can effectively shrink this goiter?

A: If a goiter is only 1 cm, then it would be barely noticeable upon palpation, and it would most likely not have any impact on her esophagus. Going ahead with an invasive procedure such as radioactive iodine ablation (RAIA) or surgical resection definitely does *not* sound necessary at this time. These procedures carry the risk of damaging the recurrent laryngeal nerve and/or parathyroid and thyroid parenchyma, and even if the procedure is successful, the goiter may grow back again anyways!

Yes, this type of simple nontoxic goiter can be effectively treated with a Shao Yang-harmonizing phlegm-dispelling, swelling-dispersing hardness-breaking, and liver-calming yang-subduing formula variant such as Wen Dan Tang, Xian Fang Huo Ming Yin, San Zhong Kui Jian Tang, or Xiao Chai Hu Tang. However, it will take a long time for this treatment regimen to produce effective results. I would say the feeling of "something in my throat" is likely a psychosomatic symptom and does *not* involve physical compression.

Case Study #14: Total Thyroidectomy Induces Generalized Edema

Q: Can the localized swelling and weight gain that often follows total thyroidectomy be identified as yang vacuity?

A: Weight gain may follow total thyroidectomy due to the resulting hypothyroid state the patient is left in. Western medicine will typically administer thyroid replacement therapy (L-thyroxine) to compensate. Yes, in TCM this can be identified as qi and yang vacuity pattern, requiring administration of a spleen-fortifying qi-supplementing formula such as Bu Zhong Yi Qi Tang adding yang-supplementing medicinals; and if the swelling is severe, then add The Four Lings.

Case Study #15: Postsurgical Elevated TSH and FT4

Q: After undergoing a total thyroidectomy, a 32 y/o female incurred chills and fever, generalized weakness, finger tremor, sunken and heavy pulse, dizziness, cramping, numbness in the extremities, nausea, and vomiting. Lab tests showed *extremely elevated* TSH 703 (0.5–6 uU/ml), *slightly elevated* FT4 levels, and *elevated* TgAB 122 (< 20 IU/ml).

At first, I tried administering Ban Xia Tian Ma Bai Zhu San and then Xiao Chai Hu Tang, but her symptoms did not improve. Finally, I tried Gan Mai Da Zao Combining Ban Xia Hou Po Tang adding Gan Jiang, Fu Zi, and Huang Qin (8 qian each), and Rou Gui (10 qian). That's when her symptoms started improving! Is this an example of where *elevated* TSH and FT4 levels can be identified as true cold and false heat pattern?

A: Following total thyroidectomy, it is common for patients to develop hypothyroidism (in 50% of patients this condition will remain longstanding) and hypoparathyroidism and hypocalcemia (typically resolve with administration of vitamin D and calcium supplementation). Rarely, thyroid storm (thyrotoxic crisis) may arise, which requires the addition of great yang-supplementing medicinals into your main formula.

Yes, I would identify this pathocondition as true cold and false heat pattern. I like your formula selection! It's an optimal application of the Shen Fu Tang and Qi Fu Tang approach, a wonderful variant on Zao Fu Tang. You should write this case up and publish it. This treatment alone will make your name renowned worldwide and possibly even placed in the annals of TCM history!

The thyroid is not the only part of the body that secretes thyroxine—muscle, fat, the heart, lungs, liver, kidneys, marrow, and brain also contain cells that secrete this hormone. In a nutshell, great yang-supplementing medicinals simply function to awaken these "thyroid embryonic stem cells."

VIII. HEAD DISORDERS

Section 1: Eye Disorders

The head is home to the five offices (五官 wǔ guān) and the seven orifices (七窍 qī qiào). In this section, common clinical cases involving the eyes, ears, and mouth will be presented.

Case Study #1: "Lacrimal Duct Laxation"

Q: A 50 y/o female patient has frequent tearing from her left eye and you can see a tear drop pooling in the inner canthus. Others around her notice this, inquire about it, and express their concern, which she says adds to the physical distraction. Results of a medical examination ruled out nasolacrimal duct obstruction, and her doctors didn't give her a diagnosis. I think this may be a qi-vacuity pattern pathocondition and am considering prescribing Bu Zhong Yi Qi Tang variant. Please offer your advice and guidance.

A: It sounds to me like a simple case of "lacrimal duct laxation"—a term that I use to describe laxity of the lacrimal ducts that results in a compromised capacity to regulate the flow of tears produced in the lacrimal gland and causes excessive tearing (epiphora). The most common causes of epiphora are: 1) "lacrimal duct laxation" and 2) nasolacrimal duct obstruction (dacryostenosis).

1) "Lacrimal duct laxation" can be treated in the same way as tearing on exposure to wind (i.e., allergic rhinitis) and thus can be identified as either kidney yang vacuity or spleen yang vacuity with exterior pattern. For kidney yang vacuity with exterior pattern, I would prescribe You Gui Yin adding Ma Huang, Bai Zhi, Xi Xin, Bai Guo, and Ren Shen; and for spleen yang vacuity

with exterior pattern, I would prescribe Bu Zhong Yi Qi Tang adding Ma Huang, Bai Zhi, Xi Xin, and Bai Guo.

2) Nasolacrimal duct obstruction can be identified as stomach heat pattern, thus requiring the administration of a formula variant such as Qing Wei San, Huang Lian Jie Du Tang, Liang Ge San, Qing Shang Fang Feng Tang, or Ge Gen Qin Lian Tang.

Case Study #2: Dry Eye Syndrome

Q: A 56 y/o male patient has had symptoms of dry eyes for over two years, which worsen when he is fatigued. He has been administered traditional Korean medicine (TKM) treatment in the past with poor results, so he has to resort to artificial tears. His stool, urine, and blood pressure are all normal. What would you do for this patient?

A: Dry eye syndrome (DES) (keratoconjunctivitis sicca (KCS)) can be identified as yin vacuity heat with dryness or blood desiccation pattern. Dust and pollution are the most common potential irritants. This pathocondition most commonly occurs in women and patients who are active outdoors (e.g., air pollution, wind). You should advise patients with this pathocondition to thoroughly rinse their eyes with water when they come in from outside and to *not* wear makeup (a potential irritant as well). And for patients who spend long hours in front of the computer screen, advise them to take a break every half hour and rinse their eyes.

Also, explain to the patient that excessive application of artificial tears (specifically the antioxidants contained within) can irritate the eyes leading to blurred vision and blood congestion, which correlates with red-thread mark (紅絲赤縷 hóng sī chì lǚ) described in classical TCM texts. When artificial tears are applied to eyes that are already irritated by proteinaceous buildup, this establishes an environment susceptible to mycotic (fungal) infestation which causes further irritation (e.g., itchiness and burning).

As for treatment, I would prescribe a heat-clearing toxin-resolving, yin vacuity-heat clearing yin-enriching, and blood-nourishing dryness-moistening formula such as (Yu Sheng) Hyperactive Immune Formula, Huang Lian Jie Du Tang, Wen Qing Yin, or Ying Gan San; Zhi Bo Di Huang Tang, Xue Ku Fang, or Sheng Yu Tang; or Bai He Gu Jin Tang or Ba Xian Chang Shou Wan. Make sure to include yin-nourishing medicinals such as Tian Men Dong, Mai Men Dong,

Sha Shen, Xuan Shen, Sheng Di Huang, and Tian Hua Fen in your formula. These medicinals will promote the production of the body's own "natural" moisturizing and lubricating fluids instead of artificial tears. Also, bleed Zan Zhu (UB2) and Si Zhu Kong (SJ23); and needle Bai Hui (GV20), Da Zhui (GV14) (above, on, and below), He Gu (LI4), San Yin Jiao (SP6), Tai Chong (LV3), Yin Ling Quan (SP9), Xue Hai (SP10), and Shen Men (HT7). This approach will relieve symptoms and effectively treat the pathocondition.

Case Study #3: Sjogren's Syndrome – Dry Eyes

Q: Based on my understanding, Sjogren's syndrome (SS) is an autoimmune disorder that can result in symptoms of dry, gritty, itchy, and burning eyes; and keratoconjunctivitis sicca (dry eye syndrome (DES)) is caused by either accelerated tear evaporation due to poor tear quality or inadequate tear film volume, resulting in similar symptoms as SS. Are these symptoms a result of spasm in the vasculature surrounding the eye sockets?

A: Sjogren's syndrome (SS) is an autoimmune disorder involving lymphocytic infiltration of the exocrine gland and secondary gland dysfunction. This infiltration results in atrophy of the secretory epithelium of the lacrimal glands and causes desiccation of the cornea and conjunctiva. This may compromise blood flow to the vasculature and innervation of the nerves surrounding the eyes. SS can be classified as yin vacuity heat with dryness pattern.

My therapeutic regimen typically includes the administration of Hyperactive Immune Formula; bleeding Zan Zhu (UB2), Si Zhu Kong (SJ23), Da Zhui (GV14) (above, on, and below), and Tai Yuan (LU9); and needling Feng Chi (GB20), Tian Zhu (UB10), He Gu (LI4), San Yin Jiao (SP6), and Yin Ling Quan (SP9). Also, if the patient's eyes feel dry and gritty and/or itch and burn, then advise the patient to gently rub the eyelids, massage around the eye sockets, and rinse the eyes with water.

Remember! Encourage the patient to apply artificial tears *only* when absolutely necessary! This will prevent dependency on the artificial tears from developing, ensure the optimal efficacy of the drops, and reduce the potential for side effects, while the TCM therapeutic regimen gradually regulates the patient's constitution and eventually resolves the underlying inflammatory pathocondition.

Case Study #4: Meibomian Gland Dysfunction – Dry Eyes

Q: A patient of mine was diagnosed with meibomian gland dysfunction (MGD) by an ophthalmologist and presented with dry eyes. The artificial tears he was prescribed do *not* seem to be providing effective relief. What's the best approach for treating this patient?

A: For the general population in South Korea, your first consideration in all cases of dry eye syndrome (DES), including MGD, is blood desiccation (血枯 xuè kū), whereas in Taiwan it is an overactive immune system (autoimmune disorder). This may in part be influenced by the traditional Korean habits of eating spicy foods, drinking hard liquor, and sleeping on kang bed-stoves. The combination of these dietary and lifestyle factors makes Koreans susceptible to damage to fluids (津液毫傷 jīn yè háo shāng), fluid depletion (津液虧損 jīn yè kuī sǔn), insufficiency of essence-blood (精血不足 jīng xuè bù zú), and essence-blood failing to pour into the eyes (精血不能上注於目 jīng xuè bù néng shàng zhù yú mù)—almost like the tears dry up and evaporate right in front of the eyes! In excess, the antioxidants and lipids in artificial tears will irritate the eyes, and the lipid saturation provides a spawning pool for mycotic infestation.

Here is a 4-step therapeutic regimen to effectively treat blood desiccation pattern dry eyes:

1) Administer (Yu Sheng) Blood Desiccation Formula adding The Three Great Yang-Supplementers and Huang Qin.
2) Acupuncture (warm needle) Feng Chi (GB20), Tian Zhu (UB10), He Gu (LI4), and Zu San Li (ST36), and apply adhesive moxa cones on Zan Zhu (UB2), Yu Yao (EX-HN4), and Si Zhu Kong (SJ23).
3) Advise patients to avoid the use of cosmetics, especially near the eyes (since this might be an irritant as well!), thoroughly rinse the eyes and around the eyes numerous times each day, and massage the eyes, eyelids, and around the eyes.
4) Get 8 to 10 hours of sleep every day.

For overactive immune system (autoimmune disorder) patients that are typical here in Taiwan, this can be identified as upper burner (head and eye) wind-heat with yin vacuity or yin vacuity heat with dryness pattern. Thus, I would prescribe a heat-clearing toxin-resolving and yin vacuity-heat clearing yin-enriching formula such as (Yu Sheng)

Hyperactive Immune Formula or a heat-clearing toxin-resolving and fire-draining blood-cooling formula such as Huang Lian Jie Du Tang, Liang Ge San, or Qing Shang Fang Feng Tang adding yin-enriching medicinals. And I would also bleed Da Zhui (GV14) (above, on, and below), Zan Zhu (UB2), Si Zhu Kong (SJ23), and Tai Yuan (LU9); and needle Feng Chi (GB20), Tian Zhu (UB10), He Gu (LI4), San Yin Jiao (SP6), Yin Ling Quan (SP9), and Tai Chong (LV3).

Case Study #5: Watery Eyes

Q: One month ago, a 54 y/o male patient went hiking in the cold, blustering wind, and since then his eyes have been tearing excessively. I diagnosed this patient with watery eyes (epiphora) and prescribed You Gui Yin combining Xiao Qing Long Tang. Recently, the patient has developed a red rash with flaking suggestive of seborrheic dermatitis, so I changed to the stomach-clearing fire-draining blood-cooling formula Qing Wei San adding Huang Bo, Huang Qin, Jin Yin Hua, and Pu Gong Ying. What do you think about this approach?

A: You are on the right track! You can continue prescribing Qing Wei San variant, but I would also consider adding Ma Huang and Bai Zhi or possibly even Xi Xin, Ban Xia, and Wu Wei Zi. Once the heat (i.e., erythematous plaques with patchy scaling) clears up, then you can add small doses of Gan Jiang and Fu Zi. In cases where yin vacuity pattern presents, you can also consider adding Qing Hao, Zhi Mu, and Di Gu Pi; and if these yin-nourishing medicinals cause sloppy stool, then add Cang Zhu, Fu Ling, and Ze Xie.

Hiking in cold, windy weather will commonly bring on tearing on exposure to wind (迎風落淚 yíng fēng luò lèi), and the best way to prevent this is by wearing a warm hat and covering the nose and mouth with a scarf. Indeed, if the patient simply presented with watery eyes (i.e., tearing on exposure to wind), then your original formula of You Gui Yin combining Xiao Qing Long Tang would be the right approach!

Case Study #6: Macular Edema

Q: A 32 y/o male patient experienced distorted vision, prompting a visit to the ophthalmologist for an examination. Tests revealed macular edema and he was diagnosed with central serous chorioretinopathy (CSC). After several months of Western medicine treatment, his condition seemed to stabilize until two weeks ago, when he suddenly experienced distorted vision, black spots in the field of vision, and dry eyes.

I am considering prescribing Di Gu Pi Yin combining Wu Ling San, but this is the first time I have treated this kind of pathocondition, so I am not sure about pattern identification, treatment regimen, and prognosis. Please offer your guidance and instruction.

A: Elevation of neurosensory retina by clear fluid (macular edema) and possibly shallow detachment is a sign that hemorrhage may occur if the condition continues to deteriorate. The black spots are likely exudates and if a large patch of blackness appears this correlates with sudden blindness (暴盲 bào máng) and clear-eye blindness (青盲 qīng máng) described in classical TCM texts.

Your idea about prescribing Di Gu Pi Yin combining Wu Ling San is a good approach. However, I think it would be better to use The Four Lings instead of Wu Ling San (you don't need Gui Zhi (Rou Gui)!) and add Huang Qin, Huang Lian, Zhi Zi, and Chuan Qi (powder). This formula will promote rapid absorption of exudates and resolve the black spots. CSC correlates with indistinct vision (視瞻昏渺 shì dān hūn miǎo) and eye fog (視霧 shì wù) described in classical TCM texts. Once the fluid (macular edema) has been resorbed, then the patient will regain normal vision. Remember! TCM can effectively treat ophthalmological pathoconditions, but it takes time and requires patience.

Case Study #7: Scarring Following *Swelling* of the Optic Disc

Q: A couple of months ago, a patient presented with papilledema, and at that time, I prescribed Di Gu Pi Yin combining Huang Lian Jie Du Tang adding the The Four Lings. After administering this formula for 2 months the swelling resolved, but there is still scarring (revealed under microscopic examination). Now, I want to prescribe Ru Mo Si

Wu Tang adding Huang Qin, Fu Ling, Ze Xie, and Chuan Qi (powder). Do you think this formula will effectively treat this condition?

A: Remember! Optic disc edema and papilledema have completely different etiologies. *Optic disc edema* refers to *swelling* of the optic disc induced by factors such as infection, inflammation, hypertension, and metabolic disorders; whereas *papilledema* refers to *swelling* of the optic disc, specifically caused by increased intracranial pressure (ICP). Regardless of the etiology, s*welling* is a precursor to detachment, and if it isn't adequately treated, can result in sudden blindness (暴盲 bào máng) or clear-eye blindness (青盲 qīng máng).

That's a great formula for this condition. It is imperative to prescribe a blood-quickening stasis-resolving formula such as Ru Mo Si Wu Tang variant once the swelling has resolved. You are on the right track!

Case Study #8: Retinitis Pigmentosa

Q: Two years ago, a 58 y/o female patient began having night vision problems and loss of acuity in peripheral vision, prompting her to get it checked out. Following a thorough ophthalmological examination, she was diagnosed with retinitis pigmentosa. Western medicine treatment has not improved her condition, but it hasn't gotten worse either. However, the patient is very worried that one day this pathocondition will lead to debilitating vision loss. What can I do for this patient?

A: As long as there isn't metabolic waste buildup along the microvasculature that induces inflammation and leads to retinal vascular degeneration, then eye pathoconditions such as this can be identified as liver blood insufficiency and liver heat pattern. You can prescribe formulas such as Ru Mo Si Wu Tang, Sheng Yu Tang, Xue Ku Fang, and Qi Bao Mei Ran Dan adding Qian Li Guang, Mi Meng Hua, Fu Ling, Ze Xie, Tian Ma, She Tui, and Chan Tui. If there is blood heat, then add Mu Dan Pi and Zhi Zi.

Case Study #9: Uveitis

Q: Twenty days ago, a middle-aged male patient suddenly experienced blurred and distorted vision. He went to see an ophthalmologist, who diagnosed him with uveitis. The patient received 20 rounds of steroid injections. Right now, his vision has almost returned to normal, but he wants to try TCM treatment as well. Do you have any advice or suggestions on this case?

A: Conjunctivitis and keratitis can typically be identified as *exterior wind-heat* pattern. Treatment for this pathocondition requires administration of The Three Yellows (clears heat and resolves toxin), along with either exterior-effusing with cool and acrid medicinals (e.g., Jing Jie, Fang Feng, Jin Yin Hua, and Lian Qiao) or exterior-effusing with warm and acrid medicinals (e.g., Ma Huang and Gui Zhi)—depending on the extent of heat (inflammation), and the eye orifice conductors Qian Li Guang and Mi Meng Hua.

Both hordeolum (stye) and chalazion can be identified as *stomach exterior* or *visceral heat (inflammation)* pattern, requiring treatment with formulas such as Huang Lian Jie Du Tang, Qing Wei San, Fang Feng Tong Sheng San, or Liang Ge San. They both can be treated with hot compresses, topical washes, TCM formula administration, and if necessary, incision and curettage (using a disposable sterile blood lancet). For patients with pronounced stomach heat (inflammation) pattern, rinse the eyes with a topical wash composed of decocted Huang Lian, Mang Xiao, and sodium chloride (table salt).

Most cases of scleritis, episcleritis, and iritis can be identified as *blood-aspect stasis heat* pattern, requiring formulas such as Ru Mo Si Wu Tang, Di Gu Pi Yin, or Zhi Bo Di Huang Tang adding Qian Li Guang, Mi Meng Hua, Huang Qin, Huang Lian, Mu Dan Pi, and Zhi Zi.

Uveitis and choroiditis can be identified as *blood heat* and *blood aspect stasis heat* pattern; and opacity of the lens (cataracts) can be identified as *blood heat* pattern. For these pathoconditions, you can also prescribe Ru Mo Si Wu Tang, Di Gu Pi Yin, or Zhi Bo Di Huang Tang adding the appropriate combinations of the The Eye Brighteners (Qian Li Guang, Mi Meng Hua, She Tui, and Chan Tui), Tian Ma, Gou Ji, and Fu Ling.

Macular edema, macular degeneration, and various types of vitreous opacities (e.g., floaters) can be identified as *blood heat* and *blood aspect stasis heat* pattern. For these pathoconditions, you can also prescribe Ru Mo Si Wu Tang, Di Gu Pi Yin, or Zhi Bo Di Huang Tang adding Qian Li Guang, Mi Meng Hua, Dan Shen, and Chuan Qi (powder); and if swelling (edema) presents, then add The Four Lings.

And in cases where optic nerve degeneration has occurred, you can prescribe qi- and blood-supplementing formulas such as Bu Yang Huan Wu Tang, Sheng Yu Tang, or Ru Mo Si Wu Tang adding Chuan Qi (powder).

Case Study #10: Central Serous Retinopathy and Dry Eye Syndrome

Q: A 44 y/o male patient had a 10-year history of central serous retinopathy (CSR) and dry eye syndrome (DES). Four months ago, I began prescribing this patient Ru Mo Si Wu Tang adding Qing Hao, Zhi Mu, and Di Gu Pi. After administering this formula for 1 month, he stopped taking the medicinals, and instead, he ate lots of legumes and nuts (omega-3 fatty acids, antioxidants, and trace minerals), fish (omega-3 fatty acids), and leafy green vegetables (carotenoids (lutein and zeaxanthin)). Three months later, he contacted me saying that his eye condition had completely resolved! Do you think that this is possible?

A: There is no direct correlation between central serous retinopathy (CRS) and dry eye syndrome (DES). CRS is defined as serous retinal detachment at the posterior pole of the eyeball (at the macula or in the perimacular region) due to a defect in the pigment epithelium.

However, both of these pathoconditions can be precipitated by stress and unhealthy lifestyle and typically will spontaneously resolve within a few months. It sounds to me like the patient was more conscious of reducing stress and trying to lead a healthy lifestyle (e.g., diet, exercise, adequate sleep), which is the best way to promote healing and foster health. This gives testimony to a fundamental principle in TCM ophthalmology: "Rest the eyes and cultivate a healthy lifestyle and your vision will be free of disease."

Case Study #11: Uveitis – Induced By Overfatigue

Q: A 45 y/o female patient suffered from uveitis induced by overfatigue. After 2 weeks of Western medicine treatment (corticosteroid eye drops) the pathocondition resolved. However, during autumn of the following year it recurred and this time Western medicine treatment was not effective. My idea is to prescribe Ru Mo Si Wu Tang adding The Three Yellows and The Four Lings. Do you think this approach will be effective?

A: Yes, that formula will effectively treat uveitis. However, you should also bleed Zan Zhu (UB2), Si Zhu Kong (SJ23), Da Zhui (GV14) (above, on, and below), and Wei Zhong (UB40); and needle Feng Chi (GB20), Tian Zhu (UB10), He Gu (LI4), Tai Chong (LV3), San Yin Jiao (SP6), and Shen Men (HT7). Depending on the clinical presentation and pattern identification, other formula variants that I might consider prescribing are Zhi Bo Di Huang Tang and Wen Dan Tang.

The focus of treatment for uveitis is **on** reducing inflammation and resolving toxin. So continue prescribing your formula that contains heat-clearing toxin-resolving, blood-quickening stasis-transforming, and dampness-disinhibiting by bland percolation medicinals. Remember! TCM treatment of eye pathoconditions typically takes some time to achieve complete resolution. You may need to administer the therapeutic regimen anywhere from 3–6 months before the photophobia, ocular pain, glare, and decreased vision return to normal. This will ensure that the metabolic waste from the inflammatory response completely resolve, thus preventing recurrence and also minimizing the possibility of complications such as cataracts, glaucoma, and neovascularization.

Case Study #12: Epidemic Keratoconjunctivitis ("Pinkeye")

Q: My son caught a cold this summer and had a persistent runny nose and sneezing. Two months later he began having itchy eyes, but at the time we didn't pay too much attention to it. Then, one day the upper and lower eyelids swelled up, the whites of his eyes turned red (hyperemia), and now the conjunctiva are so swollen (chemosis) that it looks like his eyes are going to burst. It looks horrible!

I prescribed Wen Dan Tang combining (Yu Sheng) Tearing on Exposure to Wind Formula adding Jin Yin Hua, but it wasn't effective. In addition to the conjunctival symptoms, he also has nasal congestion (clear to white color) and occasionally sneezes. It worries me. What can I do for him?

A: Based on your description, I am not sure if this is a case of heaven-current red eye (天行赤眼 tiān xíng chì yǎn) with eye discharge, if it's swelling and inflammation of the eyelid as in eyelid swollen like a ball (胞腫如毬 bāo zhǒng rú qiú) and eyelid swollen like a peach (胞腫如桃 bāo zhǒng rú táo), or if the pupil is normal in the presence of swollen conjunctiva (chemosis). You may need to further clarify and/or get it examined by an ophthalmologist. I can provide this bit of advice:

The pathocondition *heaven-current red eye* with *eye discharge* described in TCM classical texts correlates with what is now called epidemic keratoconjunctivitis (EKC) or *"pinkeye"* for short, which is a highly contagious conjunctival infection caused by adenoviruses. *Eyelid swollen like a ball* refers to a round, soft swelling on the eyelid, and *eyelid swollen like a peach* refers to a reddish inflamed swelling on the eyelid and correlates with orbital cellulitis. *Conjunctival edema* may present without eyelid swelling.

Heaven-current red eye and *eyelid swollen like a peach* can both be identified as heat with exterior pattern pathoconditions; *eyelid swollen like a ball* can be identified as spleen qi vacuity or spleen qi vacuity with yang vacuity pattern; and *conjunctival edema* can be identified as water amassment pattern. If there is *sticky yellow eye discharge*, then this can be identified as exterior wind-heat-damp pattern.

For heat pattern pathoconditions, you should bleed Zan Zhu (UB2), Si Zhu Kong (SJ23), and Da Zhui (GV14) (above, on, and below); and needle Feng Chi (GB20), Tian Zhu (UB10), Wan Gu (GB12), and He Gu (LI4). He Gu (LI4) is particularly effective for relieving the feeling of heaviness and congestion in the eyes. If the pathocondition has already entered the chronic stage, then warm needle He Gu (LI4). As for TCM medicinals, you should focus on effusing the exterior, abating heat, and extinguishing wind with a formula such as Yang Dan Tang, Ge Gen Tang, or Ma Huang Tang adding heat-clearing toxin-resolving medicinals like the The Three Yellows or Jin Yin Hua, Pu Gong Ying, and Lian Qiao. You could also consider prescribing Ge Gen Qin Lian Tang, Huang Lian Jie Du Tang, Fang Feng Tong Sheng San, Liang Ge San, Qing Shang Fang Feng Tang, or Qing Yin Li Ge San.

For the *eyelid swollen like a ball* pathocondition, you can prescribe formulas such as Bu Zhong Yi Qi Tang, Gui Qi Jian Zhong Tang, or Sheng Yu Tang adding large doses of Huang Qi (possibly even adding

The Three Great Yang-Supplementers and Huang Qin); and acupuncture (warm needle) He Gu (LI4) and Zu San Li (ST36). For *conjunctival edema*, you can prescribe a formula such as Wu Ling San, Ling Gui Zhu Gan Tang, or Gui Zhi Tang adding Cang Zhu, Fu Ling, Ze Xie, Ma Huang, and Ge Gen; and if *sticky yellow eye discharge* presents, then add The Three Yellows or Jin Yin Hua, Pu Gong Ying, and Lian Qiao.

Once the more pronounced symptoms have stabilized and the brunt of the heat has resolved (e.g., *sticky yellow eye discharge* becomes whitish), the pathocondition may evolve into the chronic stage. At this time, you can consider prescribing Wen Dan Tang adding Bai Zhi, Lai Fu Zi, Ma Huang, Ci Ji Li, and Zao Jiao Ci. If *clear, watery eyes* (epiphora) present, then this can be classified as tearing on exposure to wind (迎風落淚 yíng fēng luò lèi), requiring the addition of The Three Great Yang-Supplementers and Huang Qin, or change the formula to You Gui Yin adding Ma Huang, Bai Zhi, Xin Yi, and Xi Xin. The best treatment for tearing on exposure to wind is to get out in the sunshine!

Case Study #13: Recurrent Hordeolum (Stye)

Q: I have a 10 y/o girl patient who has developed 1 or 2 styes (sometimes on the left and other times on the right side) almost every month ever since she was about 3 years old. I identified this as damp-heat pattern and thus prescribed Long Dan Xie Gan Tang adding Jin Yin Hua. Do you think this is the right approach?

A: *Hordeolum (stye)* is an acute inflammation of the Moll's or Zeis glands (aka *external* hordeolum) or the meibomian glands (aka *internal* hordeolum) caused by infection that can occur on both the upper and lower eyelids. A *chalazion* is a focal swelling of the meibomian glands (aka *deep* chalazion) and Zeis glands (aka *superficial* chalazion) caused by obstruction. Over time, a *stye* may develop into a *chalazion.*

Both of these pathoconditions can be identified as stomach heat pattern. In the acute stage, presenting with concomitant exterior wind-heat, you can consider prescribing an exterior-interior heat-clearing formula variant such as Ge Gen Qin Lian Tang or Qing Shang Fang Feng Tang. In the post-acute stage, when heat is *still* pronounced, you can prescribe a stomach-clearing fire-draining and heat-clearing toxin-resolving formula such as Huang Lian Jie Du Tang, Qing Wei San, or Liang Ge San. And if the nodule-like swelling *fails* to resolve over an extended period of time and heat is *not* pronounced, then you can consider prescribing a heat-clearing toxin-resolving, swelling-dispersing hardness-breaking, and blood-quickening pain-relieving formula variant such as Xian Fang Huo Ming Yin.

Continue administering your formula for 3–5 months after the lesion has healed. If there has not been a recurrence after this period of time, then you can discontinue administration. As for acupuncture, you can needle He Gu (LI4), Feng Chi (GB20), Tian Zhu (UB10), and Zu San Li (ST36).

Case Study #14: Syringoma

Q: A 42 y/o female patient has a history of syringomas on both lower eyelids. It's possible to squeeze out watery fluid with the fingers. Over the past 5 years she has received periodic laser treatment with minimal efficacy; not long after treatment the little bumps will come back again. Can TCM treat this condition?

A: Syringomas are harmless eccrine sweat duct tumors. You can prescribe Ma Xing Yi Gan Tang or Wen Dan Tang adding Ma Huang, Xing Ren, and Yi Yi Ren. It is also possible to use the tip of an acupuncture needle to pierce the lesion and evacuate the matter, but if there are a lot of sweat ducts affected this may be very time consuming and ultimately may not resolve the underlying problem.

Your best bet is to prescribe TCM medicinals and advise the patient to give a low cholesterol diet a try for a while. In some patients (not all!) who have an excessively high cholesterol diet (e.g., duck fat, pork belly), reducing the intake will offer positive results in resolving this purely cosmetic skin condition.

Case Study #15: Glaucoma

Q: A 48 y/o male patient was diagnosed with glaucoma upon examination by an ophthalmologist. Results showed that 90% of the optic nerve in his right eye has already been damaged, but the eye pressure is normal. He doesn't have diabetes or hypertension. What is the best approach for treating this type of glaucoma?

A: Glaucoma correlates with the pathocondition thunder head wind (雷頭風 léi tóu fēng) described in classical TCM texts. Remember! About 1/3 of all patients with glaucoma do *not* have elevated intraocular pressure (ocular hypertension). The average range of ocular pressure is 11 to 21 mm Hg.

If the ocular pressure is below 12 (*low-tension glaucoma*), then you can prescribe a qi- and blood-supplementing with yang-supplementing formula variant such as Sheng Yu Tang, Bu Yang Huan Wu Tang, Qi Bao Mei Ran Dan, Xue Ku Fang, Shen Qi Wan, or You Gui Wan. Just make sure to include Gan Jiang and Fu Zi in your formula.

If ocular pressure is between 11 and 20 (*normal-tension glaucoma*), then prescribe a qi- and blood-supplementing with blood-quickening stasis-transforming formula such as Ru Mo Si Wu Tang, Sheng Yu Tang, or Bu Yang Huan Wu Tang adding Huang Qin, Huang Lian, and Chuan Qi (powder).

If ocular pressure is over 21 (*ocular hypertension*), then prescribe a formula such as Wen Dan Tang combining Zhi Bo Di Huang Tang, Qin Lian Ru Mo Si Wu Tang, Di Gu Pi Yin, or Jian Ling Tang adding Qian Li Guang, Mi Meng Hua, She Tui, Chan Tui, Fu Ling, and Chuan Qi (powder). If headache and orbital pain presents, then add Bai Zhi and Tian Ma; and if vomiting presents add Ban Xia.

And if disease progression has already resulted in extensive optic nerve atrophy and possibly visual impairment, then the TCM treatment for this pathocondition can follow the same approach as for wind strike (stroke) (中風 zhòng fēng).

Case Study #16: Nasolacrimal Duct Obstruction (Dacryostenosis)

Q: A 64 y/o female patient with a history of nasolacrimal duct obstruction (dacryostenosis) has already undergone four dacryocystorhinostomies (a surgical procedure that creates a passage between the lacrimal sac and the nasal cavity) and one conjunctivo-dacryocystorhinostomy (C-DCR) (a tube is inserted leading from the caruncle into the nasal cavity). The tube was subsequently removed because of recurring obstruction.

Now, she is awaiting her second tube insertion procedure and has been experiencing nasolacrimal duct infection (dacryocystitis). I am planning on prescribing Gui Zhi Fu Ling Wan combining Huang Lian Jie Du Tang adding Chuan Qi (powder). What do you think?

A: Dacryostenosis (nasolacrimal duct obstruction) can be identified as stomach heat pattern. That formula may provide relief of symptoms (e.g., excessive tearing (epiphora)). But remember! You simply need to prescribe medicinals that will abate stomach heat. Thus, if it were me, I would consider prescribing a formula such as Ge Gen Qin Lian Tang, Qing Wei San, Liang Ge San, Qing Shang Fang Feng Tang, or Qing Yin Li San adding Ci Ji Li and Zao Jiao Ci (tear duct channel conductors). All of these formulas will provide effective treatment.

Case Study #17: Epiphora

Q: This female patient has a 10-year history of excessive tearing (epiphora). Examination revealed right-sided nasolacrimal duct obstruction, prompting her doctors to perform a surgical procedure to unblock the passageway (dacryocystorhinostomy). However, obstruction recurred following surgery and now she has continuous tearing. I prescribed Gui Zhi Fu Ling Wan variant, but this was not effective.

A: Excessive tearing (epiphora) can be identified as stomach heat or phlegm heat pattern, requiring administration of a formula such as Wen Dan Tang, Qing Wei San, Huang Lian Jie Du Tang, or Ge Gen Qin Lian Tang.

Case Study #18: Cataract – Postsurgical Dry Eye Syndrome

Q: I have a 68 y/o female patient with a history of dry eye syndrome (DES) and a cataract in her left eye. Due to a worsening of visual acuity, her ophthalmologist recommended she undergo surgery. Following the surgery, she has been experiencing severe eye dryness. She is currently being administered corticosteroid treatment, but the symptoms have not improved. What is the best approach for treating this condition?

A: Eye dryness is a common postsurgical complication of cataract surgery, and in patients with preexisting dry eye syndrome (DES), it can be even more troublesome. Corticosteroids are administered following surgery to reduce the risk of inflammation that could lead to other serious complications, but they also suppress mucous secretions, while other drugs, such as NSAIDS, may damage the ocular surface. These drugs may cause an "iatrogenic" exacerbation of DES.

As for TCM treatment, DES can be identified as hyperactive yang with Shao Yang heat pattern. Thus, you should bleed Zan Zhu (UB2), Yu Yao (EX-HN4), Si Zhu Kong (SJ23), Da Zhui (GV14), and Tai Yuan (LU9); needle acupoints such as Feng Chi (GB20), Tian Zhu (UB10), Wan Gu (GB12), Zan Zhu (UB2), Yu Yao (EX-HN4), Yu Wei (EX-HN37), He Gu (LI4), Zu San Li (ST36), Tai Chong (LV3), San Yin Jiao (SP6), and Yang Ling Quan (GB34); and prescribe formulas such as Hyperactive Immune Formula (including large doses of The Three Yellows). In chronic cases, you should add Dan Shen or consider changing to a blood-nourishing dryness-moistening and yin-enriching steaming bone-eliminating formula such as Xue Ku Fang or Zhi Bo Di Huang Tang, making sure to include Huang Qin, Huang Lian, Qing Hao, and Di Gu Pi.

Case Study #19: "Pain in the Eye"

Q: A 38 y/o male experienced pain in his right eye and was admitted into the hospital, where he has been receiving corticosteroid injections for 1 week now, but the pain has not subsided. There are *no* signs or symptoms of inflammation. Please offer your guidance and suggestions on this case.

A: Well, based on the limited amount of information you have given, it's tough to give you any specific advice. Do you mean pain in the eyeball or eye socket? Is visual acuity affected? How about ocular pressure? Are there any flashes or visual field disturbances? Are the pupils constricted? I suspect it may be iritis, and if so, then you can prescribe Ru Mo Si Wu Tang (including a large dose of Chi Shao) adding The Three Yellows, Bai Zhi, and Tian Ma.

Another pathocondition that comes to mind is cockscomb clam flesh (雞冠蜆肉 jī guān xiàn ròu), which can cause pain in the lower eyelid or eye socket (innervated by the maxillary nerve (CNV2)!). Cockscomb clam flesh is described in the classical TCM text *The Golden Mirror of Medicine* and includes a formula to treat this pathocondition called Chou Feng Tang (Tugging Wind Formula). If pain persists, then bleed the well acupoints of the foot and hand Yang Ming channels and needle the acupoints Feng Chi (GB20), Tian Zhu (UB10), Wan Gu (GB12), Ting Gong (SI19), He Gu (LI4), Zu San Li (ST36), and Shou San Li (LI10).

Section 2: Ear Disorders

Case Study #1: Tinnitus – "Mosquitoes Buzzing Around"

Q: About 10 years ago, a 51 y/o female began experiencing tinnitus after incurring an episode of the common cold. Now, anytime she feels fatigued or catches a cold, she will have symptoms of copious phlegm and tinnitus, which she says sounds like "mosquitoes buzzing around" and occurs both night and day. She also has shortage of qi and laziness to speak (懶言 lǎn yán), slightly low blood pressure, and *feels* overall physical decline. Stool and urine are normal. Many people say that tinnitus is very difficult to treat and that there really aren't any effective TCM medicinals or Western medicine drugs available. What do you think about it?

A: Tinnitus really is a complicated pathocondition to treat, but it isn't always as difficult as you may think. Typically, tinnitus is caused by a disorder involving the cochlea or Eustachian tubes. In TCM, tinnitus can be identified as either phlegm-rheum with static blood, phlegm heat, stasis heat with qi vacuity static blood, phlegm-rheum with hyperactive yang, or phlegm-rheum with yin vacuity pattern.

Based on the specific pattern identification, you could consider prescribing formula variants such as Xiao Ban Xie Jia Fu Ling, Er Chen Tang, Wen Dan Tang, Di Tan Tang, Zhi Bo Di Huang Tang, Xiao Chai Hu Tang, Bu Yang Huan Wu Tang, Huang Lian Jie Du Tang, or Jian Ling Tang.

A typical formula I may prescribe to brighten the eyes and sharpen the hearing for the treatment of tinnitus is Xiao Chai Hu Tang adding Long Gu, Mu Li, Lai Fu Zi, Ge Gen, Mai Men Dong, and Cang Er Zi; and if vertigo presents, then add Tian Ma. Additionally, I like to acupuncture the following acupoints: Feng Chi (GB20), Wan Gu (GB12), Yi Feng (SJ17), Ting Gong (SI19), He Gu (LI4), San Yin Jiao (SP6), Tai Chong (LV3), Tai Yang (EX-HN5), and Bai Hui (GV20).

If the patient is in the acute stage of otitis media presenting with redness, swelling, heat, and pain in the middle ear, then bleed Ting Gong (SI19), Er Men (SJ21), Tai Yang (EX-HN5), Da Zhui (GV14) (above, on, and below), and Tai Yuan (LU9). To find out more about my approach to treating tinnitus and other ear disorders, you can reference my *Chinese-Western Integrated Medicine Theory and Practice (I)* book.

Case Study #2: Tinnitus, Vertigo, and Hearing Impairment

Q: Over the past half year, I have treated over 20 patients with tinnitus and vertigo. Most of them have been qi vacuity pattern tinnitus presenting with poor circulation in the inner ear and hearing impairment (some nearly deaf!). What is your approach to treating tinnitus, vertigo, and hearing impairment?

A: First, you must differentiate. Does this case involve hearing impairment, tinnitus, or vertigo? Is there *aural fullness* (pressure or clogged sensation in the ears)? If there is *aural fullness*, when the patient swallows or speaks there will be a "residual echoing sound" in the ears. This may be caused by *Eustachean tube dysfunction (ETD)* (blockage or failure to open properly), which can be identified as phlegm-heat pattern.

Continuous, enduring tinnitus, which tends to fade in crowds of people or noisy environments and intensifies in the quiet of the night, is typically caused by *cochlear hypoxia* (*poor circulation*). This pathocondition can be identified as either phlegm-rheum or qi vacuity with depression pattern, requiring the administration of a formula variant such as Wen Dan Tang, Xue Fu Zhu Yu Tang, Bu Yang Huan Wu Tang, and Yi Qi Cong Ming Tang.

Most cases of vertigo are caused by *disorders of the vestibular system* (e.g., semicircular canal imbalance, crystals in the otolith organs become dislodged), whereas complete deafness primarily involves *auditory nerve damage* (for treatment you can reference wind strike sudden deafness).

Otitis media can also cause pus and mucus to build up in the Eustachian tube, clogging the passageway and leading to sudden hearing loss. For this pathocondition, you can prescribe Wen Dan Tang combining either Bu Yang Huan Wu Tang or Ru Mo Si Wu Tang.

Remember! Regardless of the underlying cause, in patients who present with symptoms of vertigo, you should always add Tian Ma (calms the liver and extinguishes wind and frees the network vessels)!

Case Study #3: Tinnitus – Elderly Patients

Q: What's the best way to treat tinnitus in elderly patients?

A: If tinnitus is the chief complaint, then I would typically consider prescribing either a heat-clearing phlegm-transforming formula, such as Wen Dan Tang, or a kidney-enriching yin-nourishing liquid-engendering formula, such as Ba Xian Chang Shou Wan, making sure to include Ge Gen, Mai Men Dong, Tu Si Zi, and Dang Gui in your formula.

Remember! The key here is to encourage the patient to get adequate rest and sleep: Sleep is the most effective treatment for tinnitus!

Case Study #4: Sudden Deafness

Q: One week ago, a 31 y/o patient incurred sudden deafness. His otologist diagnosed the condition as sudden sensorineural hearing loss (SSNHL) and prescribed drug treatment, but it hasn't proven effective. Do you have any advice or suggestions for this case?

A: Sudden hearing loss is commonly caused by *blockage of the Eustachian tube* or viral infection (particularly involving herpes simplex), autoimmune disease, and acute microvascular occlusion that affect the *auditory nerve*. A good way to perform a general differential diagnosis is as follows: if there is blockage of the *Eustachian tube*, then there will be a "residual echoing sound" in the ears when the patient speaks and swallows, like you feel when flying in an airplane; and if the *auditory nerve* is affected, then there won't be any residual sound at all. It is important to make this distinction, because the therapeutic approach for these pathoconditions is different.

Blockage of the Eustachian tube (Eustachian tube dysfunction (ETD)) can be identified as phlegm-rheum pattern, requiring administration of Wen Dan Tang variant. An *auditory nerve disorder* (sudden sensorineural hearing loss (SSNHL)) can be identified as blood stagnation with heat toxin and water swelling pattern. If corticosteroids have been administered, then this can be identified as yang vacuity pattern, requiring the administration of a formula variant such as Bu Yang

Huan Wu Tang, Ru Mo Si Wu Tang, or Sheng Yu Tang. If water swelling presents, then add Bai Zhu, Fu Ling, and Ze Xie; and if heat presents, then add The Three Yellows. If the patient has been receiving long-term administration of aspirin and/or anticoagulants (e.g., Warfarin), then you can approach this as you would wind strike (stroke), making sure to include The Three Great Yang-Supplementers, Huang Qin, and Ren Shen/Chuan Qi Powder into your formula.

Case Study #5: Auricular Chondritis

Q: A few years ago, a 30 y/o female patient began having inflammation in the cartilage of her right ear. She has received treatment from a dermatologist, but nothing has been effective. On observation you can see a millet-sized pustule covered by a scaly plaque that is difficult to rupture, no fluid or pus drains once ruptured, and it is extremely itchy. Can this be identified as Shao Yang heat pattern? Can I prescribe Xiao Chai Hu Tang variant to treat this pathocondition?

A: For this type of auricular chondritis, I would first consider two potential therapeutic approaches based on presentation and detailed pattern identification:

1) Treat as if it were eczema, prescribing Ma Xing Yi Gan Tang adding Sheng Shi Gao (clears heat and drains fire) and Zao Jiao Ci (quickens the blood and disperses swelling and expels pus).

2) Treat as if it were lichen (tinea) (癬 xiǎn), prescribing Blood Desiccation Formula adding Ma Huang, Xing Ren, Yi Yi Ren, Huang Qin, and Sheng Shi Gao. And if these approaches are not effective, then I would change to a heat-clearing toxin-resolving, swelling-dispersing hardness-breaking, and blood-quickening pain-relieving formula variant such as Xian Fang Huo Ming Fang.

Section 3: Periodontal Disease

Case Study #1: Gingivitis, Periodontitis, and Temporomandibular Joint Disorder

Q: A 60 y/o female patient presented with receding, swollen, and inflamed gums, and locking of the jaw. I prescribed Huang Lian Jie Du Tang (including large doses of The Three Yellows), but this treatment was not effective.

Troubled by these symptoms, she was admitted into the hospital for treatment. After a 10-day stay, she was released, but still had problems with locking of the jaw, and now her gums are even more painful and inflamed than before. How should I approach this case?

A: Swollen, inflamed gums and locking of the jaw are two completely separate pathoconditions.

Receding, swollen, inflamed gums indicate gingivitis or periodontitis, which left untreated, will become purplish in color, form pockets between the gum and bone where infection sets in and pus forms, and eventually the teeth loosen and fall out. Periodontitis correlates with galloping gan of the teeth and gum (走馬牙疳 zǒu mǎ yá gān) described in classical TCM texts and is also commonly known as centipede flat-abscess (蜈蚣疽 wú gōng jū).

In the early stage, it can be identified as stomach heat pattern, requiring administration of a stomach-clearing fire-draining formula such as Qing Wei San adding Niu Xi, Xu Duan, and Gu Sui Bu once the brunt of the heat resolves. In the post-acute stage, it can be identified as stomach yin vacuity pattern, requiring administration of an yin-nourishing dryness-moistening formula such as Gan Lu Yin or Zhi Bo Di Huang Tang adding Niu Xi, Xu Duan, and Gui Sui Bu. And in the chronic stage, it can be identified as spleen, stomach, heart, and kidney vacuity-detriment, requiring administration of a dual qi- and blood-supplementing and yin-enriching kidney-boosting formula such as Huan Shao Dan.

Locking of the jaw indicates temporomandibular joint (TMJ) disorder that may be caused by many factors such as chronic inflammation, trauma, malocclusion, and teeth grinding (bruxism). These conditions may cause TMJ joint inflammation resulting in adhesions and fibrosis of surrounding tissue that inhibit normal joint function. For heat pattern, you can prescribe Huang Lian Jie Du Tang; bleed the affected TMJ site (approximately located at Xia Guan (ST7)); and needle perpendicularly into the affected TMJ. However, if adhesions and fibrosis have already set in, then you must supplement qi and yang by adding The Three Great Yang-Supplementers and Huang Qin.

If pronounced swelling, pain, and heat present, then you must consider the possibility of trigeminal neuralgia as well. If there is just moderate pain and swelling, then you can prescribe either Huang Lian Jie Du Tang or Zhi Bo Di Huang Tang; and if the pain is severe, then add medicinals such as Gu Cui Bu, Bai Zhi, Xu Duan, Pu Huang, and The Three Insects. In addition to the local TMJ acupoint, you can also needle distal body acupoints such as He Ge (LI4), Zu San Li (ST36), Hou Xi (SI3), Yang Ling Quan (GB34), and Nei Ting (ST44).

This therapeutic regimen will provide effective treatment for both periodontitis and TMJ disorder.

Case Study #2: Alveolar Pyorrhea (Compound Periodontitis)

Q: A 55 y/o male patient has suffered from periodontitis for about 10 years. During the past year the condition has worsened, with the presence of severely painful and swollen gums and purulent inflammation. Pus pockets have formed between a number of his teeth, and over the past two weeks, his dentist has drained them twice. He has been taking antibiotics for the past 25 days now, but the swelling and pain have only decreased a little bit. What is the best approach for treating this patient?

A: Alveolar pyorrhea (compound periodontitis) correlates with galloping gan of the teeth and gum (走馬牙疳 zǒu mǎ yá gān) and bone trough wind (骨槽風 gǔ cáo fēng) described in classical TCM texts. As for treatment, I would prescribe a heat-clearing toxin-resolving formula variant such as Huang Lian Jie Du Tang to be administered orally. And also separately administer packets of Da Huang (powder), instructing the patient to mix together with rock salt (戎鹽 róng yán) (aka halite, the mineral (natural) form of sodium chloride (NaCl)) to form a toothpaste solution that provides potent heat toxin-clearing, swelling-dispersing, and pain-relieving actions.

Remember! The patient's gums are too tender to use a toothbrush right now so instruct him to rub this solution on the gums using his fingers. After the solution has been thoroughly rubbed into the gums, it can be swallowed or spit out. As you know, Da Huang also has strong laxative actions so make sure the patient is aware of this and doesn't swallow too much.

IX. MALE GENITOURINARY DISORDERS

Case Study #1: Yin Wilt, Yang Wilt, and Failure to Rise – Impotence

Q: I have a question about treating impotence (erectile dysfunction (ED)), otherwise known as yin wilting (陰痿 yīn wěi), yang wilting (陽痿 yang wěi), or failure to rise (不舉 bù jǔ) in TCM classical texts. In my clinical experience I have discovered there are many different manifestations of impotence. For the treatment of almost all types, I have had positive initial results through the administration of Yin Yang Huo (1 liang), but these effects are usually only temporary. What is your experience in treating this condition?

A: In the past, for the treatment of yin wilting, yang wilting, and failure to rise, I commonly prescribed either the yin and yang neutrally-supplementing and subduing and settling formula Gui Zhi Jia Long Gu Mu Li Tang or a kidney yang-supplementing formula such as Shen Qi Wan and You Gui Yin. Then, for a period of time, I liked to prescribe the blood-quickening qi-supplementing formula Bu Yang Huan Wu Tang adding Lu Rong, Hai Long, Hai Ma, and Ge Jie. In recent years, I have further modified this formula to Bu Yang Huan Wu Tang adding Gan Jiang, Rou Gui, Huang Bo, Ren Shen/Chuan Qi Powder, Lu Rong (powder), and Yu Sheng Wan, which has provided more effective results overall.

In cases where the underlying cause is emotional depression, then I will typically prescribe the spleen- and stomach-supplementing, phlegm-damp transforming, and wind-stabilizing formula Ban Xia Tian Ma Bai Zhu San (including a large dose of Huang Qi) adding Gan Cao and Long Yan Rou (longan flesh). You can also consider using the entire Long Yan (longan), crushing the Long Yan Ke (longan shell) and Long Yan He (longan seed) along with the flesh, or adding in crushed seeds such as Ju He (tangerine seeds), Shan Zha (hawthorn flesh with seeds), and Li Zhi He (litchi seeds). For these types of patients, this approach has proven particularly effective.

Case Study #2: Erectile Dysfunction – Diabetes Patients

Q: A 43 y/o male diabetes patient has suffered from erectile dysfunction (ED) ever since he began taking medication to treat his hyperglycemia. The patient has tried numerous treatment approaches including Viagra, Cialis, acupuncture injection therapy, and bee venom therapy, but nothing has proven ultimately effective. He is able to attain a partial erection, but unable to maintain it, and has a strong libido, but explains that he is physically "not up for the task." What would you do for this patient?

A: For diabetes patients with ED, I would prescribe blood-, qi-, and yang-supplementing medicinals such as Bu Yang Huan Wu Tang adding The Three Great Yang-Supplementers Huang Bo, Sang Bai Pi, and Ren Shen/Chuan Qi Powder. At first, you must make sure the patient continues taking the anti-diabetic medications and over time this integrative TCM and Western medicine approach will resolve the ED issues.

In the future, you can see if the patient wants to continue using other TCM formula variants, such as Zhi Bo Di Huang Tang, in order to gradually wean away from, and eventually, completely discontinue the Western medicine drugs currently needed to control hyperglycemia.

Case Study #3: Erectile Dysfunction – Bu Yang Huan Wu Tang Variant

Q: Recently, I have been treating many yang wilting patients (陽痿 yang wěi), but the results have not been as pronounced as these patients would like. I have tried formula variants such as You Gui Yin, Gui Zhi Jia Long Gu Mu Li Tang, and Bu Yang Huan Wu Tang without much success. Please offer your advice and guidance.

A: First, try to determine the cause of the erectile dysfunction (ED) and identify the pattern. You will have better results if you add The Three Great Yang-Supplementers, Ren Shen/Chuan Qi Powder, and Huang Bo into those formulas you mentioned. You can also consider adding Fu Ling, Ze Xie, Bai Zhu, and Yu Sheng Wan (starting out at 1 pill/day, and over time, increasing to 2 pills/day). Some patient's may require adding Lu Rong (powder).

What I would do is prescribe Bu Yang Huan Wu Tang variant decocted in 4 1/2 bowls (900 ml) water and 1 1/2 bowls (300 ml) soju [a clear, distilled Korean liquor traditionally made from rice, wheat, or barley] to ensure quicker results. Soaking the medicinals in a mixture of soju and water prior to decocting will enhance the liver- and kidney-warming and -supplementing, blood-quickening network vessel-freeing, and wind-dispelling cold-dissipating actions of these medicinals.

Case Study #4: Erectile Dysfunction Differential Diagnosis – "Morning Erections"?

Q: A 51 y/o male patient with a 10-year history of diabetes recently began experiencing serious erectile dysfunction (ED) problems. The patient read up on pathoconditions that correlated with his symptoms in the classic TCM text *Precious Mirror of Eastern Medicine* (東醫寶鑑 dōng yī bǎo jiàn) and used this information to prescribe a formula on his own. He prescribed Liu Wei Di Huang Wan (Supplemented Six-Ingredient Rehmannia Pill) in efforts to treat his diabetes, but it didn't provide any noticeable effects in lowering blood sugar levels or his ED issues. What do you think the best approach is for treating this patient?

A: First, you need to ask this diabetes patient if he has "morning erections (nocturnal penile tumescence)," and *if so*, then this suggests the cause of his ED is likely sexual fatigue—having sex with the same partner over a long period of time will often result in reduced interest, and overindulgence over an extended period of time can lead to loss of interest.

If the patient does *not* have "morning erections," then you can more confidently make the diagnosis of diabetes induced ED, with the pathomechanisms involving disruption of the stimulant centers in the brain and/or downstream innervation through the spinal cord, lumbar, sacrum, and penile nerve pathways. To promote innervation of the downstream motor neurons, you can prescribe medicinals that quicken the blood, supplement qi and yang, and free the network vessels such as Bu Yang Huan Wu Tang adding Di Long, Ma Huang, The Three Great Yang-Supplementers, Huang Bo, and Yu Sheng Wan.

If blood sugar levels and HbA1C levels are elevated, then add Sang Bai Pi. Depending on specific cases and respective pattern identifications, you can also consider adding Ren Shen/Chuan Qi Powder and Lu Rong (powder); or combine You Gui Yin or Shen Qi Wan with your original formula selection. Yu Sheng Wan improves nerve conduction and promotes innervation.

Case Study #5: Is There Really a TCM Penis Enlargement Elixir?

Q: Many *men* wish there penis was larger and some even go as far as surgery. In the past, I have prescribed formulas focused on penis enlargement, but results have been poor. Please share your experience and ideas on this "condition."

A: *Here* is a To-Do List for penis enlargement and sensual enhancement:

- To enlarge the girth of the shaft and engorge the tip like a viper, you can try prescribing formulas such as Bu Yang Huan Wu Tang, Gui Qi Jian Zhong Tang, and Sheng Yu Tang adding The Three Great Yang-Supplementers, Huang Bo, Ren Shen/Chuan Qi Powder, and Lu Rong (powder). Ren Shen is optional, but Chuan Qi (quickens blood and transforms stasis) and Lu Rong (invigorates kidney yang, boosts essence blood, strengthens sinew and bone, regulates thoroughfare and controlling vessels) are essential!
- To increase the intensity and pleasure of ejaculation, add Tu Si Zi, She Chuang Zi, and Sha Wan Zi.
- To tauten the ejaculatory ducts and prevent premature ejaculation, add Long Gu, Mu Li, Da/Xiao Jin Ying, and Bai Guo.

- To subdue the sensitivity of the penis tip (glans), add Zhi Mu, Huang Bo, and Mu Li.

Remember! You should explain to your patients that "prowess" is not necessarily determined by *size*. The most important aspect is normal "function." They should think long and hard before trying to change what is already a good thing!

Case Study #6: Autologous Fat Injections – It's Not Worth It!

Q: For a while autologous fat injections were popular for female breast augmentation and male girth enhancement. But it turned out that results were often not so good. After receiving these fat grafts, males commonly experienced erectile dysfunction (ED) (e.g., ability to maintain only partial erections and inability to remain erect for adequate durations). For the treatment of ED, I have tried administering Bu Yang Huan Wu Tang variant without consistent results. Please offer your ideas and suggestions.

A: *Autologous* fat injections are easily absorbed by the body. Whether it is performed for breast augmentation, penis enlargement, or cosmetic surgery on the face, it is likely to only last from 6 months to 1 year. It's really not economically affordable, nor is it a viable solution. It's also possible for scarring to occur at the injection sites, resulting in pain during erection as well as vascular and lymphatic obstruction leading to poor blood circulation and fibrosis.

Obviously, these risks far outweigh the ephemeral benefits. Despite your initial results, I would continue prescribing Bu Yang Huan Wu Tang adding The Three Great Yang-Supplementers and Ren Shen/Chuan Qi Powder. If you want to increase the intensity and pleasure of erection, then try adding Lu Rong (powder); and if you want to extend erection duration and frequency, then add She Chuang Zi and Yu Sheng Wan (start out with 1 pill/day, and if necessary, gradually increase to 2 pills/day).

Case Study #7: "Pain In the Neck" After Ejaculation

Q: I *have* a 26 y/o male patient who is physically attractive and has been very active sexually since high school. He mentioned that after ejaculating, he often feels "pain in the neck" that lasts about 10 minutes, and asked me if this was anything to be concerned about. How would you explain this? And is there any way, or need, to treat this condition?

A: *Actually*, this is something that many people experience, especially if fatigued, stressed out, or sleep deprived. If necessary, you can try prescribing an yin-enriching fire-downbearing formula such as Zhi Bo Di Huang Tang adding Ge Gen and Tian Ma.

Remember! There is the possibility this could be caused by cerebral aneurysm, and the only way to rule out this possibility is for the patient to get a thorough medical examination (CT scan, MRI, angiogram). Naturally, you don't want to scare the patient, but he should be made aware of this potential danger and decide for himself whether he wants to get tests done just to make sure.

Case Study #8: Vasectomy – Postsurgical Testicular Hematoma (Hematocele)

Q: A 30 y/o male patient underwent vasectomy. Following the procedure, a testicular hematoma (about 2.5 cm) developed in his left testicle, and he felt a dragging, aching sensation in his right testicle. Do you think Ru Mo Si Wu Tang combining Gui Zhi Fu Ling Wan will effectively treat this condition?

A: Yes, the blood-quickening stasis-dispelling and network vessel-freeing channel-regulating formula Ru Mo Si Wu Tang will most definitely provide effective treatment for postsurgical testicular hematoma. And for the dragging, aching sensation in his right testicle, you can add Long Yan He (longan seeds), Li Zhi He (litchi seeds), and Ju He (tangerine seeds).

Remember! You should also add Chuan Qi (powder) (quickens blood and transforms stasis); Huang Qin and Huang Bo (clears heat and resolves toxin); and Fu Ling, Bai Zhu, and Ze Xie (disinhibits water, percolates dampness, and drains heat).

Case Study #9: Benign Prostatic Hyperplasia – TCM Pattern Types

Q: A 49 y/o patient has been troubled by symptoms of an enlarged prostate (benign prostatic hyperplasia (BPH)). I prescribed (Yu Sheng) Wu Ling San (Nephritis Formula), which has greatly improved symptoms, but he still has problems with urinary frequency and hesitancy. Can you recommend any changes to the formula I prescribed that would provide better treatment for this patient?

A: Based on the patient's presenting signs and symptoms, BPH can typically be identified as one of the following patterns:

1) Water-damp collecting internally with kidney yang vacuity pattern—Wu Ling San (Nephritis Formula).
2) Kidney yang vacuity pattern—Shen Qi Wan.
3) Heat toxin with damp-heat pattern (usually presents in younger people whose enlarged prostate tends to be caused by infection)—Er Miao San, San Miao Wan, Si Miao San, Zhi Bo Di Huang Tang, Qing Xin Lian Zi Yin, Wu Lin San, or Ba Zheng San.
4) Qi vacuity with blood vacuity pattern—Bu Zhong Yi Qi Tang, Bu Yang Huan Wu Tang, Gui Qi Jian Zhong Tang, and Xue Fu Zhu Yu Tang.
5) Vacuous qi failing to ensure containment pattern—Wu Zi Yan Zong Wan adding Da/Xiao Jin Ying, Bai Guo, Long Yan He, and Li Zhi He.

Case Study #10: Benign Prostatic Hyperplasia – Drug Side Effects

Q: Six years ago, a 58 y/o male patient was diagnosed with enlarged prostate (benign prostatic hyperplasia (BPH)). Since then, he has been taking Western medicine drugs, but his symptoms of incomplete voiding, frequency, urgency, hesitancy, poor and intermittent stream, and terminal dribbling have not improved. Side effects of this medication have resulted in decreased libido, breast enlargement (gynecomastia), dribbling following ejaculation (i.e., 5α-reductase inhibitors interfere with the metabolism of testosterone), constipation (i.e., anticholinergics), and lower abdominal distention and pain.

I prescribed (Yu Sheng) Long Dan Xie Gan Tang including large doses of Huang Qin, Fu Ling, and Ze Xie (8 qian each). Do you think this is the right approach?

A: Long Dan Xie Gan Tang can effectively treat liver channel depressed heat (肝經鬱熱 gān jīng yù rè), damp-heat brewing and binding (濕熱蘊毒 shī rè yùn jié), and damp-heat pouring downward (濕熱下注 shī rè xià zhù) pattern pathoconditions. But enlarged prostate presenting with incomplete voiding, frequency, urgency, hesitancy, poor and intermittent stream, terminal dribbling, and lower abdominal pain does not seem to correlate too well with that pattern.

Typically, a BPH patient presenting with incomplete voiding, frequency, urgency, hesitancy, poor and intermittent stream, and terminal dribbling can be identified as qi vacuity pattern. I think of qi vacuity as a "slackening" or "laxation" of the glandular tissue. In these patients, dribbling will commonly present following ejaculation. As for treatment, you can prescribe a qi-supplementing yang-upbearing formula such as Bu Zhong Yi Qi Tang or a qi- and blood-supplementing formula such as Bu Yang Huan Wu Tang adding The Three Great Yang-Supplementers (incrementally increasing the dose up to a maximum of 5–8 qian each), Huang Bo, Da/Xiao Jin Ying, Bai Guo, and Wu Wei Zi.

However, since your patient is also taking Western medicine drugs that are causing the undesirable side effects of abdominal pain and distention and constipation, I would consider going ahead and prescribing either Tao Ren Cheng Qi Tang (quickens the blood and transforms stasis and precipitates stasis heat), Di Dang Tang (attacks and expels static blood), or Huang Long Tang (clears heat and induces draining precipitation and boosts qi and nourishes the blood). Resolving the constipation should also relieve the pain. If constipation does *not* present, then I would consider prescribing Gui Zhi Fu Ling Wan (quickens the blood and transforms stasis and disperses accumulations and concretions) or Dang Gui Shao Yao San (nourishes the blood and regulates the liver and fortifies the spleen and disinhibits dampness) to directly relieve the pain.

The patient should consult with his Western medical physician about changing the dosage and/or types of drugs, as well as the possibility of gradually weaning away from these drugs altogether.

Once the underlying condition improves, the patient will eventually not have to rely on the Western medicine drugs anyways, thus alleviating these side effects!

Case Study #11: Enlarged Prostate – Liver Channel Depressed Heat & Damp-Heat Brewing Into Heat Toxin Pattern

Q: For patients with enlarged prostate (benign prostatic hyperplasia (BPH)), my first-line formula is Long Dan Xie Gan Tang variant, which effectively resolves inflammation and inhibits the metabolism of testosterone into androgen dihydrotestosterone (DHT) (i.e., antiadrenergic actions). If results are limited or unsatisfactory, then I will apply your "prostate gland laxation" treatment approach adding qi- and yang-supplementing medicinals such as Ren Shen (powder), Rou Gui (powder), and Tu Si Zi. This has proven effective, especially for resolving dribbling urinary incontinence and urinary retention. However, I am not sure how to determine when the patient has been effectively cured and when I should discontinue treatment. How long should I prescribe this TCM formula regimen?

A: BPH can be differentiated into 3 basic pattern types:

1) Qi vacuity ("prostate gland laxation") pattern—This type tends to manifest in older patients with a history of taking libido-boosting supplements (e.g., kidney yang-supplementing TCM medicinals, folk herbs, Western medicine drugs), an active sex life, poor nutritional intake, and a preference for spicy foods. Typically, the presenting symptoms are incomplete voiding, frequency, urgency, hesitancy, poor and intermittent stream, and terminal dribbling, but *no pain.*

2) Depressed blood obstruction pattern—This type tends to manifest in young and middle-aged people who have abstained from sex for long periods of time, enjoy applying pressure on the urethra or perineum during intercourse in order to prolong or restrict ejaculation, or have the habit of sustaining an erection for long durations without ejaculation. In addition to the above symptoms, these patients may also present with *aching* or *distention* in the *perineum.*

3) Liver channel depressed heat (肝經鬱熱 gān jīng yù rè), damp-heat brewing and binding (濕熱蘊毒 shī rè yùn jié), and damp-heat pouring downward (濕熱下注 shī rè xià zhù) pattern—This type tends to manifest in young and middle-aged people who take libido-boosting supplements (e.g., kidney yang-supplementing TCM medicinals, folk herbs, Western medicine drugs), maintain an active sex life, and have a preference for spicy foods. In addition to the above symptoms, these patients may also present with an *aching sensation* in the *ureter*.

Remember! For the treatment of BPH patients presenting with dribbling urinary block (癃閉 lóng bì) the first-line treatment for both TCM (e.g., cold and bitter medicinals) and Western medicine (e.g., alpha-blockers, 5-alpha-reductase inhibitors) involve draining and suppressing. So if you come across a patient who has been administered these types of medicinals and/or drugs for a long period of time, and they either do not or no longer show efficacy, then you must consider the possibility of true cold and false heat pattern.

The onset and progression of this pathocondition varies from patient to patient and may also be dependent upon a healthy lifestyle and diet. Once your patient's symptoms have resolved, then you can begin gradually reducing the dosage of your formula. For instance, you can prescribe 1 packet of decocted medicinals to be taken over a 2 or 3-day period for a couple of weeks and then 1 packet over a 4 or 5-day period for a couple more weeks, continuing in this manner up until complete discontinuation.

In the future, if the patient begins to notice any signs or symptoms, then advise him to come in for a "booster" regimen, which will depend on the severity of the symptoms. If the symptoms are mild, then you can approach it as regulating the constitution, prescribing the reduced dosages as just explained above; but if symptoms are more pronounced, then you may need to go ahead and prescribe the full dosage for a while to get him back on the right track.

Case Study #12: TKM Prostate Lavage Therapy – Be Careful Not to Damage Urethra!

Q: On a related note, there is a Traditional Korean Medicine (TKM) prostate lavage therapy in South Korea that is popular right now and I've heard some people say it is effective. I have not tried this approach because I am concerned about the direct exposure of medicinals irritating the sensitive mucous membranes. What is your opinion on this method?

A: I have not read up on this popular TKM prostate lavage therapy, so I really don't know too much about it. If you do try it clinically, then make sure to carefully monitor the concentration and pH level in order to prevent the potential of damaging the mucous membrane of the urethra. Another thing is you'd have to learn how to irrigate the urethral canal all the way through to the prostate gland, which doesn't sound very easy or pleasant for that matter. Does it require intubation? If so, repeated intubation may cause urethritis. You would have to be very cautious!

Case Study #11: Benign Prostatic Hyperplasia (BPH) – Nocturia

Q: A 52 y/o male patient with enlarged prostate (benign prostatic hyperplasia (BPH)) has to get up to urinate at least 10 times every night and the post-micturition dribbling is so bad that it's like he wets his pants. He is really having a tough time with this. After taking Western medicine drugs, these symptoms improved some to the point where he only has to get up 3–4 times each night to urinate, but he still has pronounced dribbling after voiding.

I prescribed Long Dan Xie Gan Tang adding Bai Jiang Cao, which resulted in resolution of nocturia, but post-micturition dribbling was still present in the daytime. Is this an indication that the prostate remains enlarged and continues obstructing the urethra and urine flow? What is the best approach for this condition?

A: Enlarged prostate (BPH) can be broadly categorized into the following three patterns: qi vacuity, stasis swelling, and heat (i.e., inflammation). The people of South Korea and Taiwan share similar lifestyles (e.g., nutritional intake, societal pressures) and environmental factors (e.g., pollutants containing estrogens and androgens), which can readily lead to inflammation, stasis, depression, and obstruction.

I would continue prescribing Long Dan Xie Gan Tang adding combinations of medicinals such as Cang Zhu, Fu Ling, and Ze Xie; Pu Gong Ying, Lian Xu, and Huang Bo; and Da Huang, Tao Ren, and

Mu Dan Pi. In some cases, you could also consider adding blood-quickening stasis-resolving medicinals like Chuan Qi, Niu Xi, and Chi Shao.

Remember! The key is to accurately identify the pattern, but as you have found in the majority of cases when the onset of BPH occurs at a relatively younger age (< 60 y/o) it can be identified as heat pattern, but when onset occurs in older people (> 60 y/o), you must consider the greater likelihood of either qi vacuity or yang vacuity pattern. The logic here is that those with earlier onset BPH are more likely to have a genetic predisposition, making them more susceptible to the effects of lifestyle habits and environmental factors, which tend to result in heat pattern. Conversely, the etiology of those with later onset more likely result from simple mechanical breakdown, which can be identified as qi or yang vacuity pattern.

Case Study #12: Inguinal Pain

Q: A 43 y/o male patient experienced pain in his left inguinal region that extends over towards the hip area. He went for an examination, but the results of the x-ray and CT scan were inconclusive. Both urine and stool are normal. I prescribed Ru Mo Si Wu Tang adding Ju He, Chuan Lian Zi, Yan Hu Suo, and Mu Xiang. However, I am not really sure about this case and have also considered the possibility of sciatica or a hip (coxofemoral) joint problem. Please offer your guidance and advice on this case.

A: It sounds to me like this is a case involving inguinal hernia or possibly varicocele.

If this is a case involving *varicocele*, you can consider the following therapeutic approaches. For slowly evolving and/or chronic varicocele, presenting with a swollen and hard scrotum, you can prescribe a qi-moving pain-relieving and hardness-softening bind-dissipating formula such as Ju He Wan adding Long Yan He and Li Zhi He. For paroxysmal varicocele of relatively rapid onset, you can prescribe a liver and gallbladder repletion fire-draining and lower burner damp-heat-clearing formula such as Long Dan Xie Gan Tang adding Ju He and Li Zhi He. And during acute flare-ups, presenting with pronounced swelling and heat, subtract The Three Great

Yang-Supplementers (Gan Jiang, Fu Zi, and Rou Gui) and add Long Dan Cao and Huang Qin.

Inguinal hernia (as well as other types of abdominal hernias) may also present with pain radiating downwards to the testicles or upwards over the abdomen into the chest, for which you can prescribe a qi-supplementing yang-upbearing formula such as Bu Zhong Yi Qi Tang (including large doses of Huang Qi) adding Long Yan He, Li Zhi He, Ju He, Wu Zhu Yu, Shan Zha, Huang Qin, and Chuan Lian Zi; or a kidney-warming cold-dispelling, qi-moving liver-coursing, and hernia-dispersing pain-relieving formula such as San Ceng Hui Xiang Wan adding Huang Qi, Yuan Hu, Mu Xiang, Long Yan He, Li Zhi He, and Shan Zha.

In times of antiquity, when physical activity and labor were the norm, hernias were a very common malady! In our modern day, *hernia* is much rarer and usually only occurs in weightlifters or movers. For these types of patients, a blood-nourishing blood-quickening, stasis dispelling pain-relieving, and network vessel-freeing channel-regulating formula such as Ru Mo Si Wu Tang, Ge Xia Zhu Yu Tang, or Xun Qi Huo Xue Tang will provide effective treatment.

Ru Mo Si Wu Tang variant will also effectively treat *varicocele*, especially if it results from overexertion such as in weightlifters, martial artists who practice Iron Crotch exercises (swinging weights from their testicles!), and even those who consciously restrain ejaculation upon erection. If there is pronounced heat (upon palpation or the patient feels heat and distention), then add Huang Qin, Huang Bo, Long Dan Cao, Zhi Zi, Bai Zhu, Fu Ling, and Ze Xie.

Even if further examination confirms *hip joint inflammation* (*synovitis*) or *sciatica*, the broad-spectrum actions of TCM medicinals (e.g., blood-quickening stasis-transforming, heat-clearing toxin-resolving, and water-disinhibiting by bland percolation) will provide effective treatment for these pathoconditions as well.

X. SKIN DISORDERS

This chapter will discuss the most common skin disorders—rashes, warts, seborrheic dermatitis, atopic dermatitis, eczema, and pruritis.

Section 1: Rashes

Case Study #1: Urticaria vs. Pityriasis Rosea

Q: Are there any differences in the treatment of urticaria and pityriasis rosea?

A: *Urticaria* is a hypersensitivity (allergic) reaction presenting as well-circumscribed superficial plaques (wheals) or angioedema (swelling), which may be either pale (白疹 bái zhěn) or red (erythema) (赤疹 chì zhěn), itchy, and prickly with a burning sensation. Typically, the skin manifestations resolve spontaneously anywhere from a few minutes to 72 hours.

Pityriasis rosea is a self-limiting rash likely of viral origin that typically presents with prodromal symptoms (i.e., flu-like) and a single coin-shaped "herald patch" (pink-colored macule) a couple of weeks prior to the subsequent eruption of pink-colored oval, scaly macules and plaques over the entire trunk, which may or may not be itchy (pruritis). Once these macules and plaques have resolved many patients will be left with a postinflammatory hypopigmentation or hyperpigmentation that looks like tinea versicolor, which may spontaneously resolve in a few months time.

At the onset, both pathoconditions can be identified as exterior wind-heat pattern, and in the chronic stage, *urticaria* may be identified as blood desiccation pattern, unlike *pityriasis rosea* which seldom presents as blood desiccation pattern unless the patient has been administered oral and/or topical corticosteroids or autoimmune suppressants. For *pityriasis rosea*, you should also prescribe topical TCM medicinal pastes (ointments) and administer the therapeutic regimen up until there aren't any more plaques remaining. In both pathoconditions, the administration of TCM medicinals will ensure a faster and more complete resolution of symptoms.

Case Study #2: Urticaria – I Got It At the Spa!

Q: One week ago, a 52 y/o female went to the spa and by the time she got home red wheals (hives) appeared all over her body. She went to a dermatologist who prescribed oral and topical medication that wasn't effective.

I prescribed Da Qing Long Tang adding Huang Qin and Bai Xian Pi. After 1 week of administration the color of the wheals had lightened. How long do you think it will take to treat this pathocondition?

A: Urticaria can be identified as an exterior wind-heat pattern, and it's not difficult to treat at all. You can consider prescribing a sweat-effusing exterior-resolving and lung-diffusing wind-dispelling formula such as Da Qing Long Tang, Yue Bi Tang, Yang Dan Tang, Gui Zhi Ma Huang Ge Ban Tang, or Bai Hu Tang. Typically, it takes about 1 week for the redness to lighten and 2–3 weeks before the lesions completely fade.

Case Study #3: Dormant Papules (Chronic Intermittent Urticaria)

Q: About 6 months ago this patient developed itchy wheals (hives) that appeared sporadically and randomly dispersed over the body. The patient's dermatologist diagnosed her with chronic intermittent urticaria. During flare-ups, the patient would take oral antihistamines or receive a shot, which would resolve the symptoms for a few days, but then recur again. I prescribed Gui Zhi Ma Huang Ge Ban Tang and Da Qing Long Tang, which only provided temporary results just like the Western medicine treatment. Please offer your guidance and advice on this case.

A: Dormant papules (隱疹 yǐn zhěn), also known as wind papules (urticaria) (風疹 fēng zhěn) and wind pimples (風疙瘩 fēng gē da), correlates with chronic intermittent urticaria. Based on your description, it sounds like your patient's pathocondition can be identified as blood desiccation with exterior wind-cold pattern. Thus, you can prescribe (Yu Sheng) Blood Desiccation Formula adding Gan Jiang, Fu Zi, Huang Qin, Ma Huang, and Gui Zhi. If severe pruritis presents, then bleed Da Zhui (GV14) (above, on, and below) and needle Feng Chi (GB20), Tian Zhu (UB10), San Yin Jiao (SP6), Yin

Ling Quan (SP9), and Xue Hai (SP10). You should also remind the patient to keep the body warm!

Case Study #4: Generalized Dormant Papules

Q: A 35 y/o female patient, who has taken daily dosages of aspirin for many years, first began presenting with intermittent generalized dormant papules (chronic intermittent urticaria) 2 years ago following the common cold (external contraction). Ever since then, whenever she catches a cold with a fever or her body temperature rises, a rash with itchy wheals of various sizes will present, and after scratching, they will spread and merge into larger lesions. She tried taking Western medicine drugs, but complained of side effects involving knee pain, so she discontinued treatment.

The edematous plaques (wheals (hives)) are pinkish colored. When she eats spicy foods or adds certain seasonings she becomes lethargic and feels stiffness and pain in the nape and neck (right side). I want to prescribe Huang Lian Jie Du Tang adding Pu Gong Ying. Do you think this will be effective?

A: Common side effects of aspirin are rash, GI tract problems (e.g., ulcerations, pain, heartburn), and drowsiness. If the rash you describe is indeed a side effect of the aspirin, I would identify this as blood heat pattern and prescribe a blood-nourishing yin-enriching formula variant such as Di Gu Pi Yin. However, it would appear unlikely that after all these years of taking aspirin this normally mild drug would suddenly induce previously non-existent side effects.

A skin rash resulting from external contraction (i.e., microbial infection) can be identified as exterior wind-heat with blood heat pattern. For this pattern type, you can administer a sweat-effusing exterior-resolving and lung-diffusing wind-dispelling formula such as Da Qing Long Tang, Yue Bi Tang, Yang Dan Tang, Gui Zhi Ma Huang Ge Ban Tang, or Bai Hu Tang. Just make sure to include Huang Qin, Sheng Shi Gao, Zhi Mu, Qing Hao, Di Gu Pi, and Lian Qiao in your formula.

A pink-colored rash suggests blood desiccation pattern. If spicy foods and seasonings trigger this type of rash, then it can similarly be identified as blood desiccation with blood heat pattern. Remember!

Winter itch (xerotic eczema) is another possibility for patients in northern temperate climates, as well as elderly patients in subtropical and tropical coastal climates during the winter months. For this pattern type, you can administer a blood-nourishing yin-enriching dryness-moistening formula such as (Yu Sheng) Blood Desiccation Formula adding Gan Jiang, Fu Zi, Huang Qin, Sheng Shi Gao, Ma Huang, and Gui Zhi (or Jing Jie and Fang Feng); and if blood heat pattern is more pronounced, then add Qing Hao, Zhi Mu, Di Gu Pi, and Lian Qiao.

Sometimes patients with a combination of different symptoms and pathoconditions—a "potpourri," if you will, try to link everything together into a compelling storyline that fits their own diagnostic narrative. You should listen to this story and entertain all possibilities, but don't put too much credence into its veracity! The physician must carefully evaluate the patient's history, signs and symptoms, and diagnostic indicators to conduct accurate pattern identification as the basis for determining treatment. Remember! You must be confident in your own judgment and decisions. Don't just let others lead you around by the nose!

Case Study #5: Body Temperature Increase Induces Red, Itchy Wheals and Papules

Q: A 20 y/o female has a history of developing red, itchy wheals and papules on her skin every time she exercises, takes a hot shower, or eats hot soup—basically anytime her body is exposed to heat or her body temperature rises. During these eruptions, if she scratches her skin, the rash will expand into larger-sized pink-colored welts. Recently, she said that red wheals covered her entire body, erupting intermittently and resolving spontaneously.

She is aware of foods that commonly trigger allergic reactions in people so she avoids these foods. The patient half-jokingly told me that her condition is so annoying that "Sometimes, even when I kiss my boyfriend I get a skin rash!" I really don't know what to prescribe for this case. I was considering Yue Bi Tang adding Jing Jie and Fang Feng. Do you think this would be a good approach?

A: This sounds like a case of blood desiccation with blood heat pattern. I would consider prescribing a blood-nourishing yin-enriching dryness-moistening formula such as Blood Desiccation Formula adding Qing Hao, Zhi Mu, and Di Gu Pi (or Lian Qiao, Pu Gong Ying, and Jin Yin Hua); an yin-enriching blood-cooling formula such as Di Gu Pi Yin or Xi Jiao Di Huang Tang; or a Shao Yang-harmonizing formula such as Xiao Chai Hu Tang adding Qing Hao, Zhi Mu, and Di Gu Pi. If itchiness (pruritis) is pronounced, then you can add Zao Jiao Ci (quickens the blood, disperses swelling, and expels pus), Ji Li Zi (calms and courses the liver and dispels wind), and Lu Lu Tong (expels wind and frees the network vessels and disinhibits water and eliminates dampness). If exterior wind-cold (or wind-heat) pattern present, then add medicinals such as Ma Huang, Rou Gui, and Sheng Shi Gao or Jing Jie (effuses the exterior and dissipates wind and outthrusts papules and heals sores) and Fang Feng (effuses the exterior and dissipates wind and overcomes dampness and relieves pain).

Additionally, in cases presenting with severe pruritis, you should bleed Da Zhui (GV14) (above, on, and below), Wei Zhong (UB40), and Cun Kou (Tai Yuan (LU9)); and then needle Feng Chi (GB20), Tian Zhu (UB10), He Gu (LI4), Qu Chi (LI11), Chi Ze (LU5), Zu San Li (ST36), San Yin Jiao (SP6), and Kun Lun (UB60).

For these types of patients with *urticaria*, you could also try the lung-diffusing heat-draining and water-dissipating swelling-dispersing formula Yue Bi Tang or the sweat-effusing exterior-resolving with internal heat-clearing formula Da Qing Long Tang adding Jing Jie and Fang Feng. This may be an effective approach for treating the wind-cold exterior repletion with interior heat pattern that many South Korean patients may present with as a result of living in a cold, temperate climate, eating spicy foods, and drinking hard liquor.

This is similar for *atopic dermatitis* patients who typically present with exterior wind-heat pattern at the onset or during acute flare-ups and blood desiccation pattern (e.g., blood desiccation with heat, blood desiccation with exterior wind-heat or exterior wind-heat-damp, blood desiccation with cold, blood desiccation with exterior cold and yang vacuity) in the post-acute and chronic stages.

Remember! Skin pathoconditions can be tricky, especially if they evolve into the chronic stages, during which true cold and false heat (真寒假熱 zhēn hán jià rè) pattern may present, so you must closely examine and evaluate the patient to accurately identify pattern identification.

Case Study #6: Urticaria – Types and Patterns

Q: Are there any distinguishing differences between wind papules, dormant papules, and urticaria? What triggers these eruptions? In my clinical experience, it seems to be that certain foods, drug reactions, and the common cold precipitate flare-ups; and sometimes there is no identifiable precipitating factor (idiopathic origin). Western medicine will prescribe antihistamines, which may initially resolve the pathocondition, but often 1–2 days later the rash will recur. What's the best way to treat urticaria?

A: Wind papules (風疹 fēng zhěn), dormant papules (隱疹 yǐn zhěn), and wind pimples (風疙瘩 fēng gē da) are among the terms described in TCM classical texts that correlate with urticaria. Here in Taiwan, most patients with urticaria can be identified as blood desiccation with yang vacuity and a bit of exterior pattern. Patients with this pattern typically present with pink papules, wheals, or patches; or pinkish to white-colored lines appearing when the surface of the skin is scratched (dermatographia).

For this pathocondition, I typically prescribe Xue Ku Fang adding The Three Great Yang-Supplementers and Huang Qin; and after administration, if subsequent scratching results in mild redness and serous exudate, then I will add Sheng Shi Gao. If external contraction (i.e., microbial infection) was the initial precipitating factor and the urticaria subsequently recurs, then I would prescribe a sweat-effusing exterior-resolving and lung-diffusing wind-dispelling formula such as Gui Zhi Ma Huang Ge Ban Tang or Da Qing Long Tang adding Huang Qin and Sheng Shi Gao.

Spontaneous bleeding of the skin (urticarial vasculitis) can be identified as blood heat pattern for which you can prescribe a blood-nourishing yin-enriching formula such as Di Gu Pi Yin, Jia Wei Xiao Chai Hu Tang, or Xi Jiao Di Huang Tang; or possibly an outthrusting the exterior with coolness and acridity and heat-clearing toxin-resolving formula such as Yin Qiao San adding Qing Hao, Zhi Mu, and Di Gu Pi.

In the majority of cases, the cause is likely unknown (idiopathic). However, if it happens to be a manifestation of inflammatory connective tissue disease (e.g., systemic lupus erythematosus, Sjogren syndrome), then you should prescribe the heat-clearing toxin-resolving and yin vacuity-heat clearing yin-enriching formula (Yu Sheng)

Hyperactive Immune Formula (including large doses of The Three Yellows) adding up to 8 liang of Sheng Shi Gao.

In Taiwan, unlike South Korea, we must consider the possibility of dengue fever; and particularly the severe symptoms resulting from becoming infected with the virus a second time, which may lead to dengue hemorrhagic fever (DHF)—purpuric lesions (petechiae, purpura, and ecchymoses), bleeding gums, hematemesis, melena, shock, and circulatory failure. If dengue fever is diagnosed, then you must add Ma Huang, Xing Ren, Di Long, Bai Zhu, Fu Ling, and Ze Xie into the Hyperactive Immune Formula mentioned above. In these severe cases, Western medicine treatment involves administration of corticosteroids, intravenous immunoglobulins, intubation, and plasmapharesis. Fortunately, South Korea doesn't have the dengue virus so you don't need to worry about this!

Case Study #7: Antihistamines Discontinued – Rash Returns

Q: Two months ago, a generalized rash suddenly developed over a 43 y/o female patient's entire body. There was *no* specific herald patch as in pityriasis rosea; instead, small papules first appeared which then developed into large wheals. She was administered antihistamines which relieved symptoms for a while, but the rash returned after discontinuing the medication.

I prescribed Da Qing Long Tang adding Huang Qin (8 qian). The patient felt that the TCM regimen has provided better overall efficacy than Western medicine, but the small papules still come back. Can you suggest a better approach for treating this pathocondition?

A: The key to pattern identification for wind papules (urticaria) is coloration. Red or pink-red colored papules, macules, and wheals can be identified as *exterior wind-heat* pattern. Pink or flesh-colored macules and wheals and pinkish or white-colored dermatographia can be identified as *blood desiccation* pattern.

South Koreans eat lots of hot-spicy acrid foods (e.g., chili, garlic, seasonings) and enjoy drinking hard liquor. People whose diet consists of excessive consumption of hot-spicy and hot acrid foods over a long period of time are naturally predisposed to developing yang vacuity constitutions with insufficiency of essence-blood (精血不足 jīng xuè bù zú) and insecurity of the defensive exterior (衛表不固 wèi biǎo bù gù). This type of yang vacuity tends to *not* be responsive to highly acrid and highly hot kidney yang-supplementing medicinals (e.g., The Three Great Yang-Supplementers) and often requires adding warm acrid orifice-opening medicinals (e.g., Chuan (Hua) Jiao, Xi Xin, Wu Zhu Yu) into the formula as well. I attribute this phenomenon to warm acrid cell membrane receptors within the body "getting used to" and "building up a tolerance for" the constant warm acrid stimulation from the diet. Eventually they even become unresponsive to the actions of warm acrid yang-supplementing medicinals, requiring medicinals that "open the orifices" with warmth and acridity. Thus, based on this observation alone, I would expect that many of your patients could be identified as *blood desiccation with yang vacuity and exterior wind* pattern. You can consider the following therapeutic approaches:

In cases of *exterior wind-heat* (or *wind-heat-damp*) and *externally contracted wind-heat* pattern, patients will incur a sudden eruption of red wind papules (urticaria) or hives on the skin. For these patients, you can prescribe a sweat-effusing exterior-resolving and lung-diffusing wind-dispelling formula such as Ma Huang Gui Zhi Ge Ban Tang, Da Qing Long Tang, Yue Bi Tang, Jing Fang Bai Du San, or Ren Shen Bai Du San adding Sheng Shi Gao and Huang Qin. If itch (pruritis) is pronounced, then add Zao Jiao Ci, Ci Ji Li, and Lu Lu Tong. If swelling (e.g., hives, angioedema) and heat (i.e., red or pink-red colored) are pronounced, then make sure to include large doses of Sheng Shi Gao and Huang Qin; bleed Da Zhui (GV14) (above, on, and below), Cun Kou (Tai Yuan (LU9)), Shang Yang (LI1), and Li Dui (ST45); and needle Feng Chi (GB20), Tian Zhu (UB10), He Gu (LI4), Zu San Li (ST36), Wei Zhong (UB40), and Hou Xi (SI3).

In cases of *blood desiccation with yang vacuity and exterior wind* pattern, you can prescribe Blood Desiccation Formula adding Ma Huang, Gui Zhi, Jing Jie, and Fang Feng. If dermatographia presents, you should add large doses of Gan Jiang and Fu Zi, and if necessary, medicinals that "open the orifices" with warmth and acridity such as Chuan (Hua) Jiao, Xi Xin, and Wu Zhu Yu. And if itch (pruritis) is pronounced, then add Zao Jiao Ci, Ci Ji Li, and Lu Lu Tong. Also, warm needle the acupoints He Gu (LI4), Shou San Li (LI10), Zu San Li (ST36), San Yin Jiao (SP6), Yin Ling Quan (SP9), and Xue Hai (SP10).

Encourage patients receiving long-term administration of antihistamines to gradually discontinue those drugs, and make sure your formula includes Ma Huang and Rou Gui (promote sweating and resolve the exterior, diffuse the lung and calm panting, disinhibit water and dispersc swelling, free the nasal orifice, outthrust papules, and relieve itch). The actions of Ma Huang and Rou Gui will provide an effective alternative to antihistamines and in combination with the other medicinals in the formula composition will resolve symptoms, treat the root, and regulate the constitution to ensure the pathocondition is cured.

Remember! For those patients with unresolved *exterior wind-heat pattern* whose wind papules (urticaria) reemerge or those who incur a subsequent external contraction, the wind papules (urticaria) are more likely to affect the trachea and bronchi, causing swelling of the mucosa (angioedema) that may induce asthma and possibly even be life-threatening if the airway becomes obstructed.

Case Study #8: Wind Papules and Heat Hives – Can I Prescribe The Three Great Yang-Supplementers?

Q: Towards the end of spring, a middle-aged female patient suddenly developed small red and itchy plaques that later enlarged and spread into more diffusely distributed wheals after being scratched. She has been taking antihistamines on and off since then, but every time she discontinues the medication, the rash comes back again.

I identified this as blood desiccation with yang vacuity and exterior pattern and originally had considered prescribing Blood Desiccation Formula adding Sheng Shi Gao, Huang Qin, Ma Huang, Gan Jiang, Fu Zi, and Rou Gui. The problem is that she also happens to be hypersensitive to heat. Any time she gets in the sunshine, feels hot, and sweats a lot, red plaques and wheals (heat hives (aka cholinergic urticaria)) appear on her skin. Thus, I am concerned that prescribing The Three Great Yang-Supplementers will further exacerbate the "heat" of her pathocondition.

A: Yes, in this case it might be better to forgo the blood-nourishing yin-enriching dryness-moistening Blood Desiccation Formula adding The Three Great Yang-Supplementers! Instead, I would consider prescribing the fleshy exterior-harmonizing and evil-expelling itch-relieving formula variant Gui Zhi Ma Huang Ge Ban Tang. If severe itch presents, then add Zao Jiao Ci; and if serous exudate presents, then add Sheng Shi Gao and Huang Qin. Advise the patient to continue taking the antihistamines at first, but then gradually discontinue. If the Gui Zhi Ma Huang Ge Ban Tang does *not* offer noticeable efficacy, then add in small doses of Gan Jiang, Fu Zi, and Huang Qin.

Typically, South Korean patients who live in a cold weather climate and eat lots of spicy foods would present as exterior wind-cold with a tendency towards yang vacuity pattern, requiring administration of yang-supplementing medicinals. However, the key factor here is the *heat-to-cold* ratio, meaning that you must seek the optimal balance between the *heat* medicinals and *cold* medicinals.

In this patient with both wind papules and heat hives (cholinergic urticaria), it may be good to play it on the safe side. And if it is necessary to prescribe yang-supplementing medicinals, then start out with low doses of Gan Jiang and Fu Zi (1 qian each) along with your choice of The Three Yellows (a total of 3 qian). If heat is pronounced, then bleed to drain heat, and needle acupoints that resolve the exterior (do *not* select acupoints that supplement blood or nourish blood!).

Case Study #9: Accumulated Heat Results in Eruption of Papules – Miliaria

Q: A 19 y/o male patient of mine explained that he works at a Chinese restaurant, which is really hot inside with poor circulation. Last winter, after getting off work one afternoon, he went to exercise at the gym. Immediately after his workout, small, rice-sized red papules erupted over his entire body along with severe itch. A dermatologist prescribed medication, which helped resolve the itch a bit until the rash spontaneously resolved, but hasn't been effective at preventing subsequent repeated episodes. Now, this winter is even worse, with these papules erupting even upon mild heat. Despite it being winter, it looks a lot like heat rash to me. What do you think?

A: Yes, this does sound like a case of miliaria (aka heat rash or prickly heat). For this type of accumulated heat resulting in an eruption of papules, or any type of wind papules for that matter, you must observe the color. Typically, patients living in cold weather climates who like eating spicy foods that present with this type of rash can be identified as exterior wind-heat with yang vacuity pattern. For this pattern type, you should bleed Da Zhui (GV14) (above, on, and below) and prescribe a fleshy exterior-harmonizing and evil-expelling itch-relieving formula such as Gui Zhi Ma Huang Ge Ban Tang adding Huang Qin and Sheng Shi Gao (if heat is more pronounced) or Gan Jiang and Fu Zi (if cold is more pronounced).

Remember! People with high-strung (nervous) personalities tend to have a more intensified reaction to stimulus. This specific mechanism may involve the free nerve endings, which extend into the mid layers of the dermis and surround the hair follicles. Thus, for these patients, I would also consider adding in large doses of blood-nourishing spirit-calming medicinals such as Da Zao and Long Yan Rou.

Case Study #10: Alcohol and Spicy Foods Induce Itchy Wind Papules and Maculopapular Eruptions

Q: About 3 months ago, after a night out partying and drinking alcohol with friends, the next day this 29 y/o female patient began feeling a prickly, painful sensation on her scalp. She went to see a dermatologist who prescribed medication which relieved the symptoms.

Not long afterwards she went abroad and faced a lot of pressure, and the red macules (erythematous rash) recurred, presenting as itchy red spots on her head, face, torso, arms, and legs, every time she drank alcohol or ate spicy foods. I administered Blood Desiccation Formula adding Huang Qin and Sheng Shi Gao, but it was not effective at all. Do you think Di Gu Pi Yin variant would be better? Please offer your advice and consultation.

A: You should first make sure to clearly examine whether the skin lesions are macules (flat skin lesions differing in color from the surrounding skin), papules (small, palpable skin lesion < 1 cm in diameter), vesicles (small fluid-containing blister), bullae (large fluid-containing blister), pustules (vesicles filled with pus), wheals (hives), or plaques (palpable, usually raised lesion > 1 cm). Also, is the skin itchy?

Based on the prickly, painful sensation in her scalp, it sounds to me like a case of itchy wind papules (風疹搔癢 fēng zhěn sāo yǎng) and maculopapular eruptions (班疹 bān zhěn), which can be identified as exterior wind-heat pattern. If the papules are bright red in color, then this can further be classified as construction-defense disharmony (營衛不和 yíng wèi bù hé).

As for treatment, I would prescribe a fleshy exterior-harmonizing and evil-expelling itch-relieving formula such as Gui Zhi Ma Huang Ge Ban Tang adding Sheng Shi Gao or a sweat-effusing exterior-resolving and lung-diffusing wind-dispelling formula such as Da Qing Long Tang or Yue Bi Tang; bleed Da Zhui (GV14) (above, on, and below), Wei Zhong (UB40), and the well points of the three yang channels on the hands and feet; and needle Feng Chi (GB20), Tian Zhu (UB10), He Gu (LI4), Zu San Li (ST36), Wei Zhong (UB40), and Hou Xi (SI3).

Case Study #11: Pruritic Maculopapular Eruptions

Q: I have a 37 y/o male patient with idiopathic pruritis that develops into maculopapular eruptions (a mix of macules (flat) and papules (raised)) after scratching and then spontaneously resolves. I do*n't* think this rash is a result of hypersensitivity to food, clothing, or environmental factors; and the patient does*n't* have night sweating or late afternoon tidal heat. For these reasons, I decided to prescribe Di Gu Pi Yin variant, which helped relieve the symptoms, but did not completely cure the pathocondition.

A: That's a good formula. However, the blood-nourishing and -cooling yin-enriching actions of Di Gu Pi Yin are more directed at treating dark red (purple or black) macules or lesions (e.g., petechiae, purpura, ecchymoses), whereas vesicular and papular eruptions can be identified as exterior wind-heat pattern. Thus, I would also consider adding Qing Hao, Zhi Mu, Ma Huang, and Gui Zhi along with Zao Jiao Ci (quickens the blood, disperses swelling, and expels pus), Ji Li Zi (calms and courses the liver and dispels wind), and Lu Lu Tong (expels wind and frees the network vessels and disinhibits water and eliminates dampness) to resolve the itchy papules. If heat is pronounced, then add Sheng Shi Gao and Bai Xian Pi; and if intense itching presents, then add She Tui (treats all types of skin sores) and Chan Tui (courses wind, dissipates heat, outthrusts papules and relieves itch).

Case Study #12: Is It Recurrent Herpes Zoster?

Q: A 51 y/o female patient has a history of recurrent herpes zoster that appears on her left arm during times of fatigue. The lesions present as vesicular eruptions with burning and prickly pain that last for 1–2 weeks and then spontaneously resolve.

A: It doesn't sound to me like the recurring vesicles on your patient's left arm would be herpes zoster, but it may be herpes simplex. For recurrent herpes simplex (HSV-1) try prescribing a heat-clearing toxin-resolving, swelling-dispersing hardness-breaking, and blood-quickening pain-relieving formula such as Xian Fang Huo Ming Yin adding Huang Qin and Pu Gong Ying.

Case Study #13: Dyshidrotic Eczema (Pompholyx) – Acute and Subacute vs. Chronic Stages

Q: I prescribed Xian Fang Huo Ming Yin combining Ma Xing Yi Gan Tang to treat a patient diagnosed with subacute dyshidrotic eczema (pompholyx). This has not proven ultimately effective, as the condition seems to get better for a while and then worsens again. I am considering adding a small dose of Xiong Huang (0.8 g/day). Please offer your advice on this case.

A: In the acute and subacute stages of pompholyx and palmoplantar pustulosis (PPP) presenting with pruritic vesicular eruptions, I will have the patient soak their feet in (Yu Sheng) Athlete's Foot/Pompholyx Infusion (contains Xiong Huang) and prescribe oral administration of Ma Xing Yi Gan Tang. If this isn't effective, I will consider adding Huang Qin, Lian Qiao, Zao Jiao Ci, Lu Lu Tong, and Ci Ji Li. Typically, unless it is a case involving sexually transmitted diseases (STDs), I only prescribe Xiong Huang for topical application (as I have done here) due to its high toxicity.

If the patient has been administered corticosteroids, antibiotics, or other immunosuppressive drugs for long periods of time and/or the pathocondition has entered the chronic stage, presenting with pronounced thickening of the cornified layer (stratum corneum) down to the translucent layer (stratum lucidum) with a clear or pearly white appearance and scaling, then this can be identified as blood desiccation pattern. Thus, you should prescribe a blood-nourishing yin-enriching dryness-moistening formula variation such as (Yu Sheng) Blood Desiccation Formula, perform acupuncture (warm needling) on the corresponding channels of the affected hands and feet, and have the patient topically apply Purple Cloud Ointment or sesame oil to the thickened cracked skin.

Remember! In the acute and subacute stages, soaking in Athlete's Foot/Pompholyx Infusion *will* provide effective relief for these types of vesicular and suppurative eruptions presenting in pompholyx, PPP, or dermatophyte infection (i.e., tinea pedis (aka athlete's foot or Hong Kong foot)), but *not* in the chronic stages!

Case Study #14: Recalcitrant Dyshidrotic Eczema – Exterior Wind Damp-Heat

Q: About 1 year ago, a 27 y/o female patient felt severe fatigue prior to incurring a sudden eruption of fluid-filled vesicles on her hands and feet that produce serous exudate after breaking. She went to see a dermatologist who prescribed topical and oral corticosteroids and ultraviolet light therapy (psoralen and ultraviolet A (PUVA)). At the onset, the skin on the palms of her hands and soles of her feet were red colored, but after receiving over 8 months of Western medicine treatment the skin is now pink.

At first, I prescribed Xian Fang Huo Ming Yin variant, which resulted in the vesicles completely disappearing in a short period of time. But 10 days later the vesicles abruptly erupted again! It's been 3 months now and this cycle of remission and recurrence has continued, with both hands (cheiropompholyx) and feet (pedopompholyx) intensely itchy when the vesicles begin to reappear.

Over the past year, I have tried a number of different formulas: Xian Fang Huo Ming Yin adding Long Dan Cao (8 qian), Ci Ji Li (1 liang), Huang Qin (1 liang), and even small doses of Xiong Huang; (Yu Sheng) Seborrheic Dermatitis Formula adding Long Dan Cao, Ci Ji Li, and Huang Qin; and recently I have switched over to Blood Desiccation Formula combining Ma Xing Yi Gan Tang adding Long Dan Cao. However, the recurrent cycle continues—vesicles suddenly appear in procession every 3–4 days, clear fluid (serous exudate) oozes after breaking, blisters peel off, and the skin turns a pinkish-red and becomes dry with painful fissures opening up (especially in cold winter months).

A: This sounds like a case of recalcitrant dyshidrotic eczema (recalcitrant palmoplantar pompholyx or chronic pompholyx). This pathocondition can be identified as exterior wind-damp-heat pattern, which has not entered the blood desiccation level yet.

Thus, I would prescribe Xian Fang Huo Ming Yin (including a large dose of Sheng Shi Gao) adding Ma Huang, Xing Ren, Yi Yi Ren, and Huang Qin (large dose). In addition, you should bleed Da Zhui (GV14) (above, on, and below), Cun Kou (Tai Yuan (LU9)), and the well points on the hands and feet; soak the affected areas in (Yu Sheng) Athlete's Foot/Pompholyx Infusion; and needle exterior-resolving acupoints (e.g., Feng Chi (GB20), Tian Zhu (UB10), He Gu (LI4), Wai Guan (TB5), Zhong Zhu (TB3), Hou Xi (SI3), Chi Ze (LU5), Kun Lun (UB60), Di Wu Hui (GB42), and Tai Chong (LV3)).

Continue with this regimen until there have been no recurring exacerbations for 3–5 months and/or after incurring 2–3 external contractions (common colds) without any exacerbations. That's when you can gradually discontinue treatment and consider this pathocondition cured!

Case Study #15: Damp Papules

Q: This patient has suffered from damp papules (eczema) for more than 10 years. It looks a bit like athlete's foot (tinea pedis). The soles of both feet are covered with layers of scabby plaques, but with *no* itching, and for the most part, *no* pus, except for a bit at the center of the scabs where pustules form, and when the pustules break open, the scabby area enlarges.

The patient has tried using many different types of oral and topical medications, but none have proven effective. In fact, these medications have seemed to exacerbate the spread of the crusty, scabby plaques. Histologic examination revealed a special type of skin disease that I have never studied about before. Can you offer any suggestions or advice about this patient's condition?

A: Eczema is a broad term that denotes any type of inflammation of the skin. Based on your description, I would prescribe the topical (Yu Sheng) Athlete's Foot/Pompholyx Infusion (patient soaks the affected area in an infusion of water and medicinal solution) and an oral TCM formula decoction.

If the affected lesions *present* with a rancid odor, then I would prescribe a heat-clearing toxin-resolving, swelling-dispersing hardness-breaking, and blood-quickening formula such as Xian Fang Huo Ming Yin adding Ma Huang, Xing Ren, and Yi Yi Ren; bleed the foot well points; and needle Tai Chong (LV3) and Di Wu Hui (GB42).

If there is *no* rancid odor, then I would prescribe a blood-nourishing yin-enriching dryness-moistening formula such as Blood Desiccation Formula adding Ma Huang, Xing Ren, Yi Yi Ren, Gan Jiang, Fu Zi, and Huang Qin; and acupuncture (warm needle) acupoints on channels that correspond with the site of the lesions such as Tai Chong (LV3), Di Wu Hui (GB42), Tai Bai (SP3), Gong Sun (SP4), Ran Gu (KI2), Tai Xi (KI3), Jin Men (UB63), and Kun Lun (UB60).

You mentioned that the "histologic examination revealed a special type of skin disease." This suggests the possibility of palmoplantar pustulosis (PPP), which shares similarities to psoriasis, or it may be some type of rare fungal infection. Regardless, the TCM therapeutic approach will be the same.

Case Study #16: Is It Pompholyx?

Q: A pediatric patient of mine presented with itchy vesicles and occasional oozing of foul-smelling discharge (purulent exudate) on his hands and feet that looks like dyshidrotic eczema (pompholyx). I prescribed Xian Fang Huo Ming Yin adding Huang Qin (1.5 liang) and Sheng Shi Gao (2 liang), but it wasn't effective. Then, I switched to (Yu Sheng) Seborrheic Dermatitis Formula, administering it for 2 months without any noticeable efficacy.

Do you think this could be atopic dermatitis, folliculitis, or nummular dermatitis? Would pompholyx get worse during the winter? Would pompholyx present with skin eruptions extending up to the wrists and ankles?

A: Dyshidrotic eczema (pompholyx) may occur all year round. In my clinical experience, extremes of cold or hot weather do *not* necessarily exacerbate this condition, though some patients may be more sensitive to seasonal changes than others. You might as well try prescribing an exterior-resolving dampness eliminating and lung qi-diffusing and disinhibiting formula such as Ma Xing Yi Gan Tang adding Sheng Shi Gao, Huang Qin, Zao Jiao Ci, Lu Lu Tong, and Ci Ji Li. The treatment approach involves first expressing and expelling pus outward and relieving itch. No itch means no scratching, which will minimize the chances of secondary infection.

If indeed your patient has atopic dermatitis, then you can consider prescribing Blood Desiccation Formula adding The Three Great Yang-Supplementers, Ma Huang, Xing Ren, Yi Yi Ren, Sheng Shi Gao, and Huang Qin. In my experience, atopic dermatitis *does* tend to get worse during the winter months.

Case Study #17: Pompholyx – Toes

Q: A 28 y/o female patient has had eruptions of itchy vesicles on her toes for the past 6 months. She was diagnosed with dyshidrotic eczema (pompholyx) by a dermatologist and has tried topical corticosteroids and ultraviolet light among other therapies, but nothing has worked. After she scratches these vesicles, foul-smelling pus oozes out and it becomes extremely itchy.

I prescribed Xian Fang Huo Ming Yin combining Ma Xing Yi Gan Tang along with the (Yu Sheng) Athlete's Foot/Pompholyx Infusion foot soak. Do you think this is a good approach?

A: Yes, this should effectively treat her condition. If you want to speed up the process, then bleed Da Zhui (GV14) (above, on, and below), and the foot well points on the affected side(s); and needle the Toe Crevice Acupoints (four acupoints located on the dorsal aspect of the foot at the proximal V-shaped bases between the 1st, 2nd, 3rd, 4th, and 5th metatarsal bones) on the affected side(s), along with Shen Men (HT7) and Chi Ze (LU5) contralaterally.

Section 2: Warts

Case Study #1: Common Warts – They Keep Coming Back!

Q: This 20 y/o female patient began having recurring warts growing on the fingers and dorsum of her left hand during her first year of high school. She has tried laser therapy and surgical removal, but they continue growing back. The warts appear dark red colored and she has no other symptoms.

A: Common warts (verruca vulgaris) can be identified as exterior damp with heat toxin and blood heat pattern. I would prescribe Ma Xing Yi Gan Tang adding Mu Dan Pi or Zhi Zi, and possibly even Wan Ling Dan; and apply the moxa wool cauterization method just as you would for corns. This will provide effective treatment for most patients.

Case Study #2: Flat Warts and Seborrheic Dermatitis

Q1: This 25 y/o female patient began having white translucent flat warts appearing on both sides of her face near Tai Yang (EX-HN5). She also has a history of seborrheic dermatitis for which she had received Western medicine treatment for 1 1/2 years and also 3–4 months of traditional Korean medicine (TKM) treatment. None of these treatments has provided a complete cure, and she still feels mild itch in those affected areas of her face and scalp. I prescribed Blood Desiccation Formula combining Gui Zhi Ma Huang Ge Ban Tang adding Sheng Shi Gao and Huang Qin. Do you think this is the right approach?

A: The formula you prescribed should provide effective treatment for both seborrheic dermatitis and flat warts. However, I would also add Yi Yi Ren (disinhibits water and percolates dampness and clears heat and expels pus), which will complement your formula composition with the exterior-resolving dampness-eliminating and lung qi-diffusing and disinhibiting actions of Ma Xing Yi Gan Tang as well.

Q2: Three years ago, a 28 y/o female patient incurred an outbreak of flat warts near Tai Yang (EX-HN5) on both sides of her face. She underwent over 1 year of Western medicine immunotherapy, which was not effective; and in fact, the dispersion of the warts actually expanded. Now, these warts cover nearly 2/3 of her face. The warts are densely distributed, slightly raised, brownish colored, and vary in size, and her skin is dry and mildly itchy.

I prescribed Blood Desiccation Formula combining Ma Xing Yi Gan Tang adding Zhu Ru, Zhi Shi, Ban Xia, and Ma Chi Xian for oral administration, and also a decoction of Ku Shen, Xia Ku Cao, Zi Cao, Ma Chi Xian, and Da Qing Ye for topical application as a facial wash.

A: Typically, flat warts (verruca plana) that itch and have dark pigmentation can be identified as phlegm, and specifically, exterior damp-phlegm or phlegm-rheum pattern. Thus, I would prescribe a heat-clearing phlegm-transforming formula such as Wen Dan Tang adding Zao Jiao Ci and Ci Ji Li (8 qian each); and if the itch persists, then add Cang Bai Pi, Sheng Shi Gao, and Huang Qin. This should relieve the itching and gradually resolve the pathocondition.

Remember! Closely examine the coloration, differentiating between purplish-colored static blood pattern types and red-colored dry (desiccation) pattern types. If the skin is red-colored, then this indicates heat pattern, requiring the administration of formulas that clear lung heat and resolve exterior dampness.

Case Study #3: Recurrent Juvenile Warts Following Laser Therapy – Exterior Wind-Heat Pattern

Q: Three years ago, juvenile warts (verruca plana juvenilis) began growing on the left cheek of this female patient (now 21 y/o). She had them removed with laser therapy, but not long after they came back. Now, she has itchy, bright red papules on her face that ooze serous exudates after scratching, and continue to spread.

I have treated flat warts on the face of a young woman before by prescribing Blood Desiccation Formula adding The Three Great Yang-Supplementers, Huang Qin, and Zi He Che. After one month of administering this formula, the warts had completely vanished. However, this case seems to be a completely different pattern type.

How would you treat this patient?

A: Itchy, bright red papules with serous exudate can be identified as exterior wind-heat pattern. This type of pathocondition requires administration of an exterior-resolving dampness eliminating and lung qi-diffusing and disinhibiting formula such as Ma Xing Yi Gan Tang adding Sheng Shi Gao or Ma Xing Gan Shi Tang adding Sheng Shi Gao and Huang Qin; a sweat-effusing exterior-resolving and lung-diffusing wind-dispelling formula such as Da Qing Long Tang, Yue Bi Tang, or Gui Zhi Ma Huang Ge Ban Tang adding Sheng Shi Gao and Huang Qin; a sweat-effusing exterior-resolving and wind-dissipating dampness-dispelling formula such as Jing Fang Bai Du San adding Sheng Shi Gao and Huang Qin; or a heat-clearing toxin-resolving, swelling-dispersing hardness-breaking, and blood-quickening formula such as Xian Fang Huo Ming Yin adding Huang Qin and Pu Gong Ying.

If intense itch presents, then add Ci Ji Li, Zao Jiao Ci, and Lu Lu Tong. And in addition to the prescribing a formula decoction for this pathocondition, I would also bleed Da Zhui (GV14) (above, on, and below), Cun Kou (Tai Yuan (LU9)), and Wei Zhong (UB40); and needle Feng Chi (GB20), Tian Zhu (UB10), He Gu (LI4), and Zu San Li (ST36).

Case Study #4: Flat Warts – Therapeutic Modalities

Q: Over the past 3 months, I have been treating another case of flat warts with Ma Xing Yi Gan Tang adding Zi He Che, and surprisingly, this has not been effective. I've even tried adding The Three Great Yang-Supplementers, Huang Qin, and Huang Lian, but still no positive results. In the past, I've always had success with this formula, but for this case it's just not working. Do you have any suggestions?

A: Flat warts (verruca plana) are caused by a viral infection that spreads via direct skin-to-skin contact from someone else (or object) or from another part of one's own body. There are also many different treatment modalities you can apply: oral decoctions, topical applications, wart needling (needle into the wart and around the perimeter), moxibustion on ginger, moxibustion on garlic, moxibustion on medicinal cake, and the moxa wool cauterization method.

Ma Xing Yi Gan Tang is one formula that may be effective for certain cases, and depending on the type of pattern identified, you may also consider prescribing Xian Fang Huo Ming Yin, Blood Desiccation Formula, Dang Gui Si Ni Jia Wu Ju Yu Sheng Jiang Tang, Chong He Tang, and Jing Fang Bai Du San. For some cases, the long-term administration of Sheng Yu Tang and Dang Gui (powder) may also be effective. If heat presents, then add Sheng Shi Gao and Huang Qin. Western medicine typically treats viral warts (common warts, plantar warts, plane warts) with topical applications of salicylic acid, 5-flourouracil, or retinoic acid, and if that doesn't work, then with cryotherapy or surgery.

Section 2: Seborrheic Dermatitis

Case Study #1: Seborrheic Dermatitis – Red Patches Suddenly Appear on Neck

Q: I have a 34 y/o female seborrheic dermatitis patient with the following history: 2 years ago red patches suddenly appeared on her neck. A dermatologist diagnosed the patient with seborrheic dermatitis and prescribed medication that initially resolved the symptoms, but not long after, it recurred. Now, she presents with red patches on her neck and upper chest and mild itch, and her condition worsens during menstrual cycles. She does *not* have any greasy, yellow scaling, crusting, or burning sensation.

I have prescribed (Yu Sheng) Seborrheic Dermatitis Formula and (Yu Sheng) Blood Desiccation Formula variants on different occasions and neither have proven effective in completely resolving symptoms and curing the condition. Please share your experiences in treating this type of pathocondition.

A: People who drink hard liquor, eat garlic and chili peppers, don't drink enough water, sweat profusely, stay up late, don't get enough sleep, and are exposed to wind tend to be more susceptible to developing seborrheic dermatitis. In these types of patients, it is common for skin eruptions (erythematous plaques) to arise after catching the common cold, which can be identified as externally contracted exterior pattern. Males with a higher frequency of sexual activity, and females during menstruation and ovulation, tend to present with more severe cases.

If the exterior-resolving dampness eliminating, lung qi-diffusing and -disinhibiting, heat-clearing toxin-resolving, and wind-dispelling action of Seborrheic Dermatitis Formula is *not* initially effective, then try adding Huang Qin (or Pu Gong Ying); bleeding Da Zhui (GV14) (above, on, and below); and needling Feng Chi (GB20), Tian Zhu (UB10), He Gu (LI4), and Zu San Li (ST36). You can also advise the patient to lick her fingers with her own saliva and rub the saliva into the affected areas, especially if it is on the face. If greasy, yellow scaling (purulent exudate) and crusting present, then consider including 2–4 liang of Sheng Shi Gao and adding The Three Yellows; and in cases where purulent exudate is so excessive that it causes dizziness and lethargy, then add Gan Jiang, Fu Zi, Ren Shen, and Yu Sheng Wan.

Remember! Once seborrheic dermatitis enters the chronic stage and/or the patient has been administered *topical* antifungals or corticosteroids for extended periods of time and/or *oral* antifungals (inhibit cortisol synthesis) for even a short duration, then it can be identified as exterior wind-heat with yin vacuity pattern. Thus, you should administer a vacuity-heat clearing yin-enriching and blood-nourishing dryness-moistening formula such as Bai He Gu Jin Tang, Zhi Bo Di Huang Tang, or Ba Xian Chang Shou Wan. And make sure to include Tian Men Dong, Mai Men Dong, Zhi Mu, Yuan Shen, Sha Shen, and Jie Geng in your formula. This therapeutic regimen will effectively relieve symptoms, cure the condition, and ensure that it doesn't recur.

Case Study #2: Seborrheic Dermatitis – Exterior Wind-Heat-Damp Pattern

Q: Red patches (erythematous plaques) suddenly appeared about 2 to 3 cun above the hairline on the back of a 38 y/o female's head and on her upper chest and back. The red patches are slightly raised, rough-textured, and range from a mild itch to a burning sensation at the site of lesions. She has tried taking Western medicine, which did relieve the symptoms, but not long afterwards, red patches reappeared.

I prescribed (Yu Sheng) Seborrheic Dermatitis Formula (including Sheng Shi Gao (2 liang) and Jin Yin Hua (1 liang)) without much success. She's had these red patches for 2 months now, and during ovulation and menses, the burning sensation on her skin intensifies.

A: Seborrheic dermatitis can be identified as exterior wind-heat-damp pattern that typically only presents down as far as the crease below the breasts and may also appear on the upper back. People who are exposed to wind, sweat profusely, stay up late, don't get enough sleep (less than 8 hours/day), eat a lot of spicy foods and garlic, and don't drink enough water tend to be more susceptible to seborrheic dermatitis. Catching a cold (external contraction) also tends to induce flare-ups in certain people.

You should advise seborrheic dermatitis patients to keep the head, face, chest, neck, and upper back areas clean with water, rinsing between 5–10 times every day and using a towel to dry the skin, or possibly a wet towel to dab the face clean. No cosmetics or washing products should be used, including soaps, lotions, and moisturizers. If the skin is too dry, then you can advise the patient to wet the fingers with saliva (like a "medicinal tonic") and rub the affected site (especially effective for the face!). If a hydrocortisone cream or more potent topical steroid has been administered, resulting in swollen and tight facial muscles, then advise the patient to massage (or pressure massage) the head and face until the muscles feel fatigued and mildly sore (2–3 times/day).

Additionally, you can advise the patient to eat lots of high water content and mucilaginous foods such as water chestnuts, legumes, asparagus, pears, persimmons, melons, cucumbers, okra, Chinese yams, lotus root, chia seeds, sea cucumbers, jellied pig's feet, pork rind, and fish gelatin. And recommend cooking with yin-nourishing lung heat-abating medicinals such as Sha Shen, Ge Gen, Mai Men Dong, and Jie Geng.

For patients with *severe* seborrheic dermatitis, your therapeutic regimen should include bleeding Da Zhui (GV14) (above, on, and below), Cun Kou (Tai Yuan (LU9)), and the well point of the stomach meridian; needling Feng Chi (GB20), Tian Zhu (UB10), He Gu (LI4), and Zu San Li (ST36); and adding The Three Yellows to your main formula. If female patients have exacerbations during ovulation and menses, then add blood-cooling medicinals such as Mu Dan Pi, Zhi Zi, Sheng Pu Huang, Chi Shao, and Sheng Di Huang.

Case Study #3: Seborrheic Dermatitis Formula

Q: About 5 or 6 years ago, this 48 y/o female patient was diagnosed with seborrheic dermatitis on her neck and upper chest. Her condition still fluctuates with periodic flare-ups of red patches that itch and feel prickly when she sweats. I prescribed Xian Fang Huo Ming Yin (including large doses of Sheng Shi Gao and Jin Yin Hua) adding Huang Qin. How would you treat this condition?

A: Seborrheic dermatitis commonly presents on creases in the face, eyebrows, hairline, behind the ears, neck, upper chest, and in the inframammary folds (the creases under the breasts), wherever there is a high density of seborrheic glands. It is speculated that normal skin organisms (i.e., *Malassezia ovale*) may play a role in causing this pathocondition. Sweating will result in a hot, prickly, and itchy sensation, and when the person scratches, purulent exudate (greasy yellow scaling) and bleeding may occur at the irritated site with subsequent crusting. South Koreans like spicy foods, garlic, and hard liquor, making them more susceptible to developing this pathocondition. And once it develops, it is not that easy to completely cure.

For treatment, you could prescribe Xian Fang Huo Ming Yin, but if it were me, I would go ahead with an exterior-resolving dampness eliminating, lung qi-diffusing and -disinhibiting, heat-clearing toxin-resolving, and wind-dispelling formula such as (Yu Sheng) Seborrheic Dermatitis Formula adding Huang Qin, Huang Bo, and Zhi Mu (or Sheng Mu Li, Qing Hao, and Zi He Che) and Yu Sheng Wan. This approach will be more effective. You should also bleed Da Zhui (GV14) (above, on, and below), Cun Kou (Tai Yuan (LU9)), and the well points of the stomach and spleen channels; and needle Feng Chi (GB20), Tian Zhu (UB10), Zu San Li (ST36), Tai Chong (LV3), San Yin Jiao (SP6), and Chi Ze (LU5).

Case Study #4: Wandering Wind of the Face and Glossy Scalp Wind

Q: A 35 y/o male civil servant has had seborrheic dermatitis for the past 7 years. The affected areas include the chest (near Dan Zhong (RN17)), eyebrows, neck, forehead, and the nasolabial folds. During flare ups he has redness over his entire face, papules in the nasolabial folds and eyebrows, crusting, scaling, and raised plaques on his forehead.

I prescribed (Yu Sheng) Seborrheic Dermatitis Formula adding Zhi Mu (1 liang) and Pu Gong Ying (1 liang). It's already been 1 month, but I haven't seen any noticeable results. Please offer your advice and suggestions.

A: Seborrheic Dermatitis Formula will be effective for cases of seborrheic dermatitis that can be identified as exterior wind-heat-damp pattern. If there is pronounced heat, then it can be classified as wandering wind of the face (面游風 miàn yóu fēng) and glossy scalp wind (油風 yóu fēng) as described in classical TCM texts. For the presentation of this pathocondition, you should bleed Da Zhui (GV14) (above, on, and below), Cun Kou (Tai Yuan (LU9), and Wei Zhong (UB40); needle Feng Chi (GB20), Tian Zhu (UB10), He Gu (LI4), and Zu San Li (ST36); and add Sheng Shi Gao, Huang Lian, and Huang Bo to the formula.

Remember! You should also advise seborrheic dermatitis patients to wash the affected area frequently throughout the day (5–10 times) with *just* water (they do *not* need to use cleansers!) and then dab dry with a towel. After washing, if the skin feels tight or too dry, then advise the patient to massage (or pressure massage) the affected area and/or wet the fingers with their own saliva (like a "medicinal tonic"), using a rubbing and gliding method to massage the affected area (especially effective for the face!). This regimen will quickly relieve the symptoms. Also, it's a good idea for patients with seborrheic dermatitis to file down their fingernails to avoid inadvertently scratching their face and causing further irritation.

Cosmetics (*even* moisturizers!) are anathema to seborrheic dermatitis patients. During the winter season, patients must stay warm and avoid exposure to wind, and if they are exposed to wind, then wear a face mask, scarf, or visor. Patients should rinse their face after sweating, cut back on spicy foods (e.g., chili, garlic), don't stay up late, drink lots of liquids, and eat lots of fruits with high water content and mucilaginous vegetables, fish, and meats.

It has been my experience that male patients who stay up late "burning the midnight oil" and engaging in frequent sexual intercourse are also more susceptible to developing dry front teeth (齒燥 chǐ zào), along with the wandering wind of the face and glossy scalp wind. For these patients, you can also consider adding heat clearing fire-draining, yin-enriching dryness-moistening, and blood-cooling steaming bone-eliminating medicinals such as Zhi Mu, Huang Bo, Qing Hao, Di Gu Pi, Yuan Shen, Tian Men Dong, Mai Men Dong, and Sheng Di Huang to the main formula.

Case Study #5: Seborrheic Dermatitis – Signs of Therapeutic Efficacy

Q: Right now I have a very compliant seborrheic dermatitis patient with a lot of patience who has tried the gamut of Western medicine treatment. She came to see me about 1 month ago seeking TCM treatment, which included a prescription of an orally administered formula, bleeding, and acupuncture. Over the past 1 month of this therapeutic regimen, at first the scaling increased, then the skin color turned from dark red back to its normal coloration and the thickened plaques resolved, with the resiliency of the skin returning. This seems to be a sign of efficacy. What do you think?

A: Being able to shed the old skin and rejuvenate new growth in just 1 month's time is quite impressive. This is definitely a sign that you are on the right path! However, this pathocondition usually takes some time to completely cure, so don't be surprised if some flare-ups occur along the way.

Here are some other things to remember in case this patient has a flare-up or when you treat other patients with this pathocondition. In the acute stage or during flare-ups, which can typically be identified as exterior wind-heat-damp pattern, I like to prescribe Seborrheic Dermatitis Formula. If heat is pronounced in any stage and/or during severe flare-ups (e.g., red colored itchy skin), then add combinations of heat-clearing toxin-resolving and fire-draining medicinals such as The Three Yellows, Pu Gong Ying, and Sheng Shi Gao into the formula; and bleed Da Zhui (GV14) (above, on, and below) and Cun Kou (Tai Yuan (LU9). Additionally, in the acute stage and during flare-ups, I would perform acupuncture on acupoints such as Feng Chi (GB20), Tian Zhu (UB10), He Gu (LI4), Zu San Li (ST36), and San Yin Jiao (SP6); and in the chronic stage, add Yin Ling Quan (SP9) and Xue Hai (SP10).

In classical TCM texts this pathocondition correlates with wandering wind of the face (面游風 miàn yóu fēng) and glossy scalp wind (油風 yóu fēng). To prevent the potential for further irritation and secondary infection, urge your patient to restrain from scratching the affected site. A good way for damping the desire to scratch is having the patient wet his/her fingers with saliva and apply pressure message instead. After the initial acute phase (or subsequent flare-up) has resolved, which can be identified as effulgent yin vacuity fire or lung-kidney yin depletion, you can consider prescribing a vacuity-heat clearing yin-enriching and blood-nourishing dryness-moistening formula such as Zhi Bo Di Huang Tang, Ba Xian Chang Shou Wan,

Bai He Gu Jin Tang, or Qing Zao Jiu Fei Tang.

You can be confident that this pathocondition has been cured after the patient has either incurred 2–3 external contractions (common colds) or gone through a full winter without a flare-up. If these patients happen to catch a cold, it is essential for them to immediately get it treated and under control, thus preventing another flare-up. You should also advise these patients to abstain from drinking hard liquor and eating spicy foods, and don't overdo the raw garlic. Regulating the constitution consists of a healthy lifestyle, getting plenty of sleep, and eating lots of yin-enriching foods with high water and mucilage content.

Remember! Seborrheic dermatitis patients should get adequate amounts of sleep, drink lots of water, frequently rinse their face with water, and eat lots of high water-content fruits and mucilaginous vegetables such as turnips, pears, legumes, water chestnuts, asparagus, and legumes. These types of patients should *not* apply makeup or use any type of cosmetic products, and after they go outside, work up a sweat, or are exposed to dusty environments, they must make sure to wash their faces with water afterwards.

Case Study #6: Atopic Dermatitis Resolves But Acne and Folliculitis May Appear

Q: Over the past 6 months, I have been treating a 24 y/o male patient with atopic dermatitis. At the onset, the skin on his face, neck, and flexor surfaces of the arms and legs was thickened (almost like elephant's skin!).

Right after I started treating him with Blood Desiccation Formula, he decided (did *not* discuss with me!) to *abruptly* stop using the topical corticosteroids prescribed by his dermatologist. Not long after that, he had a "flare-up" with his face swelling up and profuse scaling.

Thus, I began prescribing Huang Lian Jie Du Tang variant, and about 3 months later, these symptoms gradually resolved, as his skin rejuvenated back to its normal texture and suppleness. The Huang Lian Jie Du Tang variant seems to be working well. Do you think I should continue prescribing this formula?

A: Both seborrheic dermatitis and atopic dermatitis are exacerbated by external contraction wind evil that may lead to flare-ups. So if the patient catches a cold (external contraction) make sure he gets it treated and resolved.

Once the manifestation of symptoms (e.g., eczema, pruritis) of atopic dermatitis resolve, adolescents and young adults in particular have a tendency to incur breakouts of acne and folliculitis. This is simply a therapeutic response (瞑眩反應 míng xuàn fǎn yìng) as the underlying heat toxin at the root of the pathocondition is being drawn out and effused from the body. For patients with these "breakouts," I would prescribe Xian Fang Huo Ming Yin variant (clears heat and resolves toxin, disperses swelling and breaks hardness, and quickens the blood).

The heat-clearing toxin-resolving formula Huang Lian Jie Du Tang may be effective at clearing the heat in the short term, but if it is prescribed for long durations it has a tendency to cause sloppy stools and poor food intake in many patients. Instead, I would consider prescribing a blood-nourishing yin-enriching, exterior-resolving wind-dispelling, and spleen- liver- and kidney-supplementing formula such as Atopic Dermatitis Formula or a blood-nourishing yin-enriching dryness-moistening adding The Three Yellows (clear heat and resolve toxin). These formulas will provide effective results without the gastrointestinal side effects.

Case Study #7: Seborrheic Dermatitis – Movement and Qi Theory

Q: Many seborrheic dermatitis patients in South Korea can be identified as blood desiccation with blood heat pattern and that's why I frequently prescribe (Yu Sheng) Blood Desiccation Formula adding Sheng Di Huang and Huang Qin. Please share your thoughts and perspectives about this pathocondition.

A: TCM diagnosis and pattern identification as the basis for determining treatment encompasses an understanding of the environment, climate, demographics, religious beliefs, customs, eating habits, dress, and lifestyles of the patient. This is the clinical application of the movement and qi theory (運氣醫學 yùn qì yī xué) in a nutshell!

Koreans are a strong and courageous people with a principled character and upright nature who like to eat spicy foods and drink hard liquor. South Korea also shares the same cold and wet temperate climate as northeastern China, thus making the people naturally predisposed to cold-damp pattern pathoconditions. However, Koreans also share similarities with the people of Sichuan Province in western China in that they like eating spicy and acrid foods. These factors commonly result in pathoconditions that can be identified as true cold and false heat, exterior wind-heat, blood desiccation with blood heat, blood vacuity with yang vacuity, and other complex patterns

Case Study #8: Seborrheic Dermatitis – Elderly Patient's Scalp

Q: A 60 y/o female patient has had seborrheic dermatitis on her scalp for the past 1 1/2 years. She has tried both TCM and Western medicine without effective results. Now, she presents with red, thick plaques over her entire scalp that feels prickly and itchy (*no* oozing or crusting).

A: A patient with seborrheic dermatitis presenting with these types of symptoms can typically be identified as exterior wind-heat pattern. First, I would bleed Da Zhui (GV14) (above, on, and below) and also bleed directly on the affected sites with the most pronounced itch; needle Feng Chi (GB20), Tian Zhu (UB10), He Gu (LI4), Shen Men (HT7), Yang Ling Quan (GB34), and Wei Zhong (UB40); and prescribe Seborrheic Dermatitis Formula adding Huang Qin and Pu Gong Ying (or Huang Bo and Huang Lian).

However, for elderly patients you must also take into consideration the possibility of blood desiccation itchy skin (血枯膚癢 xuè kū fū yǎng), tinea capitus (頭癬 tóu xiǎn), or erythrasma (紅癬 hóng xiǎn), because the age of onset for chronic inflammatory skin disorders such as seborrheic dermatitis and psoriasis are usually < 50 y/o. For these types of pathoconditions, you can prescribe a blood-nourishing yin-enriching dryness-moistening formula such as Blood Desiccation Formula adding combinations of heat-clearing toxin-resolving and liver-calming yang-subduing medicinals such as Sheng Shi Gao, Huang Qin, Sheng Long Gu, Sheng Mu Li, and Yu Sheng Wan.

In classical TCM texts there was not always a clear distinction made between the etiology of the various pathologic terms that include lichen (癬 xiǎn) as a part of its name. Rather, this term was often simply a physical description of the lesions that manifested on the skin. However, most of these terms—e.g., coin lichen (圓癬 yuán xiǎn), coin lichen (金錢癬 jīn qián xiǎn), dry lichen (乾癬 gān xiǎn), oxhide lichen (牛皮癬 niú pí xiǎn), and pine bark lichen (松皮癬 sōng pí xiǎn)—correlate with either tinea, eczema, dermatitis, or psoriasis.

Section 4: Atopic Dermatitis

Case Study #1: Blood Desiccation – Itchy, Lichenified Lesions

Q: Six years **ago**, this 18 y/o male patient began having itchy skin on his left wrist and lower leg and the dorsum of his right foot. The patient has been treated with both Western medicine and Traditional Korean Medicine (TKM) without noticeable efficacy. Now, he continues to use an unspecified folk remedy in addition to my orally administered formula decoction.

Initially, I prescribed Xian Fang Huo Ming Yin variant, which was not effective either. For my second formula, I decided to change over to (Yu Sheng) Blood Desiccation Formula adding The Three Great Yang-Supplementers, Huang Qin, Sheng Shi Gao, Long Yan Rou, Ban Xia, Hou Po, Ma Huang, Gui Zhi, and Xing Ren. After taking this formula for two weeks, the patient presented as follows: serous exudate (clear, sticky, odorless fluid) began oozing from the affected sites, encrustations formed (previously completely dry), there was pronounced heat upon palpation and generalized itch (only during the evening), skin coloration turned bright red (previously it was dark colored), and the stool was normal.

Based on your clinical experience in treating patients with atopic dermatitis, do you think these are positive signs of therapeutic efficacy?

A: Your second formula is the correct approach. It sounds to me like a case of chronic atopic dermatitis. Don't worry! Continued administration of your treatment will gradually relieve itch. If the lichenified lesions cover a large area with profuse oozing (i.e., serous or purulent exudate), crusting, and itching, then you can prescribe a medicinal infusion and instruct the patient to soak the affected sites (or entire body) in a tub of this solution. This will quickly relieve itching!

Over time this TCM therapeutic regimen (consisting of orally administered formula decoction and topically applied medicinal infusion) will gradually mitigate and eventually resolve the cycle of oozing, crusting, and itch. However, to ensure the pathocondition has been completely cured, it will be necessary to continue taking the oral decoction (i.e., Blood Desiccation Formula) up until the papules and pustules of acne and folliculitis present. This manifestation can be understood as a therapeutic response (瞑眩反應 míng xuàn fǎn yìng) in which the heat toxin at the root is finally being drawn out and effused from the body. At that time, you can switch over to a heat-clearing toxin-resolving, swelling-dispersing hardness-breaking, and blood-quickening formula such as Xian Fang Huo Ming Yin variant, administering this formula up until the skin has returned to its normal texture and coloration. That's when you know the pathocondition has been completely cured!

Note: The medicinal infusion for external application I just referred to is composed of the following medicinals: Feng Qiu (Lu Lu Tong), Ru Xiang, Mo Yao, Da Huang, Sang Bai Pi, Zao Jiao Ci, Gan Shi, Hua Shi, Sheng Shi Gao, and Huang Qin (2 liang each). Boil this formula in a large pot for 20–30 minutes, and once the decoction has cooled to room temperature, pour it into a tub. The patient should soak the affected site (or entire body) until the medicinals have adequately saturated the skin and absorbed into the pores. After a soaking session, this medicinal infusion should be put back into the pot and stored for reuse. The next day, the patient can reboil this same decocted medicinal infusion for about 5 minutes and proceed with the soaking process as before. This medicinal infusion can be used in this way for 3–7 days before you need to decoct a new batch of fresh raw medicinals.

Case Study #2: Atopic Dermatitis and Tearing on Exposure to Wind – Is There Any Relationship?

Q: It seems there are some similarities in the presenting symptoms of patients with atopic dermatitis and tearing on exposure to wind. Are these two pathoconditions related?

A: In my opinion, *atopic dermatitis* and *tearing on exposure to wind* (迎風落淚 yíng fēng luò lèi) are both the result of external contraction (microbial infection) evil that has either *not* been completely eliminated (邪熱未盡 xié rè wèi jìn) or *persists* as a type of external contraction post-infectious sequelae. In the first scenario, a viral infection has occurred at some time in the past, which remains dormant and undetectable in the body; and in the second scenario, the virus may have been eliminated but has disrupted the functional capacity of the body's immune system mechanisms. In both scenarios, a state of imbalance (dyshomeostasis) results, making the body easily compromised by both internal (e.g., seven affects (emotional and psychological), fatigue) and external (e.g., Western medicine drug side effects, weather, environmental irritants) factors. The patient may go through asymptomatic periods or suffer persistent and enduring manifestations.

However, the clinical picture and presenting symptoms of *atopic dermatitis* and *tearing on exposure to wind* are different. *Atopic dermatitis* manifests in the presentation of eczematous, itchy lesions on the flexural creases (e.g., elbow (antecubital), knee (popliteal fossae)), skin folds, backs of the hands, and eyelids. The classical TCM pathologic term that directly correlates with atopic dermatitis is four bends wind (四彎風 sì wān fēng), giving a physical description of the predilection for developing eczematous, itchy lesions on the "bends" (flexural creases) of the limbs. *Tearing on exposure to wind* affects the nasal cavity and tear ducts and presents with symptoms of sneezing, tearing, and runny nose. There are many causes of tearing on exposure to wind including *"lacrimal duct laxation," chronic conjunctivitis*, and *chronic rhinitis*.

Patients with *chronic conjunctivitis* often explain that it "feels like something is stuck in my eye." This pathocondition correlates with squinty eye flying silk (瞇目飛絲 mī mù fēi sī) as described in TCM classical texts. For treatment, I would prescribe a blood-nourishing yin-enriching dryness-moistening formula such as Blood Desiccation Formula or a blood- and qi-supplementing, blood-cooling stasis-dispelling, and yin-enriching formula such as Sheng Yu Tang adding Ci Ji Li; and acupuncture (warm needle) Feng Chi (GB20), Tian Zhu (UB10), He Gu (LI4), and Zu San Li (ST36).

Patients with *chronic rhinitis* typically present with white- or yellow-colored purulent nasal discharge and post-nasal drip, requiring administration of a heat-clearing phlegm-transforming formula such as Wen Dan Tang adding exterior-resolving with warmth and acridity and nasal orifice-freeing medicinals such as Ma Huang, Bai Zhi, Lai Fu Zi, Xi Xin, and Xin Yi.

Patients with *"lacrimal duct laxation"* can be treated with a spleen qi-supplementing or kidney yang-supplementing formula variant such as Shi Quan Da Bu Tang, Bu Zhong Yi Qi Tang, or You Gui Yin.

Case Study #3: Refractory Atopic Dermatitis

Q: Atopic dermatitis is a very difficult pathocondition to treat. Once it seems like you are getting it under control, it comes back again, sometimes with even more severe exacerbations. I have not found a way to completely cure it. Recently, I have been treating an 18 y/o patient who initially presented with generalized erythema, intense pruritis, xerosis over the entire body, lichenified lesions on the "four bends" (flexural creases of the knees and elbows) and thickened skin on the hands.

After being administered TCM treatment, the generalized erythema, dry skin, and intense pruritis has improved. Now, the only place that is itchy is on the "four bends," but the thickened skin on the palms remains and the fingernails (mainly the thumbs) are dry and lusterless. I have not been able to make any further progress on this patient. What would you do for this patient? Please offer your advice and suggestions.

A: Patients with a history of severe, refractory atopic dermatitis will take a long time to completely cure. As with this patient, you will find that TCM medicinals are able to readily mitigate the severity of symptoms and get the condition under control, but a cycle of remission and recurrence often persists.

Remember! Stay confident and continue administering your therapeutic regimen. You should continue prescribing either Blood Desiccation Formula (including large doses of Dang Gui, He Shou Wu, Tu Si Zi, and Sha Wan Ji Li) adding The Three Great Yang-Supplementers, Huang Qin (counterbalances the heat), and Ma Huang (large dose); or Atopic Dermatitis Formula (including large doses of Ma Huang, Dang Gui, He Shou Wu, Tu Si Zi, and Sha Wan Ji Li) adding The Three Great Yang-Supplementers and Huang Qin. Also, if heat is pronounced, then bleed Da Zhui (GV14) (above, on, and below) and Cun Kou (Tai Yuan (LU9)); and needle acupoints such as Feng Chi (GB20), Tian Zhu (UB10), He Gu (LI4), Zu San Li (ST36), Xue Hai (SP10), Yin Ling Quan (SP9), San Yin Jiao (SP6), Shen Men (HT7) (or Nei Guan (P6)), and Tai Chong (LV3). In cases of cold pattern (or when heat is *not* pronounced), it is *not* necessary to bleed; instead, you should warm needle, which will warm the channels, supplement the blood, and quiet the heart and calm the spirit.

Gradually, over time, the symptoms will resolve and a therapeutic response (瞑眩反應 míng xuàn fǎn yìng) of papules and pustules of acne and folliculitis will "break out." I interpret this as the heat toxin at the root of the pathocondition finally being drawn out and effused from the body. At that time, you can switch over to a heat-clearing toxin-resolving, swelling-dispersing hardness-breaking, and blood-quickening formula such as Xian Fang Huo Ming Yin variant, administering this formula up until the skin has returned to its normal texture and coloration. That's when you know the pathocondition has been completely cured!

Case Study #4: What is "Four Bends Wind"?

Q: During interviews and treatment sessions with some of my atopic dermatitis patients, I have mentioned the TCM term "four bends wind (四彎風 sì wān fēng)" and how it correlates with their pathocondition. Could you help me clarify the underlying meaning of this term?

A: In classical TCM texts the term "four bends wind" is used to describe a pathocondition typically caused by external contraction wind evil and presents with the symptoms of dry skin, pruritis, eczema (i.e., maculopapular, erythematous lesions that can also have scaling, crusting, oozing, and blistering), and lichenification (i.e., thickening of the skin with accentuated skin markings). At the onset and in mild cases, eczema and lichenification tends to be more prominent in the flexural creases (antecubital and popliteal fossae), skin folds, extensor surface of hands, and flexor surfaces; however, in severe cases eczema and lichenification may be generalized.

"Four bends" is a TCM classical anatomical description of the four main flexural creases, consisting of the arms (antecubital fossa (anterior aspect of elbow)) and legs (popliteal fossa (posterior aspect of knee)). "Four bends" along with the etiology of external contraction wind evil combine to form the TCM classical pathologic term "four bends wind"; and as the name implies, this pathocondition directly correlates with atopic dermatitis!

The onset of this pathocondition commonly manifests in infants, presenting with dry skin, pruritis, eczema (over the cheeks, face, head, and extensor surfaces of the extremities), Dennie-Morgan folds (increased folds below the eyes), and may follow an episode of infantile seborrheic dermatitis (aka "cradle cap"). It can also manifest in childhood and adolescence, with the presentation of eczema and lichenification as described above and severe pruritis at nighttime during sleep, resulting in intense scratching that may cause bleeding and lead to secondary infection. Though not as common, four bends wind can also manifest in adulthood.

In the acute stage and during flare-ups with secondary bacterial infection, four bends wind may present with maculopapular, erythematous lesions that ooze foul-smelling (e.g., fishy or like a corpse) purulent exudate and serosanguineous exudates. These types of cases can be identified as true heat pattern or exterior wind-heat-damp pattern, requiring administration of a sweat-effusing exterior-resolving and lung-diffusing wind-dispelling formula such as Da Qing Long Tang, Ma Xing Yi Gan Tang (adding Sheng Shi Gao and Huang Qin), and Yue Bi Tang; or a heat-clearing toxin-resolving, swelling-dispersing hardness-breaking, and blood-quickening formula such as Xian Fang Huo Ming Yin.

In the chronic stage, four bends wind typically presents with dry skin, pruritis, eczema, lichenification, and serous exudate; and can be identified as blood desiccation or blood desiccation with spleen vacuity cold phlegm pattern, requiring administration of Blood Desiccation Formula or Atopic Dermatitis Formula.

Case Study #5: Infantile Atopic Dermatitis

Q: To tell you the truth, I really don't have the heart to treat those 1–2 year old babies with atopic dermatitis. So small with such tender, supple and sensitive skin, afflicted with the torment of dry, red skin over the neck, nape, abdomen, back, ears, and the flexural creases (four bends). And it itches so badly that they often can't sleep and they scratch so hard it bleeds.

Recently, a couple brought in their baby explaining that he had symptoms resembling atopic dermatitis (*no* oozing exudate) along with a runny nose and sneezing. However, the strange thing about the dry, red itchy skin is that once the baby awakens in the mornings the skin returns to normal coloration. Does this sound like a case of atopic dermatitis to you?

A: Infants and children aged 1–2 years old tend to be afflicted with especially severe atopic dermatitis (aka four bends wind) that requires long-term treatment in order to see improvement. The atopic triad or *atopy* is commonly referred to as a genetic predisposition for any hypersensitive IgE-mediated reaction, which commonly manifests in the three pathoconditions of atopic dermatitis (eczema), allergic rhinitis, or allergic asthma, but may manifest as food allergies and allergic conjunctivitis.

My view on the etiology of *atopy* is that it results from external contraction (microbial infection) evil that has either *not* been completely eliminated (邪熱未盡 xié rè wèi jìn) or *persists* as a type of external contraction post-infectious sequelae. In the first scenario, a viral infection has occurred at some time in the past, which remains dormant and undetectable in the body; and in the second scenario, the virus may have been eliminated but has disrupted the functional capacity of the body's immune system mechanisms. In both scenarios, a state of imbalance (dyshomeostasis) results, making the body easily compromised by both internal (e.g., seven affects (emotional and psychological), fatigue) and external (e.g., Western medicine drug side effects, weather, environmental irritants) factors. The compromised immune system overreacts (i.e., hypersensitivity reaction (adaptive immune system)) and fails to protect the body against normally harmless internal and external factors, which then manifests in pathoconditions such as tearing on exposure to wind (allergic rhinitis), asthma, atopic dermatitis (four bends wind), nasal polyps, conjunctivitis, and most commonly, as wind papules (urticaria).

In the acute stage and during flare-ups, these types of pathoconditions can be identified as exterior wind-heat or exterior wind-heat-damp pattern, requiring administration of a fleshy exterior-harmonizing and evil-expelling itch-relieving formula such as Gui Zhi Ma Huang Ge Ban Tang or an exterior-resolving dampness eliminating and lung qi-diffusing and disinhibiting formula such as Ma Xing Yi Gan Tang. For infants and young children (< 2 y/o), you can prescribe granulated extract powder (approx. 0.5 g/day/for 3–5 kg baby, 0.75 g/day for 6–8 kg baby, 1 g/day for 9–12 kg, etc.), mixing it in with the infant's milk (or baby formula).

Atopy may also manifest as pathoconditions such as *dyshidrotic eczema (pompholyx)*, which can be identified as exterior wind-heat-damp pattern; *hidradenitis suppurativa* (an autoinflammatory disorder (innate immune system)), which can be identified as exterior wind-heat pattern; and *nummular (discoid) dermatitis*, which can be identified as exterior damp with stasis heat pattern. If large doses of Western medicine drugs (e.g., topical steroids, calcineurin inhibitors) have been administered, then these pathoconditions can be identified as either exterior cold with wind, blood desiccation itchy skin, or visceral agitation pattern.

For these types of *atopy* pathoconditions that have entered the chronic stage (usually later on in adolescence or adulthood), I will typically prescribe Blood Desiccation Formula adding large doses of The Three Great Yang-Supplementers, Ma Huang, Xing Ren, and Yi Yi Ren. If heat is pronounced, then you can also add Sheng Shi Gao and Bai Xian Pi. Additionally, I would advise patients with dry and lichenified skin to apply topical applications such as Purple Cloud Ointment, sesame seed oil, jellied pig's feet, or suet.

Remember! For these types of pathoconditions resulting from external contraction (microbial infection) evil that has *not* been completely eliminated or external contraction sequelae that still *persists*, TCM provides a more comprehensive and effective therapeutic regimen than Western medicine, which can only provide itch-relieving and inflammation-resolving actions.

Case Study #6: Severe, Generalized Atopic Dermatitis

Q: Recently, I have been treating several patients with severe, generalized atopic dermatitis. In all of these cases, the pattern has been similar: initially, there is noticeable improvement in their symptoms, but about 1 month into treatment, they suddenly incurred flare-ups. These flare-ups have been frustrating and tough to endure, and have obviously left the patients wondering whether TCM can *really* provide lasting efficacy. Where do I go from here?

A: Atopic dermatitis is an inherently difficult pathocondition to completely cure, especially if it has already entered the chronic stage with generalized presentation of symptoms. This condition will take time to treat, so don't fool yourself or the patient into thinking that a "miracle" will happen over night! For this type of severe, generalized atopic dermatitis presenting with itchy maculopapular, erythematous lesions, scaling, oozing, crusting, xerosis, and lichenification over the entire body, I once treated a patient for 3 1/2 years before she was completely cured.

In cases of severe flare-ups, you can prescribe a medicinal infusion for external application composed of Da Huang, Ru Xiang, Mo Yao, Sang Bai Pi, Zao Jiao Ci, Hua Shi, Lu Gan Shi, and Huang Qin. Instruct the patient to boil this formula in a large pot for 20–30 minutes, cool to room temperature, and then pour the decoction into a tub. The patient should soak the entire body in this decoction 2x/day until the skin is thoroughly saturated. After each soak, it would be optimal for the patient to let the decoction dry naturally, further allowing complete saturation into the pores. Throughout the day, sesame oil can be topically applied on the skin, which functions as a skin conditioner (hydrates and softens) and emollient (moisturizer).

For these patients, I would prescribe a blood-nourishing yin-enriching dryness-moistening formula such as Blood Desiccation Formula adding large doses of The Three Great Yang-Supplementers, Ma Huang, Xing Ren, and Yi Yi Ren. And if heat is pronounced, then also add Sheng Shi Gao and Bai Xian Pi. Additionally, I would warm needle Feng Chi (GB20), Tian Zhu (UB10), He Gu (LI4), Zu San Li (ST36), Xue Hai (SP10), Yin Ling Quan (SP9), San Yin Jiao (SP6), Shen Men (HT7), and Tai Chong (LV3); and bleed Da Zhui (GV14) (above, on, and below), Cun Kou (Tai Yuan (LU9)), and Wei Zhong (UB40). And if heat is pronounced, then also bleed the well points on the hands and feet.

Case Study #7: Atopic Dermatitis or Psychogenic "Itch"?

Q: Over the past 6 months, I have been treating a young girl with a case of mild atopic dermatitis (prescribing (Yu Sheng) Atopic Dermatitis Formula variant). The symptoms seem to resolve at times and then "flare-up" again with itching. I emphasize "flare-up" because the only noticeable sign or symptom is "the itch." There are *no* other common symptoms (e.g., erythematous lesions, xerosis, oozing, crusting, lichenification) that would typically present in a patient with atopic dermatitis.

The last time her mother brought her in, I realized that the girl only itches when her mother is by her side; otherwise, it does *not* "itch" at all. During our visits, the girl repeatedly asks her mother to buy her things or to do things together with her. I am wondering if these "flare-ups" of atopic dermatitis are in fact psychogenic. Is that a possibility?

A: It is certainly possible! In rare cases, you may come across a patient with "atopic dermatitis" of psychogenic origin. For this patient, I would try adding Long Yan Gan and Da Zao (nourish the blood and calm the spirit), Bai Jiang Can (extinguishes wind, transforms phlegm, and checks tetany), and Sheng Mu Li and Sheng Long Gu (calm the liver and subdue yang) and Yu Sheng Wan (quiets the spirit and calms the nerves) to your formula.

Case Study #8: Itch – Chronic Four Bends Wind

Q: I have a 54 y/o female patient with a 20-year history of generalized pruritis and symptoms that resemble atopic dermatitis: erythematous patches, papules, oozing, crusting, and intense pruritis on the medial aspects of her thighs and arms, neck, and upper abdomen. And these symptoms worsen during menstruation.

She has undergone a thorough examination for allergic triggers, but nothing has been identified. Recently, blood tests revealed increased T-Bil. Do you think hyperbilirubinemia could be the cause of her itch?

A: A female patient with a 20-year history of four bends wind (四彎風 sì wān fēng) sounds like atopic dermatitis and blood desiccation itchy skin (血枯膚癢 xuè kū fū yǎng) to me. Erythematous papules and vesicles with excoriations and serous exudate have evolved into thick lichenified plaques through a chronic inflammatory process of healing and relapse. It likely does not have anything to do with low T-Bil. blood-nourishing yin-enriching, exterior-resolving wind-dispelling, and spleen- liver- and kidney-supplementing

As for treatment, you can prescribe a blood-nourishing yin-enriching dryness-moistening formula such Blood Desiccation Formula or a blood-nourishing yin-enriching, exterior-resolving wind-dispelling, and spleen- liver- and kidney-supplementing formula such as Atopic Dermatitis Formula (including large doses of Dang Gui, He Shou Wu, Tu Si Zi, and Sha Wan Zi) adding The Three Great Yang-Supplementers, and Huang Qin (counterbalances the heat). And if heat is pronounced, then add Sheng Shi Gao. Technically, you don't really need to add any other medicinals for elevated T-Bil, because Dang Gui, He Shou Wu, and Tu Si Zi already have a liver-emolliating action, but if you think it's necessary, you can consider adding Sheng Zhi Zi.

I would also needle Feng Chi (GB20), Tian Zhu (UB10), He Gu (LI4), Chi Ze (LU5), Nei Guan (P6), San Yin Jiao (SP6), Yin Ling Quan (SP9), and Xue Hai (SP10); and if heat is pronounced, then bleed Da Zhui (GV14) (above, on, and below), Cun Kou (Tai Yuan (LU9)), and the spleen channel well point. During the cold weather months, if heat is *not* pronounced, you can warm needle, but during the warm weather months, simply needling *without* moxa will suffice.

Case Study #9: Four Bends Wind – Abdominal Cramps

Q: A 13 y/o female patient has had atopic dermatitis since she was 2 months old. It presents as relapsing erythematous lesions with severe itching, scratch marks (excoriations), scaling, and lichenified plaques on her face, flexural creases (four bends), abdomen, and back. The strange thing about her case is that every time she has painful abdominal cramps (*no* food stagnation) the atopic dermatitis worsens. She has tried both TCM and Western medicine *without* any significant improvement. What do you think I should do for this patient?

A: Gastrointestinal symptoms (e.g., diarrhea, regurgitation, vomiting, colic) are common in children with atopic dermatitis. It's possible your patient may have some systemic reaction to certain triggers that would cause GI tract and skin symptoms to present concomitantly. (Yu Sheng) Atopic Dermatitis Formula contains the qi-boosting spleen-fortifying and qi-moving phlegm-transforming actions of Xiang Sha Liu Jun Zi Tang (Dan Shen, Cang Zhu, Fu Ling, Mu Xiang, Sha Ren, Chen Pi, Ban Xia, and Gan Cao). Long-term administration of this formula will relieve symptoms and resolve both the skin and GI tract conditions. If necessary, you could also consider adding Yuan Hu Suo for the painful abdominal cramps.

Other than that, I would treat this as any other four bends wind case, administering the TCM therapeutic regimen up until the skin is clear and supple, and the patient has incurred 2–3 external contractions or after going through 1 winter without relapse. If the patient has already started puberty, you should administer this regimen up until the therapeutic response (瞑眩反應 míng xuàn fǎn yìng) manifestations of papules and pustules (i.e., acne and folliculitis) present. At that time, you should consider changing your formula to Xian Fang Huo Ming Yin variant, continuing administration up until the condition completely resolves. That's when you know for sure that the atopic dermatitis (and the GI tract symptoms) has been cured for good!

Case Study #10: Skin Allergies and Atopic Dermatitis

Q: A 10 y/o girl has had a history of skin allergies over the past 4 years. Every time she catches a cold (external contraction), she gets intensely itchy, pink-colored cloud-like wheals on her face, the flexural creases (four bends), abdomen, and back. Her parents mentioned that their daughter likes to eat pork fat and innards, which they think may trigger the allergic reaction. Each time these eruptions appear, her parents take her to a dermatologist who prescribes antihistamines, which has *not* had any noticeable efficacy. How should I treat this patient?

A: This sounds like atopic dermatitis to me, and correlates with four bends wind (四彎風 sì wān fēng) and blood desiccation itchy skin (血枯膚癢 xuè kū fū yǎng) described in classical TCM texts. As for treatment, I would prescribe either Di Huang Yin Zi, Qi Bao Mei Ran Dan, or Blood Desiccation Formula (nourish the blood and moisten dryness and nourish kidney and liver yin and replenish essence); or Atopic Dermatitis Formula (nourishes the blood and enriches yin, resolves the exterior and dispels wind, and supplements the spleen, liver, and kidney). If blood desiccation is pronounced, then add large doses of Dang Gui, He Shou Wu, Tu Si Zi, and Sha Wan Zi. If administration of this formula does *not* result in significant improvement, then you should also consider adding The Three Great

Yang-Supplementers and Huang Qin (counterbalances the heat).

Remember! For these types of atopy patients, the "external contraction" symptoms you referred to are often merely the manifestations of the immune system's hypersensitivity reaction (e.g., low-grade fever of 37 to 38 C°, runny nose, and malaise). If the symptoms of hypersensitivity reaction are *mild*, then you can consider simply excluding the The Three Great Yang-Supplementers and adding The Three Yellows. But if these symptoms of hypersensitivity reaction are *pronounced* or if the patient really has caught a cold (external contraction), then consider changing to a sweat-effusing exterior-resolving and lung-diffusing wind-dispelling formula such as Da Qing Long Tang, Gui Zhi Ma Huang Ge Ban Tang, Yue Bi Tang, Ma Xing Gan Shi Tang, or Ma Xing Yi Gan Tang. Once the external contraction (microbial infection) has resolved, then you can continue prescribing your original formula.

At first, the skin will still itch, but it will eventually flake off (exfoliate) and new, replenished healthy skin will grow. Once the brunt of the skin flare-ups have been mitigated, you can reduce the dosage of your original formula; for instance, instead of 1 packet/3x/day, you can administer 1 packet (approx. 600 ml) of decocted raw medicinals over a 2 to 3 day period in order to regulate the constitution.

Section 5: Blood Desiccation Itchy Skin

Case Study #1: Blood Desiccation with Exterior Wind-Heat Pattern

Q: I have a 30 y/o female patient whose skin itches upon exposure to sunlight (solar urticaria). After she scratches the itch, a red-colored rash (i.e., erythematous plaques, papules, wheals) appear over her entire body, along with a sensation of pronounced heat. Once she stops scratching, this rash will eventually spontaneously resolve. Recently, this condition has been getting worse, with erythematous plaques, papules and wheals more diffusely distributed and the sensation of heat intensified.

She has been administered corticosteroids, but it has *not* been very effective. Unfortunately, my prescription of (Yu Sheng) Blood Desiccation Formula adding Zi He Che (3 qian) has *not* offered any better results. Do you have any suggestions about treating this type of pathocondition?

A: I don't think exposure to sunlight (solar urticaria) is triggering the erythematous plaques, papules, and wheals per say. A more apt Western medicine diagnosis might be miliaria (aka prickly heat, heat rash, or sweat rash) or cholinergic urticaria (aka heat hives). Regardless, I would not worry too much about nomenclature.

These types of skin rashes can be classified as external contraction (microbial infection) evil that has *not* been completely eliminated (邪熱未盡 xié rè wèi jìn) or *persists* as a type of external contraction post-infectious sequelae. In the first scenario, a viral infection has occurred at some time in the past, which remains dormant and undetectable in the body; and in the second scenario, the virus may have been eliminated but has disrupted the functional capacity of the body's immune system mechanisms. In both scenarios, a state of imbalance (dyshomeostasis) results, making the body easily compromised by both internal (e.g., seven affects (emotional and psychological), fatigue) and external (e.g., Western medicine drug side effects, weather, environmental irritants) factors. The compromised immune system overreacts (i.e., hypersensitivity reaction (adaptive immune system)) and fails to protect the body against normally harmless internal and external factors.

Your patient's pathocondition can be identified as either blood desiccation with exterior wind-heat or exterior wind-heat pattern. But I would further examine the skin to conduct more detailed pattern identification based on the coloration (bright red, dark or purplish red, pink) and type of skin manifestations (e.g., plaques, papules, wheals). If the coloration is bright red, then prescribe Gui Zhi Ma Huang Ge Ban Tang adding Huang Qin and Sheng Shi Gao; if it is dark or purplish red, then prescribe Di Gu Pi Yin or Yin Qiao San adding Zhi Zi, Jing Jie, and Fang Feng (or Qing Hao, Zhi Mu, and Di Gu Pi); and if it is pink, then prescribe Blood Desiccation Formula adding The Three Great Yang-Supplementers, Huang Qin, Ma Huang, and Gui Zhi. If serous exudate presents, then add Sheng Shi Gao; and if chilblains (nonfreezing cold injury) presents, then add Wu Zhu Yu, Xi Xin, Mu Tong, Fu Zi, and Huang Qin. Based on your description, Gui Zhi Ma Huang Ge Ban Tang adding Huang Qin and Sheng Shi Gao might be the best choice for this case.

Case Study #2: Winter Itch in the Elderly – Blood Desiccation Itchy Skin

Q: A 75 y/o male patient began having generalized itch (pruritis) over his entire body that was more severe at nighttime. Actually, only the parts of his body that are covered with clothing itch (uncovered areas do *not*), his skin is noticeably hot upon palpation, and there are *no* purpuric lesions. He has been treated with all types of Western medicine topical and oral medication, but nothing has been effective. My idea is to prescribe Di Gu Pi Yin variant, but I am not sure. How would you treat this patient?

A: Dry, itchy skin (e.g., xerosis, xeroderma, xerotic dermatitis, desiccation dermatitis) can be identified as blood desiccation pattern. This pathocondition is particularly prevalent in cold, northern latitudes such as South Korea, where itchy skin during the winter season can be extremely severe, especially for the elderly. Typically, I would consider prescribing a blood-nourishing yin-enriching dryness-moistening formula such as Blood Desiccation Formula, Qi Bao Mei Ran Dan, or Dang Gui Yin Zi; or a qi- and blood-supplementing and flesh-resolving channel-coursing formula such as Gui Qi Jian Zhong Tang or Ge Gen Tang adding Huang Qi.

Remember! Regardless of the formula you choose, you must include Dang Gui, The Three Great Yang-Supplementers, Huang Qin (counterbalances the heat), and adequate doses of Ma Huang (the colder the temperature, the higher the dose!). If oozing and crusting present, then add Sheng Shi Gao; and if purpuric lesions (petechiae, purpura, ecchymoses) and bleeding (sanguineous exudate) present, then prescribe a blood-nourishing yin-enriching formula such as Di Gu Pi Yin. However, you said that your patient does *not* have purpuric lesions, so it's likely a simple case of blood desiccation itchy skin.

Winter itch (winter eczema) can typically be identified as blood desiccation or blood desiccation with itchy skin pattern. By conducting a more thorough examination of the patient, you should be able to determine whether or not there are any signs of concomitant exterior wind-heat, exterior wind-cold, qi vacuity, or yang vacuity pattern presenting. If exterior wind-heat presents, then add Huang Qin and Sheng Shi Gao to your formula.

For patients of all ages with dry, itchy skin during the *cold weather* months and for elderly patients with dry, itchy skin during *all seasons*, I typically will add The Three Great Yang-Supplementers and Huang Qin (counterbalances the heat). During the warm weather months, patients of all ages who present with dry, itchy skin and white or pink-colored marks on their skin after scratching (dermatographia) can also be identified as blood desiccation pattern and treated in the same way.

As for acupuncture, if exterior wind-heat pattern presents, then you can needle Feng Chi (GB20), Tian Zhu (UB10), He Gu (LI4), Chi Ze (LU5), Zu San Li (ST36), and San Yin Jiao (SP6); and if exterior wind-cold, qi vacuity, and yang vacuity patterns present, then you can warm needle He Gu (LI4), Shou San Li (LI10), Zu San Li (ST36), San Yin Jiao (SP6), Yin Ling Quan (SP9), and Xue Hai (SP10).

Case Study #3: Blood Desiccation Formula – Itchy Skin in the Elderly

Q: I have an elderly patient who gets dry, itchy skin during seasonal changes. Now, he has red plaques and wheals on his neck, and after scratching, they swell, coalesce, and enlarge. I identified this condition as blood heat pattern and prescribed Di Gu Pi Yin variant, but the results have not been very impressive. Do you think this is the wrong approach?

A: Elderly patients with dry, itchy skin (xerosis) and winter itch (winter eczema) can be identified as blood desiccation pattern, requiring administration of a blood-nourishing yin-enriching dryness-moistening formula such as Blood Desiccation Formula.

During the cold winter months, you should add The Three Great Yang-Supplementers, Ma Huang, and Huang Qin (counterbalances the heat); and warm needle He Gu (LI4), Shou San Li (LI10), Zu San Li (ST36), San Yin Jiao (SP6), Yin Ling Quan (SP9), and Xue Hai (SP10). During warmer seasons and/or if there is pronounced heat (e.g., erythema and severe itching), then bleed Da Zhui (GV14) (above, on, and below), Cun Kou (Tai Yuan (LU9)), and the three hand and foot yang channel well points; and needle Feng Chi (GB20), Tian Zhu (UB10), He Gu (LI4), Chi Ze (LU5), Zu San Li (ST36), and San Yin Jiao (SP6).

Case Study #4: Blood Desiccation and Psychogenic Itch

Q: Five years ago after giving birth to her daughter, a 43 y/o female patient developed an itching sensation over her entire body (generalized pruritis). At that time, she was diagnosed with chronic eczema, and since then, she has tried all types of treatment (TCM, Western medicine, folk medicine) and even fasting, but nothing has been ultimately effective. In fact, her condition has gotten worse over the years. The last time she came for a clinical visit, she complained of intense itching and presented with crusting and lichenified plaques dispersed over her body and oozing after scratching on the left shin and arm and dorsum of the right foot. Pulse—stringlike, rough, and rapid; stool and urine—normal; and good appetite.

I prescribed Xian Fang Huo Ming Yin variant and performed acupuncture. Initially, this treatment effectively relieved the symptoms, but 1 month later, the condition relapsed and worsened again. This is really a tough case for me. What would you do?

A: This middle-aged female patient with itchy skin sounds like a case of blood desiccation pattern, possibly with a certain degree of psychogenic influence. I would try prescribing either a blood-nourishing yin-enriching dryness-moistening formula such as Blood Desiccation Formula adding Gan Jiang, Fu Zi, Huang Qin, and large doses of Gan Cao, Da Zao, and Long Yan Gan; or a center-harmonizing agitation-calming and stagnation-dissipating phlegm-transforming formula such as Gan Mai Da Zao Tang combining Ban Xia Hou Po Tang adding Gan Jiang, Fu Zi, Huang Qin, Dang Gui, He Shou Wu, Tu Si Zi, and Sha Wan Ji Li. Regardless of the formula you choose, you should also prescribe Yu Sheng Wan (quiets the spirit and calms the nerves), starting out at 2 pills/day, and if necessary, adding 1 to 2 pills along the way.

Case Study #5: Winter Reversal Cold – Dry, Cracked Skin

Q: Every year during the winter months, a 41 y/o female patient gets dry, cracked skin on her fingertips. She has tried all kinds of topical applications (TCM, Western medicine, folk medicine), but nothing has been effective. Do you think this is an accurate diagnosis?

A: Dry, cracked fingertips in the winter time can typically be identified as either reversal cold or blood desiccation pattern. Thus, I would consider prescribing a blood-nourishing network vessel-freeing and cold-dissipating counterflow-downbearing formula such as Dang Gui Si Ni Jia Wu Zhu Yu Sheng Jiang Tang or a blood-nourishing yin-enriching dryness-moistening formula such as Blood Desiccation Formula adding The Three Great Yang-Supplementers and Huang Qin (counterbalances the heat). This will provide effective treatment.

Case Study #6: Photosensitivity Dermatitis and Contact Dermatitis

Q: About 8 years ago, a 37 y/o male patient suddenly began developing intensely itchy, small papules (needle tip to rice grain-sized) upon exposure to sunlight and was diagnosed with photosensitivity dermatitis. He has tried various TCM treatments from different doctors, but the condition has gotten worse instead of better. Now, even wearing snug-fitting clothing will make him feel itchy.

A: This doesn't sound like photosensitivity dermatitis to me, because that condition would not elicit itching upon contact exposure with clothing; or if it is, then it may involve some type of concomitant contact dermatitis. Make sure to closely examine the skin, looking for signs of folliculitis or erythrasma. If these types of exterior wind-heat-damp pattern pathoconditions do *not* present, then this can be classified as residual heat and identified as blood desiccation or blood desiccation itchy skin with mild exterior pattern.

As for treatment, I would first bleed Da Zhui (GV14) (above, on, and below), Cun Kou (Tai Yuan (LU9)), and Wei Zhong (UB40); needle Feng Chi (GB20), Tian Zhu (UB10), He Gu (LI4), Zhong Zhu (TB3), Wei Zhong (UB40), Zu San Li (ST36), and San Yin Jiao (SP6); and prescribe Blood Desiccation Formula adding Huang Qin, Sheng Shi Gao, Sang Bai Pi, Lu Lu Tong, and small doses of Ma Huang and Gui Zhi.

Section 6: Other Skin Diseases

Case Study #1: Nighttime Subcutaneous Leg Pain

Q: A 50 y/o male patient has subcutaneous leg pain at nighttime when he sleeps, which resolves once he gets up, starts moving around (e.g., walking, calisthenics) and works up a bit of a sweat. To me, this suggests a problem with the sweat glands and can be classified as construction-defense disharmony (營衛不和 yíng wèi bù hé). What is your assessment of this case?

A: Yes, this patient with nighttime subcutaneous leg pain that resolves upon perspiration can be classified as construction-defense disharmony. As for treatment, you can prescribe a fleshy exterior-harmonizing and evil-expelling itch-relieving formula such as Gui Zhi Ma Huang Ge Ban Tang. And during the cold weather season, you should add Gan Jiang, Fu Zi, and Huang Qin. Additionally, I would acupuncture (warm needle) Feng Chi (GB20), Tian Zhu (UB10), Yang Ling Quan (GB34), Yin Ling Quan (SP9), Tai Chong (LV3), and Di Wu Hui (GB42).

Case Study #2: Multiple Lipomas

Q: I have a patient with multiple lipomas (generalized lipomatosis) from head to toe over his entire body. How would you treat this patient?

A: Multiple lipomas (generalized lipomatosis) can be identified as exterior wind-damp pattern. If subcutaneous dampness is pronounced, then I would consider prescribing an exterior-resolving dampness eliminating and lung qi-diffusing and -disinhibiting formula variant such as Ma Xing Yi Gan Tang or a heat-clearing phlegm-transforming formula such as Wen Dan Tang adding Bai Jie Zi, Lai Fu Zi, Zao Jiao Ci, Chen Pi, Zhi Ke, and Ban Xia. Otherwise, I would prescribe a heat-clearing toxin-resolving, swelling-dispersing hardness-breaking, and blood-quickening formula such as Xian Fang Huo Ming Yin or a qi- and blood-supplementing and supplementation drawing formula such as Chong He Tang adding Sang Bai Pi, Jiang Pi, and Ci Ji Li.

As for acupuncture, I would needle Feng Chi (GB20), Feng Fu (GV16), He Gu (LI4), Chi Ze (LU5), Zu San Li (ST36), and Feng Long (ST40); and for the larger lipomas, you can consider directly needling into the interior of the lipoma in a radial pattern (approximately 5–8 needles depending on lipoma size) and apply moxa cones on the needle handles (at least 3 cones/needle during each session).

Remember! This pathocondition will require long-term treatment, so it is essential that both you, and the patient, have patience! Over time, the lipomas will gradually shrink in size and absolve the unsightly cosmetic stigma.

Case Study #3: Lower Leg Ulcer and Cold Extremities

Q: A 34 y/o female patient developed a lower leg ulcer and cold extremities after having a hysterectomy. She received Western medicine treatment for over 6 months, but the ulceration on her right calf worsened. At the onset, a 1 cm dark spot appeared on the skin, which then evolved into a suppurative lesion and subsequently healed, forming a scar with hardened skin and black hair growing around the perimeter of the scar.

I have not been successful at treating this type of skin ulceration in the past and am really not sure how to approach this pathocondition. Can you offer any suggestions?

A: For lower leg ulcers you must examine the coloration of the lesion (bright red, purplish red, pink, or pale) and the type of exudate (purulent, purulent crusting, serous, seropurulent, serosanguinous, or sanguinous) in order to conduct pattern identification as the basis for determining treatment. What about the odor? Does the lesion have a rancid odor like that of an animal carcass, feces, or urine?

Based on your description, the ulceration has already healed and the main symptoms now are simply cold extremities. That means all you need to do is prescribe a qi- and blood-supplementing and center-fortifying yang-supplementing formula such as Gui Qi Jian Zhong Tang or a blood-nourishing network vessel-freeing and cold-dissipating counterflow-downbearing formula such as Dang Gui Si Ni Jia Wu Zhu Yu Sheng Jiang Tang adding Fu Zi and Huang Qin.

The administration of this formula over a period of time will dramatically improve circulation, resolve cold extremities, allow the hardened skin to regain suppleness, and prevent leg ulcerations from recurring in the future.

EPILOGUE

Our aim was to provide the reader with an insider's perspective on this subject matter through the compilation of these Q&A format case studies. We sincerely hope that TCM students, scholars, practitioners, physicians, and the interested layperson alike have gleaned valuable information on both the clinical application of TCM in primary and secondary care and as a first-line therapeutic option, as well as the integrative role TCM offers in neoadjuvant, adjuvant, complementary, and palliative therapy.

This fluid introduction of a broad spectrum of pathologies intends to inspire the reader to pursue further research and explore the vast potential for broader clinical applications.

We recognize that the development and expansion of TCM clinical applications is in part influenced by prevailing cultural factors and institutional barriers existing within each respective society and nation. Amidst these dynamics, TCM's increasingly manifest scientific basis and overwhelming efficacy continues propelling this 3,000 year-old medical system to the forefront of inquiry and discovery into its promising possibilities.

We hope that *Integrative Chinese Herbal Therapy Volume II Surfaces in Motion* has piqued your interests for learning more and encourage you to continue reading *Volume I Beyond the Being* and our upcoming volume—*Volume III Roots of Life*—in the near future.

APPENDIX

DR. LEE'S MEDICINALS

This section introduces the medicinals Dr. Lee most commonly prescribes and includes details on processing, properties, actions, indications, dosage, and pharmacodynamics. The vast majority of medicinals prescribed in this text are decocting pieces of mostly raw plants, some crude minerals and shells, and rarely animal products. There are a few exceptions of pulverized medicinals that can be administered orally, either directly ingested or made into pills, or topically applied in the form of rub-on powders, ointments, washes, infusions, and suppositories.

References from TCM classical texts are included, mostly from *The Essential Herbal Foundation* (本草備要 *Ben Cao Bei Yao*), to provide insights into the foundations of Dr. Lee's medicinal applications. Contemporary sources that present commonly acknowledged medicinal attributes (e.g., flavor, nature, channel entry) and experimental findings are also included to provide examples of evidence-based biomedical support of clinical efficacy. The primary source texts for the contemporary medicinal attributes and experimental findings are *Chinese Materia Medica Grand Dictionary* (新編中藥大辭典 *Xin Bian Zhong Yao Da Ci Dian*) and *Clinical Applications of Traditional Chinese Medicine* (中藥臨牀應用 *Zhong Yao Lin Chuang Ying Yong*).

Frequently administered medicinal pairs and combinations are introduced both as single medicinals and together with their counterparts. It is important to reiterate that these profiles are intended to highlight and clarify some of the distinctive features and applications of Dr. Lee's commonly prescribed medicinals, and not an attempt to present a complete listing of every medicinal Dr. Lee utilizes in clinical practice.

Bai Guo Ye (白果葉) – refer to **Yin Xing Ye**

Bai Ji Li (白蒺藜) – refer to **Ci Ji Li**

Bai Jiang Can (白僵蠶/Bombyx Batryticatus/Silkworm/aka **Jiang Can)**

In classical literature on pharmacopoeia, it is described as follows: "[**Bai**] **Jiang** [**Can**] doesn't rot and obtains clearing and transforming qi, thus is able to treat wind and transform phlegm, and dissipate binds and move the channels...."

In contemporary texts, it is described as having a salty and acrid flavor and a balanced nature; entering the liver and lung channels; and having wind-extinguishing tetany-checking, wind-dispelling pain-relieving, and phlegm-transforming bind-dissipating actions. It is recognized as being particularly effective for treating pathoconditions involving fright-wind and epilepsy with phlegm-heat.

Traditionally, it is paired with **Quan Xie** for the treatment of infantile phlegm-heat acute fright. It can also be combined with **Quan Xie** and **Wu Gong** for the treatment of tetanus, spasm, and convulsion with arched-back rigidity, and intractable headache (e.g., migraine, cluster headache).

*For more details, refer to **The Three Insects** profile.

Bai Shao (白芍) – refer to **Chi Shao**

Bai Zhu (白朮/Rhizoma Atractylodis Macrocephalae/White Atractylodes Rhizome)

In classical literature on pharmacopoeia, it is described as follows: "**Bai Zhu** is an essential medicinal for fortifying the spleen and stomach, expelling dampness, eliminating impediment, and dispersing food. [For] vacuous and unfortified spleen, [**Bai**] **Zhu** can supplement; and [for] stomach vacuity failing to absorb, [**Bai**] **Zhu** can assist."

In contemporary texts, it is described as having a bitter and sweet flavor and a warm nature; entering the spleen and stomach channels; and having qi-supplementing spleen-fortifying, dampness-drying water-disinhibiting, sweat-checking, and fetus-quieting actions.

This medicinal contains the primary constituent atractylone as well as esters and carbohydrates (e.g., mannose, fructose) that strengthen the constitution (promote absorption of nutrients by the spleen), disinhibit urine, lower blood sugar levels, and provide anticoagulant, antimicrobial, and anti-inflammatory actions.

Ban Xia (半夏/Rhizoma Pinelliae Ternatae/Pinellia Tuber)

In classical literature on pharmacopoeia, it is described as follows: "Mobile and dissipates and dries and moistens. Harmonizes the stomach and fortifies the spleen, supplements the liver and moistens the lung, eliminates dampness and transforms phlegm, and effuses the exterior and opens depression. Precipitates counterflow qi, checks vomiting and vexation, promotes the voice, disinhibits the waterways, and rescues sudden collapse. Treats cough and counterflow dizzy head, reversal phlegm headache, brow ridge bone pain, sore throat, chest distention, cold damage cold and heat, phlegm malaria sleeplessness, and stomach reflux vomiting; and dissipates impediment, eliminates goiter, disperses swelling and checks sweating."

In contemporary texts, it is described as having an acrid flavor, warm nature, and toxicity; entering the spleen, stomach, and lung channels; and having dampness-drying phlegm-transforming, counterflow-downbearing vomiting-checking, and glomus-dispersing bind-dissipating actions. Ban Xia is recognized as an essential medicinal for drying dampness and transforming phlegm, warming and transforming cold phlegm, and checking vomiting.

Dr. Lee includes the medicinal combination comprising the essential medicinals of Er Chen Tang—**Ban Xia**, **Chen Pi**, **Fu Ling**, and **Gan Cao**—in formulas such as Ban Xia Tian Ma Bai Zhu San, Wen Dan Tang, Xiang Sha Liu Jun Zi Tang, Atopic Dermatitis Formula, Tearing on Exposure to Wind Formula, and Asthma Formula; and the medicinal combination of **Ban Xia**, **Hou Po**, **Fu Ling**, and **Gan Cao** in Ban Xia Hou Po Tang. Additionally, Dr. Lee commonly adds the medicinal combination of **Ban Xia**, **Jie Geng**, and **Gan Cao** into formulas for the treatment of upper respiratory tract (especially the throat) pathoconditions.

Cang Zhu (蒼朮/Rhizoma Atractylodis/Black Atractylodes Rhizome)

In classical literature on pharmacopoeia, it is described as follows: "Dries the stomach and strengthens the spleen, promotes sweating and eliminates dampness, and upbears and effuses yang qi in the stomach…an essential medicinal for dissipating wind-cold-damp in the treatment of wilting [pattern]. And [**Cang Zhu**] can also resolve the six depressions: phlegm, fire, qi, blood, dampness, and food."

In contemporary texts, it is described as having an acrid and bitter flavor and warm nature; entering the spleen and stomach channels; and having spleen-fortifying dampness-drying and wind-damp-dispelling sweat-promoting actions.

Cang Zhu has the spleen-fortifying action of **Bai Zhu**, along with the advantages of stomach dampness-drying and antimicrobial actions for the treatment of gastrointestinal disorders (e.g., sloppy stool, diarrhea, dysentery) and other infectious diseases. Thus, this medicinal is ideal for Taiwan's humid subtropical climate.

Dr. Lee includes **Cang Zhu** in many Yu Sheng formulas, either added into the formula or substituted in place of **Bai Zhu** (unless the patient presents with qi vacuity). The spleen-fortifying dampness-drying action of **Cang Zhu** also counteracts the potential for digestion impairment and sloppy stools some patients experience when administered formulas containing large doses of certain medicinals (e.g., heat-clearing toxin-resolving, yin-nourishing blood-supplementing, blood-quickening stasis-transforming, yin-enriching yang-subduing). Dr. Lee also prescribes this medicinal for the treatment of damp-heat pattern myasthenia gravis, which can be classified as wilting pattern.

The physiological mechanism of its dampness-drying action primarily involves its capacity to promote increased interstitial permeability of water between membranes throughout the body.

*For more details, refer to **The Four Lings** profile.

Chai Hu (柴胡/Radix Bupleuri/Bupleurum Root)

In classical literature on pharmacopoeia, it is described as follows: "Bitter [in flavor] and balanced and slightly cold [in nature], and weak flavor (味薄 wèi báo) and qi upbearing are yang," "Governs yang qi fall, conducts clear qi upward, and thus calms evil heat in the Shao Yang and Jue Yin [channels]. [**Chai Hu**] perfuses and disinhibits qi and blood and dissipates binds and regulates menstruation, and thus is [classified as] a foot Shao Yang exterior medicinal. Treats cold damage evil heat, phlegm-heat repletion binds, vacuity damage flesh heat, retching and vomiting and heart vexation, all [types of] malarial heat (fever) and [aversion to] cold, dizzy head and red eyes, chest impediment and rib-side pain, bitterness of mouth and deafness, heat entering the blood chamber in women, all [types of] antepartum and postpartum heat, pox sores in children, and five (visceral) gan (五疳 wǔ gān) surplus heat. [It] dissipates sores and flat-abscesses of the twelve channels and congeals blood and gathers qi, just like the action of **Lian Qiao**," "Treats binding qi in the heart [region], abdomen, stomach and intestines, dietary accumulations and gatherings, alternating heat (fever) and cold (chills) evil qi [e.g., evil lying depressed in Shao Yang, evil heat depressed internally, liver channel depressed heat], and removes the old and institutes the new (推陳之新 tuī chén zhī xīn)," and "In summary, **Chai Hu** is indicated for only two conditions, one is repletion heat [pattern], for patients with external evil half-interior half-exterior, [it] conducts outward [and] thus enables external evil to naturally effuse from the exterior; and another is right vacuity (正虛 zhèng xū) [pattern], for patients with clear qi falling into the yin aspect, [it] lifts and raises and returns to its residence [and] thus enables qi in the stomach to naturally revitalize."

In contemporary texts, it is described as having a bitter and acrid flavor and slightly cold nature; entering the liver and gallbladder channels; and having heat-clearing and -dissipating, liver-coursing depression-resolving, and yang-upbearing fall-raising actions.

Chai Hu is recognized as a Shao Yang pattern essential medicinal that courses and dissipates Shao Yang half-exterior half-interior evil for the treatment of evil in the Shao Yang channel presenting with symptoms of alternating cold and heat, fullness in the chest and rib-side, bitter taste in the mouth, and dry throat.

Dr. Lee includes the medicinal pair **Chai Hu** and **Huang Qin** in formulas such as Xiao Chai Hu Tang, Chai Ling Tang, and Long Dan Xie Gan Tang.

Chan Tui (蟬蛻/Periostracum Cicadae/Cicada Molt)

In classical literature on pharmacopoeia, it is described as follows: "Salty and sweet [in flavor], cold [in nature], and no toxicity," "Slightly sweet and slightly salty in flavor and slightly cool in nature," and "**Chan** embodies the transformation of earth and wood excess qi and [it] drinks wind dew, thus does not intake food. Its qi is clear and vacuous and sweet [in flavor] and cold [in nature], thus eliminates wind-heat. Its body is light and floating, thus effuses pox sores. Its nature excels at molting, thus abates eye screen and hastens delivery and aborts the fetus. Its **molt** is an exoskeleton, thus treats skin sores and dormant papules, and its sound is clear and resonant, thus treats wind strike with loss of voice. Also, [it] rings in the day and rests at night, thus checks night crying in infants."

In contemporary texts, it is described as having a sweet flavor and cold nature; entering the lung and liver channels; and having wind-coursing heat-dissipating, papule-outthrusting itch-relieving, eye-brightening screen-abating, and fright-checking actions.

Dr. Lee classifies **Chan Tui** as an exterior membrane conductor (i.e., eyes, skin) based on its innate substance as slough (shed epithelial tissue) and its inherent capacity to *peel off* the agglutinated protein build-up on the membranous surfaces of the eyes. This is an example of the classical TCM treatment method of "resembling forms treat respective body parts and resembling organs treat respective organs (以形治形、以臟治臟 yǐ xíng zhì xíng, yǐ zàng zhì zàng)."

Dr. Lee typically prescribes the medicinal pair **Chan Tui** and **She Tui** (dispels wind, disperses swelling, kills worms, abates screens, and stabilizes fright) for the treatment of ophthalmological pathoconditions, such as lens opacities (e.g., cataract) and corneal opacities (e.g., eye screen (目翳 mù yì), scarring), and for dermatological pathoconditions presenting with intense pruritis.

*For more details, refer to **The Eye Brighteners** and **The Itch Relievers** profiles.

Chi Shao (赤芍/Radix Paeoniae Rubra/Red Peony Root)

In classical literature on pharmacopoeia, the attributes of **Chi Shao** and **Bai Shao (白芍)** are described as follows: "**Bai Shao** supplements and contracts and **Chi Shao** drains and dissipates. **Bai** [**Shao**] benefits the spleen and drains water from earth [spleen]; **Chi** [**Shao**] dissipates evil and moves stagnation in the blood."

In contemporary texts, **Chi Shao** is described as having a bitter flavor and slightly cold nature; entering the liver channel; and having heat-clearing blood-cooling and stasis-dissipating pain-relieving actions. **Bai Shao** is described as having a bitter, sour, and sweet flavor and slightly cold nature; entering the liver and spleen channel; and having yin-nourishing menstruation-regulating, liver-calming pain-relieving, and yin-consolidating sweat-checking actions.

A contemporary comparison of these two medicinals is as follows: "**Chi Shao** excels at quickening the blood and dissipating stasis and **Bai Shao** is better at tranquilizing and relieving pain; both have supplementing actions with **Bai Shao** superior at supplementing blood and nourishing yin, and **Chi Shao** superior at cooling the blood and expelling stasis."

Dr. Lee explains that most traditional formulas designed in times of antiquity originally included **Bai Shao** because the clinical presentation of dual qi and blood vacuity was far more prevalent back then, thus necessitating the emphasis of this medicinal's blood-nourishing actions. Our modern lifestyle, diet, and living environs have altered people's body constitutions with blood stasis and stagnation and a predilection towards blood heat more predominant nowadays. Thus, the blood-cooling stasis expelling actions of **Chi Shao** are more suitable for patients of today, and this is the reasoning behind **Chi Shao** replacing **Bai Shao** in Yu Sheng formula compositions and variants. Dr. Lee also adds large doses of this medicinal into formulas during certain stages of cancer treatment to inhibit tumor angiogenesis (neovascularization).

Chuan Qi (川七/Radix Notoginseng/Notoginseng Root/aka **San Qi, Shan Qi)**

In classical literature on pharmacopoeia, it is described as follows: "Dissipates blood and settles pain. Treats blood ejection and spontaneous external bleeding, blood dysentery and flooding, red eyes and swollen welling-abscesses, and is an essential medicinal for knife, club, and incised wounds" and "**Chuan Qi**...excels at transforming static blood, [it] also excels at stanching the frenetic movement of blood, is an essential medicinal for blood ejection and spontaneous external bleeding, and following [treatment] and recovery no static blood is left behind in the channels and network vessels...and [it] transforms blood stasis without compromising the engendering of new blood, making it a superb blood-rectifying medicinal."

In contemporary texts, it is described as having a sweet and slightly bitter flavor and a warm nature; entering the liver and stomach channels; and having stasis-transforming blood-stanching and blood-quickening pain-settling actions.

Chuan Qi is clinically recognized as a blood-stanching and stasis-transforming essential medicinal and also has blood-quickening pain-relieving actions that can be prescribed for the treatment of pathoconditions involving a wide range of blood stasis pattern pathoconditions, such as compromised blood perfusion (e.g., cardiovascular disease (CVD), cerebrovascular disease (CVA)) and all types of bleeding and hemorrhage.

Chuan Qi is an expensive medicinal and the process of decoction diminishes potency, thus Dr. Lee typically administers it as a pulverized powder to minimize cost and maximize efficacy. This powder is either added directly into a formula after the decoction has cooled or taken separately. Since Dr. Lee prescribes **Chuan Qi** in pulverized powder form, it is omitted from Yu Sheng formula composition listings, which are decocting pieces only. This medicinal is often paired with **Ren Shen (powder)** to form **Ren Shen/Chuan Qi Powder**, one of the pillars of Dr. Lee's therapeutic approaches.

*For more details, refer to the **Ren Shen/Chuan Qi Powder** profile.

Ci Ji Li (刺蒺藜/ Fructus Tribuli/Caltrop Fruit/aka **Ji Li Zi, Bai Ji Li)**

In classical literature on pharmacopoeia, it is described as follows: "Bitter and acrid [in flavor] and warm [in nature]," "Enters the lung, liver, and kidney channels," and "Supplements the kidney with bitterness and warmth, drains lung qi with acridity and warmth, and also dissipates liver wind, and boosts essence and brightens the eyes. Treats vacuity taxation lumbar pain, seminal emission and vaginal discharge, cough counterflow and lung wilting, milk block and concretions and conglomerations, hemorrhoids and fistulas and yin depletion, diseases of the liver, kidney, and lung channels, and hastens delivery and aborts the fetus."

In contemporary texts, it is described as having a bitter and acrid flavor and balanced nature; entering the liver, kidney, and lung channels; and having liver-calming liver-coursing and wind-dispelling eye-brightening actions.

Traditionally, **Ci Ji Li** is prescribed in combination with **Chan Tui** and **Fang Feng** for the treatment of exterior wind-heat, damp-heat, and blood desiccation pattern skin pathoconditions presenting with itchy papules (e.g., urticaria, eczema (damp papules), neurodermatitis); and with **Zao Jiao Ci** and **Chan Tui** to promote the dispersion and rupture of welling-abscesses and sores and relieve itching.

Dr. Lee typically adds the medicinal pair **Ci Ji Li** and **Zao Jiao Ci** (quickens the blood and disperses swelling and expels pus and frees milk) into formula variants for the treatment of exterior wind-heat pattern ophthalmological pathoconditions affecting the tear ducts (e.g., epidemic keratoconjunctivitis ("pinkeye")) and damp-heat pattern dermatological pathoconditions (e.g., lipomas, flat warts).

Dr. Lee further classifies **Ci Ji Li**, **Zao Jiao Ci**, and **Lu Lu Tong** (expels wind and frees the network vessels and disinhibits water and eliminates dampness) as pore conductor medicinals with their capacity to regulate—*opening* and *closing* (開闔 kāi hé)—of the pores and promote dermal circulation. Thus, he also adds this medicinal combination into formula variants for exterior wind-heat (or wind-heat-damp) and blood desiccation pattern with exterior wind-heat (or with exterior wind-heat-damp) skin pathoconditions presenting with pruritic papules and maculopapular and vesicular eruptions (e.g., dyshidrotic eczema (pompholyx), palmoplantar pustulosis (PPP), wind papules (urticaria), acute stage atopic dermatitis).

Dr. Lee explains that blood-quickening stasis-transforming medicinals (e.g., **Dang Gui**, **Chuan Xiong**, **Ru Xiang**, **Mo Yao**) promote an increase of angiogenic proteins, the precursors necessary for angiogenesis, while the medicinal pair **Zao Jiao Ci** and **Ci Ji Li** has the capacity to open up pathways in the granulation tissue and collagen deposition formed during the wound healing process. The prescription of these mutually complementary medicinals reestablishes patent vasculature and perfusion at the site of the fibrous tissue (i.e., scar) formation, restores the natural skin coloration, and shrinks the size of the scar, thus improving the cosmetic appearance of both hypertrophic and keloid scars.

*For more details, refer to **The Eye Brighteners** and **The Itch Relievers** profiles.

Cu Lu Rong (粗鹿茸) – refer to **Lu Rong**

Da Huang (大黃/Radix et Rhizoma Rhei/Rhubarb Root)

This medicinal is processed in Dr. Lee's in-house processing facility. Purchased raw, it is first steeped in rice wine over a period of 10 days (in warm weather) to 2 weeks (in cold weather), oven-dried, and then cut to be used as decocting pieces or pulverized into a powder for topical application.

In classical literature on pharmacopoeia, it is described as follows: "Great bitter [in flavor] and great cold [in nature]," "Enters the foot Tai Yin [channel] and hand and foot Yang Ming and Jue Yin [channels] blood aspect," and "Its nature is upbearing and thus does not sink, and its action is mobile and thus is not static. If steeped in wine [it] can also conduct upwards, [for] application in flushing the stomach and intestines and precipitating dryness-bind to eliminate static heat. It treats cold damage seasonal disease (傷寒時疾 shāng hán shí jí), heat effusion (fever) with delirious speech, warm-heat miasmic malaria (瘴瘧 zhàng nüè), red and white dysentery, abdominal pain and urgency, jaundice and water-swelling (edema), concretions, conglomerations, accumulations and gatherings, lodged rheum and abiding food (留飲宿食 liú yǐn sù shí), distention and fullness in the heart [region] and abdomen, fecal and urinary stoppage, blood ejection and spontaneous external bleeding, blood block and blood desiccation, blood accumulation due to damage, and all [types of] repletion heat and latent heat in the blood (血分伏熱 xuè fēn fú rè). Moves water and eliminates phlegm, erodes pus and disperses swelling, and can remove the old and institute the new."

In contemporary texts, it is described as having a bitter flavor and cold nature; entering the spleen, stomach, large intestine, liver, and heart channels; and having draining and precipitating accumulation-attacking, heat-clearing toxin-resolving, fire-draining, blood-quickening stasis-transforming, and blood-stanching actions.

This medicinal is administered for patients with a wide range of pathoconditions from gastrointestinal disorders (e.g., constipation, gallstones) to elevated intracranial pressure. Its heat-clearing draining precipitation, fire-draining, accumulation-attacking, and blood-quickening stasis-transforming actions promote the removal of metabolic waste byproducts resulting from nerve cell damage and static blood; break down bile; reduce pressure of the portal vein and relax the diaphragm muscles; stimulate intestinal motility; and eliminate endothelial hyperplasia (e.g., inflammation from autoimmune disease, viral infection). For the treatment of increased intracranial pressure (ICP), initially small amounts are prescribed, increasing incrementally in 5 fen doses up to 7–8 qian until the desired draining precipitation action is achieved, which is typically 2–3 stools per day (sometimes as much as 5 stools per day depending on the pathocondition).

In addition to oral administration, **Da Huang** powder can be topically applied on open sores for its antimicrobial and blood-stanching actions. It dries and forms a protective barrier that prevents infectious agents from entering the wound and simultaneously fights infection within the lesion. For these reasons, Da Huang is often applied topically in Dr. Lee's clinic following bloodletting therapy. Da Huang can also be blended into either a petrolatum or an emulsifying hydrophilic ointment base for the treatment of inflammatory skin pathoconditions (e.g., streptococcal, staphylococcal).

Dan Pi (牡丹皮) – refer to **Mu Dan Pi**

Dan Shen (丹參/Radix Salviae Miltiorrhizae/Salvia Root)

In classical literature on pharmacopoeia, it is described as follows: "**Dan Shen** is bitter in flavor, engenders the new and dispels evil, breaks accumulations and regulates menstruation, and disperses welling- and flat-abscesses" and "…[its] actions are equivalent to Si Wu [Tang], and is an essential gynecological medicinal."

In contemporary texts, it is described as having a bitter flavor and slightly cold nature; entering the heart and liver channels; and having blood-quickening menstruation-regulating, blood-cooling welling abscess-dispersing, and spirit-quieting actions. Traditionally, it is one of the most commonly used medicinals for gynecological and obstetric pathoconditions.

Dr. Lee commonly includes **Dan Shen** decocting pieces in qi-supplementing, blood-supplementing, and stasis-dispelling formulas instead of **Ren Shen** to improve cerebrovascular, cardiovascular, and peripheral vascular circulation and diffuse depressed heat. This substitution is founded in the TCM classical theory of enduring illness results in stasis, which applies to many of Dr. Lee's patients who seek treatment for their chronic pathoconditions. Depending on the presenting signs, symptoms, and pattern, Dr. Lee may prescribe **Ren Shen** (powder) (or **Ren Shen/Chuan Qi Powder**) and **Dan Shen** together with their respective qi- and blood-supplementing actions forming a complementary medicinal combination that adheres to the TCM classical theory of qi is the commander of blood and blood is the mother of qi (氣為血之帥、血為氣之母 qì wèi xuè zhī shuài, xiě wéi qì zhī mǔ).

Dang Gui (當歸/Radix Angelicae Sinensis/Chinese Angelica Root)

This medicinal is processed in-house in Dr. Lee's own medicinal processing and decoction facility. Raw **Dang Gui** (head, body, and tail) is first washed and cleaned and then placed in barrels where it is steeped in cooking rice wine until the roots are fully saturated (anywhere from 10 days (hot weather) up to 2 weeks (cold weather)).

The saturated roots are then oven-dried at low temperatures to preserve freshness and ensure longer storage life.

In classical literature on pharmacopoeia, it is described as follows: "Supplements the blood, moistens dryness, and lubricates the intestines," "**Dang Gui** is sweet [in flavor] and warm [in nature], engenders blood and supplements the heart, supports vacuity and boosts detriment, and expels stasis and engenders the new," and "**Dang Gui** is sweet in flavor and heavy, thus specializes in supplementing blood; it is acrid [in flavor] and its qi is light, thus it also moves blood. Movement in supplementation and supplementation in movement, indeed, it is a qi-in-blood medicinal (血中氣藥 xuè zhòng qì yào) and an in-blood sage medicinal."

In contemporary texts, it is described as having a sweet and acrid flavor and a warm nature; entering the liver, heart, and spleen channels; and having blood-supplementing blood-harmonizing, menstruation-regulating pain-checking, and dryness-moistening intestine lubricating actions. Prescribed in small doses (≤ 2 qian), it nourishes blood; in large doses (3–4 qian), it has blood-quickening stasis-transforming actions.

Dang Shen (黨參/Radix Codonopsis/Codonopsis Root)

In classical literature on pharmacopoeia, it is described as follows: "Enters the hand and foot Tai Yin channel qi aspect" and "Supplements the center and boosts qi, harmonizes the spleen and stomach, and eliminates vexation-heat. [For] slight vacuity of center qi, use [**Dang Shen**] to regulate and supplement, it's the most appropriate."

In contemporary texts, this medicinal is described as having a sweet flavor and a slightly warm nature; entering the spleen and lung channels; and having center-supplementing qi-boosting, spleen-fortifying lung-boosting, and liquid-engendering actions.

Considering the comparatively high cost of **Ren Shen**, many TCM physicians will substitute **Dang Shen** for mild cases of center qi vacuity. However, for the types of severe acute diseases and chronic disorders that Dr. Lee commonly treats presenting with pronounced blood stasis and qi vacuity, **Dang Shen** is generally *not* a viable substitute. Instead, Dr. Lee will prescribe **Dan Shen** (blood-quickening stasis-transforming and blood-cooling actions) decocting pieces in place of **Dang Shen**, and either add **Ren Shen** (powder) separately for its potent qi-supplementing and nourishing actions or **Ren Shen/Chuan Qi Powder** for its qi-supplementing, nourishing, and stasis-dispelling actions. Dr. Lee *does* include **Dang Shen** in formulas such as Gui Zhi Jia Long Gu Mu Li Tang, Pu Xiao Dang Bao Tang, and Sheng Hua Tang to improve the flavor of the formula, supplement qi, fortify the stomach, and promote digestion.

Di Gu Pi (地骨皮/Cortex Lycii/Chinese Wolfberry Root Bark)

Di Gu Pi is the root bark of either *Lycium chinensis* Mill. or *Lycium barbarum* L., and the ripe fruit of the latter is **Gou Qi Zi**.

In classical literature on pharmacopoeia, it is described as follows: "Downbears latent fire in the lung and drains liver and kidney vacuity heat. Cools the blood and supplements right qi, thus treats evil heat of the five [organs] internally, blood ejection (吐血 tù xiě) and bloody urine, and cough and dispersion-thirst…Treats exterior unfixed location wind evil and corpse transmission (consumption) (傳戶 chuán hù) steaming bone with sweating."

In contemporary texts, it is described as having a sweet and bland flavor and cold nature; entering the lung, liver, and kidney channels; and having blood-cooling steam-eliminating and lung-clearing fire-downbearing actions. It is recognized as among the best medicinals for abating vacuity heat and taxation heat and treating steaming bone qi aspect pathoconditions.

Dr. Lee includes this medicinal paired with **Mu Dan Pi** (a steaming bone blood aspect medicinal) in the formula Di Gu Pi Yin and together with **Qing Hao** and **Zhi Mu** in Hyperactive Immune Formula. Additionally, he commonly adds the combination of **Qing Hao**, **Di Gu Pi**, and **Zhi Mu** into formula variants for the treatment of all types of pathoconditions presenting with symptoms such as intermittent fever, enduring heat, enduring cough, and yin vacuity dryness.

Di Huang (地黃) – refer to **Sheng Di Huang**

Di Long (地龍/Lumbricus/Earthworm/aka **Qiu Yin)**

In classical literature on pharmacopoeia, it is described as follows: "Cold in nature but descending, cold in nature thus resolves all types of heat diseases, descending thus disinhibits urine, and treats lower extremity diseases and frees the channels and network vessels. Indicated for cold damage malaria, great heat mania and vexation, urinary stoppage in adults and children, acute and chronic fright wind (急慢慄風 jí màn jǐng fēng), and joint-running wind pain (歷節風痛 lì jié fēng tòng)."

In contemporary texts, it is described as having a salty flavor and cold nature; entering the liver, spleen, and urinary bladder channel; and having heat-clearing wind-extinguishing, channel-freeing network vessel-quickening, panting-calming, and urine-disinhibiting actions.

Dr. Lee commonly pairs this medicinal with **Ma Huang** for pathoconditions affecting the respiratory and vasomotor centers in the brainstem (e.g., cerebrovascular accident (CVA), trauma, microbial infection, enduring illness) and for the treatment of wind-cold-damp impediment.

Ding Shu Xiu (丁豎杇/Scaber Elephantopus/Elephant's Foot)

In contemporary texts, it is described as having an acrid flavor and cool nature; entering the liver, kidney, stomach, and small intestine; and having urine-disinhibiting swelling-dispersing, blood-cooling toxin-resolving, phlegm-dispelling, and pain-relieving actions.

In Dr. Lee's pharmacopoeia, it is an essential medicinal for inhibiting the synthesis of blood urea nitrogen (BUN) and serum creatinine (Cr) in the treatment of pathological conditions that result from hypoperfusion of blood through functionally normal kidneys (prerenal), structural damage to the renal parenchyma (intrinsic renal), and urinary tract obstruction (postrenal).

Dr. Lee commonly prescribes **Ding Shu Xiu** paired with **Ren Dong Teng**, adding them into Wu Ling San (Nephritis Formula), Chai Ling Tang, or other formula variants based on presenting signs, symptoms, and pattern identification.

Du Zhong (杜仲/Cortex Eucommiae/Eucommia Bark)

In classical literature on pharmacopoeia, it is described as follows: "For all [types of] vacuity in the lower burner, without **Du Zhong** [one] cannot supplement; [for] dampness in the lower burner, without **Du Zhong** [one] cannot disinhibit; [for] aching in the legs, without **Du Zhong** [one] cannot eliminate, and [for] pain in the lumbus and knees, without **Du Zhong** [one] cannot eliminate…[For] supplementing the liver and boosting the kidney, [it] is indeed an essential medicinal," "Treats lumbar spine pain, supplements the center and boosts qi, hardens the sinew and bone, strengthens the mind, and eliminates genital damp itch and dribble after voiding," and

"Sweet [in flavor] and warm [in nature] [it] can supplement and mildly acrid [in flavor] [it] can moisten. The color purple enters the liver channel qi aspect, moistens liver dryness, and supplements liver vacuity. The child makes the mother replete, thus [it] also supplements the kidney. When the liver is full, the sinews are fortified and when the kidney is full, the bones are strengthened, thus enabling the sinews and bones to fix together [attach]. Treats aching lumbus and knees, genital damp itch, dribble after voiding, and fetal spotting and miscarriage."

In contemporary texts, it is described as having a sweet flavor and warm nature; entering the liver and kidney channels; and having liver and kidney-supplementing, sinew- and bone-strengthening, and fetus-quieting actions.

Dr. Lee commonly pairs **Du Zhong** and **Niu Xi** (quickens the blood and dissipates stasis, supplements the liver and kidney, and frees the channels (menstruation) and relieves pain) in the formulas You Gui Yin, Tong Jing Fang, Paralysis Formula #1, Paralysis Formula #3, and Zuo Gui Yin. Dr. Lee also pairs **Du Zhong** with **Xu Duan** (quickens the blood, stanches bleeding, quiets the fetus, and supplements the liver and kidney) in the formula Dang Gui San.

Duan Long Gu (Calcined Dragon Bone) – refer to **Long Gu**

Duan Mu Li (**Calcined Oyster Shell**) – refer to **Mu Li**

Duan Shi Gao (Calcined Gypsum) – refer to **Shi Gao**

Fu Ling (茯苓/Sclerotium Poriae Cocos/Poria)

In classical literature on pharmacopoeia, it is described as follows: "**Fu Ling** is sweet [in flavor] and warm [in nature], engenders liquid and checks thirst, abates heat and quiets the fetus, and boosts the spleen and aides yang" and "...percolates dampness and disinhibits the orifices and eliminates dampness...."

In contemporary texts, it is described as having a sweet and bland flavor and balanced nature; entering the heart, spleen, and kidney channels; and having water-disinhibiting dampness-percolating, and spleen-fortifying spirit-quieting actions. It is experimentally proven to increase the urinary excretion of electrolytes (e.g., potassium, sodium, chloride), lower blood sugar levels, and provide sedative actions.

As a general rule, if large doses of this medicinal are prescribed (≥ 8 qian), Dr. Lee will include a comparable dose of **Ze Xie** to enhance water-disinhibiting actions.

*For more details, refer to **The Four Lings** profile.

Fu Zi (附子/Radix Aconiti Lateralis Carmichaeli Praeparata/ Aconite)

In this book the medicinal referred to as **Fu Zi** is actually **Tian Xiong (天雄)**, which is the root tuber of this plant without the daughter (accessory) roots. The processing of this medicinal entails steeping in a solution of magnesium chloride ($MgCl_2$), sodium chloride (NaCl), and water, and then it is dried and sliced into small pieces.

In classical literature on pharmacopoeia, it is described as follows: "The mother [root] is **Wu Tou (烏頭)**, the [peripheral] accessory roots are **Fu Zi**, the [peripheral] extensions [of the accessory roots] are **Ce Zi (側子)**, and the long slender part [extending from the mother root] is **Tian Xiong**," "…great drying and yang returning, kidney- and life fire-supplementing, and wind-cold-damp-expelling [actions]," and "…frees the twelve channels [with] no limits beyond its reach."

In contemporary texts, it is described as having an acrid and sweet flavor, hot nature, and toxicity; entering the heart, kidney, and spleen channels; and having yang-returning counterflow-stemming, yang-reinforcing fire-supplementing, and cold-dissipating pain-relieving actions.

*For more details, refer to **The Three Great Yang-Supplementers** profile.

Gan Di Huang (乾地黃) – refer to Sheng Di Huang

Gan Jiang (乾薑/Rhizoma Zingiberis Officianalis/Dried Ginger)

This medicinal is processed by steaming **Sheng Jiang** with sulfur. In classical literature on pharmacopoeia, it is described as having "drying, yang-returning, diffusing, and vessel-freeing [actions]" and the complementary relationship between **Gan Jiang** and **Fu Zi** is expressed as follows: "**Fu Zi** is mobile [extends throughout body] and **Gan Jiang** is both mobile and static [long-lasting effect]."

In contemporary texts, it is described as having a bitter and astringent flavor and a warm nature, entering the spleen and liver channels, and having center-warming cold-expelling and yang-returning vessel-freeing actions.

*For more details, refer to **The Three Great Yang-Supplementers** profile.

Ge Gen (葛根/Radix Puerariae/Kudzu Root)

In classical literature on pharmacopoeia, it is described as follows: "Acrid and sweet [in flavor] and balanced [in nature] and light [and] buoyant [so it] upbears and effuses," "[**Ge Gen**] enters Yang Ming channel, thus can move stomach qi upwards, engender liquid and check thirst; and also enters the spleen channel, thus opens the interstices and promotes sweating and resolves flesh and abates heat. [It] is a sage medicinal for treating spleen and stomach vacuity diarrhea. Treats cold damage and wind strike, Yang Ming headache, blood dysentery and warm malaria, and intestinal wind and pox sores (痘瘡 dòu chuāng). [It] can also raise yin wind, dissipate bind fire, resolve liquor toxicity, disinhibit stool and urine, and kills the toxin of the hundred medicinals."

In contemporary texts, it is described as having a sweet and acrid flavor and cool (or balanced) nature; entering the spleen and stomach channels; and having flesh-resolving heat-abating, measles- and papules-outthrusting, liquid-engendering thirst-allaying, and yang-upbearing diarrhea-checking actions.

The main constituents of **Ge Gen** are daidzein, puerarin and other isoflavones, which function as signal carriers and defense responses to pathogenic attacks; and it also contains phytoestrogens with antioxidant properties. This medicinal has been experimentally proven to increase coronary and cerebral blood flow, reduce myocardial oxygen consumption and increase oxygen supply, directly dilate blood vessels, and inhibit platelet aggregation.

Gen Gen is the sovereign medicinal in Ge Gen Tang, which Dr. Lee commonly prescribes for pathoconditions such as externally contracted wind-cold, crick in the neck (落枕 lào zhěn) and painful stiff nape (頭項強痛 tóu xiàng qiáng tòng). Dr. Lee also combines this medicinal with **Huang Qin** and **Huang Lian** to form a variant of Ge Gen Qin Lian Tang for the treatment of exterior (evil) not yet resolved and evil heat entering the interior with heat diarrhea (or heat dysentery).

Gu Sui Bu (骨碎補/Rhizoma Drynariae/Boneknit Root)

In classical literature on pharmacopoeia, it is described as follows: "Bitterness and warmth supplement the kidney, thus [it] treats tinnitus and kidney vacuity enduring diarrhea. [Since] the kidney governs bone, [it] treats fractures and toothache. [**Gu Sui Bu**] also enters Jue Yin [channel] and can break blood and stanch bleeding."

In contemporary texts, it is described as having a bitter flavor and warm nature; entering the liver and kidney channels; and having blood-quickening injury-mending and kidney-supplementing bone-strengthening actions.

Dr. Lee commonly adds the medicinal pair **Gu Sui Bu** and **Xu Duan** (quickens the blood, joins sinews and bones, supplements the liver and kidney, and quiets the fetus) into formula variants for the treatment of skeletal bone, marrow, and dental pathoconditions (e.g., fractures, osteoporosis, periodontitis). This medicinal pair is also included among the essential medicinals in the medicinal paste Diao Fen Gao (Suspension Powder Paste). And for the treatment of both malignant and benign tumors, this medicinal pair serves as a conductor that targets hard tissue—eliminating stasis and engendering the new. The medicinal combination of **Gu Sui Bu**, **Xu Duan** and **Niu Xi** (quickens the blood and dissipates stasis, supplements the liver and kidney, and frees the channels (menstruation) and relieves pain) comprise the essential medicinals of the formula Tong Jing Fang.

Gui Zhi (桂枝) – refer to **Rou Gui**

Huang Bai (黃柏) – refer to **Huang Bo**

Huang Bo (黃柏/Cortex Phellodendri/Phellodendron Bark/aka **Huang Bai)**

In classical literature on pharmacopoeia, it is described as follows: "Drains ministerial fire and supplements kidney water," "**Huang Bo** is bitter [in flavor] and cold [in nature], drains fire and nourishes yin, and can be used [to treat] steaming bone with damp-heat and precipitation of blood," "[It is a] foot Tai Yang channel conductor medicinal," and "Combined with **Cang Zhu** [this pair] is called Er Miao Wan (二妙丸) (aka Mysterious Two Powder), [with its] heat-clearing dampness-disinhibiting actions forming an essential medicinal [pair] for treating wilting [pattern]."

In contemporary texts, this medicinal is described as having a bitter flavor and cold nature; entering the kidney, urinary bladder, and large intestine channels; and having heat-clearing dampness-drying, fire-draining toxin-resolving, and heat-abating steam-eliminating actions.

*For more details, refer to **The Three Yellows** profile.

Huang Lian (黃連/Rhizoma Coptidis/Coptis Rhizome)

In classical literature on pharmacopoeia, it is described as follows: "**Huang Lian** is bitter in flavor, drains the heart and eliminates impediment, drains heat and resolves toxin, and thickens the intestines and checks diarrhea" and "It has six actions: one, drains heart fire; two, eliminates middle burner heat; three, indispensable for [treating] all sores; four, eliminates wind-damp; five, treats fulminant fire eye (暴發火眼 bao fā huǒ yǎn); and six, checks blood in the stool."

In contemporary texts, it is described as having a cold nature and bitter flavor; entering the heart, liver, stomach, and large intestine channels; and having heat-clearing dampness-drying and fire-draining toxin-resolving actions.

The market price of this medicinal frequently fluctuates and is considerably more expensive than **Huang Qin** and **Huang Bo**. Thus, due to cost considerations, Dr. Lee tends to either prescribe smaller doses of this medicinal, or substitutes **Huang Qin** and/or **Huang Bo** instead, or prescribe a combination of all three (aka **The Three Yellows**) depending on the pattern and pathocondition being treated. Typically, larger doses of **Huang Lian** are reserved for severe heat patterns or specific pathoconditions such as vasculitis, gastrointestinal ulcers, inflammatory autoimmune disorders.

*For more details, refer to **The Three Yellows** profile.

Huang Qi (黃耆/Radix Astragali/Astragalus Root)

Dr. Lee only administers premium quality raw northern **Huang Qi**, which is distinguishable by its reddish phloem that encircles the xylem of the vascular tissue of the plant. In classical literature on pharmacopoeia it is described as follows: "**Raw [Huang Qi]** secures the exterior, effuses in the absence of sweating, checks in the presence of sweating, warms the seam of the flesh (肉分 ròu fēn), fortifies the interstices of the flesh, drains yin fire, and resolves flesh heat. **Mix-fried [Huang Qi]** supplements the center and boosts original qi, warms the triple burner, strengthens the spleen and stomach, engenders blood and flesh, expels pus and internally draws, and is a sore and welling-abscess sage medicinal."

In contemporary texts, it is described as having a sweet flavor and a slightly warm nature; entering the spleen and lung channels; and having qi-supplementing yang-upbearing, water-disinhibiting swelling-dispersing, and sore-expressing flesh-engendering actions.

For the treatment of qi vacuity pattern pathoconditions, Dr. Lee typically starts out with a dose of 1 liang and increases incrementally by 5 qian every 1–2 weeks depending on the patient's presenting signs and symptoms, eventually peaking at a maximum dose of 2.5 liang. Excessive doses of beyond 3–5 liang may cause compromised blood vessels to rupture or paroxysmal increases in intracranial pressure in the presence of arteriosclerosis, atheroclerosis, hematoma, or adhesions in the subarachnoid space of the meninges.

Dr. Lee explains that **Huang Qi** promotes accelerated exchanges across membranes throughout the body and regulates the permeability of the glomerular membrane thus inhibiting protein loss. This medicinal has been experimentally and clinically proven to eliminate nephritic proteinuria, increase myocardial contractility, contain estrogen-like effects, and provide broad-spectrum antimicrobial efficacy.

Among its bioactive constituents, astragalus saponins lower blood pressure, promote erythrocyte membrane stability, increase c-AMP concentration of blood plasma and tissues, boost immune function, and promote the regeneration of liver DNA synthesis; and astragalus polysaccharides enhance immune function, regulate blood sugar levels, protect the cardiovascular system, and accelerate regeneration of tissue growth in patients suffering from radiotherapy complications.

Huang Qin (黄芩/Radix Scutellariae/Scutellaria Root)

In classical literature on pharmacopoeia, it is described as follows: "**Huang Qin** is bitter [in flavor] and cold [in nature], bitter drains liver fire, engenders and clears the large intestine, and [treats] both damp and heat," "Bitter [flavor] enters the heart, cold [nature] overcomes heat, drains the middle burner fire [and] eliminates spleen domain damp-heat...," "[Zhu (朱)] Dan Xi (丹溪) uses **Huang Qin** to downbear phlegm as a means of downbearing fire," and "**Huang Qin** is an upper and middle burner medicinal."

In contemporary texts, it is described as having a cold nature and bitter flavor; entering the lung, stomach, gallbladder, and large intestine channels; and having heat-clearing dampness-drying, fire-draining toxin-resolving, blood-cooling blood-stanching, and heat eliminating fetus-quieting actions.

*For more details, refer to **The Three Yellows** profile.

Ji Nei Jin (雞內金/Endothelium Corneum Gigeriae Galli/Chicken Gizzard/aka **Ji Zhun Pi)**

In classical literature on pharmacopoeia, it is described as follows: "Sweet and balanced [in flavor] and astringent in nature" and "Disperses grain and water, eliminates heat and relieves vexation, and frees the small intestine and urinary bladder. Treats diarrhea and dysentery and frequent defecation, enuresis and bloody urine, flooding and vaginal discharge and intestinal wind, diaphragm dispersion and stomach reflux, and food malaria in children."

In contemporary texts, it is described as having a sweet flavor and neutral nature; entering the spleen, stomach, small intestine, and urinary bladder channels; and having food-dispersing stomach-fortifying and essence-astringing (seminal) emission- and enuresis-checking actions.

Dr. Lee commonly adds the medicinal pair **Ji Nei Jin** and **Shan Zha** into formulas (e.g., heat-clearing toxin-resolving, yin-nourishing blood-supplementing, blood-quickening stasis-transforming, yin-enriching yang-subduing) that may impair digestion and cause sloppy stools in some patients. This medicinal pair is also added into formula variants for the treatment of hyperlipidemia and hypertrigliceridemia.

Ji Li Zi (蒺藜子) – refer to **Ci Ji Li**

Jiang Can (僵蠶) – refer to **Bai Jiang Can**

Jie Geng (桔梗/Radix Platycodi/Platycodon Root)

In classical literature on pharmacopoeia, it is described as follows: "White in color and belongs to metal, enters the lung and drains heat. [**Jie Geng**] also enters the hand Shao Yin heart and the foot Yang Ming stomach channels" and "Opens and raises qi and blood, resolves exterior cold evil, clears and disinhibits head, eyes and throat, and opens stagnant qi in the chest and diaphragm. [Treats] all [types of] phlegm congestion and hasty panting, nasal congestion, and red eyes, throat impediment and sore throat, toothache and mouth sores, pulmonary welling-abscesses, and dry cough.... [It] is a boat medicinal

(舟楫之藥 zhōu jí zhī yào) that carries all medicinals upwards and conducts bitter discharging and drastic precipitating medicinals [downwards]…."

In contemporary texts, it is described as having a bitter and acrid flavor and balanced nature; entering the lung channel; and having lung-diffusing phlegm-transforming, throat-disinhibiting, and pus-expelling actions. Its balanced nature makes this medicinal suitable for use in both cold and heat pattern pathoconditions.

Dr. Lee commonly adds the medicinal combination of **Jie Geng**, **Ban Xia**, and **Gan Cao** into formulas for the treatment of upper respiratory tract (especially the throat) pathoconditions.

Ju He (橘核/Semen Citri Reticulatae/Tangerine Seed)

In classical literature on pharmacopoeia, it is described as follows: "Bitter [in flavor], balanced [in nature], and no toxicity," "Enters foot Jue Yin [channel]," "Enters the kidney and urinary bladder [channels]," and "**Ju He** is bitter [in flavor] and warm [in nature] so it can enter the kidney and urinary bladder [channels], and in addition to diseases resulting from yin cold, [it] is commonly included in formulas [for treating] mounting qi (hernia)."

In contemporary texts, it is described as having a bitter flavor and balanced nature; entering the liver and kidney channels; and having qi-moving bind-dissipating and pain-relieving actions for the treatment of mounting qi (hernia), painful swollen testicles, mammary welling-abscesses (乳癰 rǔ yōng), lumbar pain, and urinary bladder qi pain. It is commonly prescribed in combination with **Li Zhi He**, **Xiao Hui Xiang**, and **Chuan Lian Zi** for the treatment of stomach pain and mounting qi (hernia) pain.

Due to **Ju He**'s lightness in substance and relative bulkiness, Dr. Lee typically prefers to add **Li Zhe He** and **Long Yan He** into a main formula, and simply advises the patient to eat the seeds of this medicinal as dietary therapy, since tangerines are grown locally, inexpensive and easily accessible.

*For more details, refer to **The Seeds** profile.

Li Zhi He (荔枝核/Semen Litchi/Litchi Seed)

In classical literature on pharmacopoeia, it is described as follows: "Sweet and slightly astringent [in flavor] and warm [in nature]," "Enters the liver and kidney [channels]," and "Dissipates stagnant qi and repels cold evil. Treats stomach duct pain and women's blood qi pain. Its fruit [grows] double bound and the seed resembles gonads, and thus treats bulging mounting (㿗疝 tuí shàn) and swollen testicles based on its similarity of appearance. The **shell** [殼 ké] promotes eruption of pox sores (痘瘡 dòu chuāng)."

In contemporary texts, it is described as having a sweet and slightly bitter flavor and warm nature; entering the liver and kidney channels; and having qi-moving bind-dissipating, cold-dissipating pain-relieving, and liver-coursing qi-rectifying actions. It is commonly prescribed in combination with **Xiao Hui Xiang**, **Ju He**, and **Chuan Lian Zi** for the treatment of stomach pain and mounting qi (hernia) pain.

Early on in Dr. Lee's clinical practice he would also prescribe **Xiao Hui Xiang** and **Chuan Lian Zi**, but nowadays prescribes **Mu Xiang** and **Yuan Hu Suo** instead. In fact, this exemplifies a general pattern that has occurred over the years: as Dr. Lee gains clinical experience, he has gradually discontinued the usage of many medicinals with narrowly defined actions in preference for medicinals with a broader therapeutic spectrum.

*For more details, refer to **The Seeds** profile.

Long Gu (龍骨/Os Draconis/Dragon Bone)

The sources of this medicinal are the fossilized skeletal bones of mammals, such as mammoths, hipparions (an extinct genus of horse), rhinoceros, elephant, deer, and bovine. The primary constituents of **Long Gu** are calcium carbonate (CaCO3) and calcium phosphate (Ca3(PO4)2) along with small amounts of iron (Fe), magnesium (Mg), aluminum (Al), potassium (K), sodium (Na), chlorine (Cl), and sulfate (SO4).

In classical literature on pharmacopoeia, it is described as follows: "Sweet and astringent [in flavor] and slightly cold [in nature]," "Enters the hand Shao Yin and Yang Ming and foot Jue Yin channels," and "Promotes contraction of floating away right qi (浮越之正氣 fú yuè zhī zhèng qì) and astringes the intestines and boosts the kidney, quiets the soul and settles fright, and repels evil and resolves toxin. Treats profuse confused dreaming, fright epilepsy and malarial dysentery, blood ejection and spontaneous external bleeding, and seminal emission and prolapse of the rectum [anal desertion]. Disinhibits the small and large intestines, secures essence and checks sweating, stabilizes panting and closes sores, and astringes, checks, and stems [all types of] desertion (脫 tuō)."

In contemporary texts, it is described as having a sweet and astringent flavor and balanced nature and entering the heart, liver and kidney channels. **Sheng Long Gu (生龍骨/Crude Dragon Bone)** subdues yang and quiets the spirit for the treatment of yin-vacuity hyperactive yang, vexation, agitation and irascibility, palpitations and insomnia, dizzy head and vision, mania, withdrawal, and fright. **Duan Long Gu (煅龍骨/Calcined Dragon Bone)** astringes and secures for the treatment of seminal emission and premature ejaculation, vaginal discharge and flooding and spotting, vacuity sweating and enduring diarrhea, damp sores and itchy papules, sores that fail to close, and bleeding due to external injury. Traditionally, **Duan Long Gu** is ground into powder for use as a topical application in the treatment of damp sores with discharge (i.e., transudation, exudation) that fail to heal over a prolonged period of time.

Despite its superior astringing and wound-healing efficacy, **Duan Long Gu** also causes *intense* skin and tissue irritation (e.g., stinging pain) lasting up to an hour after topical application. Based on clinical experience, Dr. Lee believes **Sheng Long Gu** provides adequate astringing efficacy with the potential for only *mild*, *if any*, skin irritation, thus he prescribes the crude form for both internal and external administration.

*For more details, refer to the **Long Gu and Mu Li** medicinal pair profile.

Long Gu and Mu Li

This is one of Dr. Lee's commonly prescribed medicinal pairs. **Long Gu** has a sweet and astringent flavor and balanced nature, predominantly enters the *liver channel*, and thus excels at settling fright and quieting the spirit. **Mu Li** has a salty and astringent flavor and cold nature, predominantly enters the *kidney channel*, and thus excels at securing the lower orifices and clearing heat to preserve yin and check diarrhea. Both **Long Gu** and **Mu Li** have astringent properties and spirit-quieting stirring palpitation-checking actions. **Mu Li** also *has* hardness-softening bind-dissipating actions, whereas **Long Gu** does *not*.

This medicinal pair has liver-calming yang-subduing, fright-settling spirit-quieting, and yin-constraining and -astringing actions for the treatment of disquieted heart and spirit, fright palpitations, forgetfulness, vacuity sweating and seminal emission, vacuity efflux desertion (滑脫 huá tuō), enduring dysentery and enduring diarrhea, flooding and spotting and vaginal discharge, clouded head and flowery vision resulting from vacuity yang straying upward (上越 shàng yuè), rib-side distention and pain, and persistent coughing of blood and blood ejection (吐衄 tǔ nǜ).

Dr. Lee utilizes the actions of **Long Gu and Mu Li** in Jian Ling Tang and Gui Zhi Jia Long Gu Mu Li Tang and also commonly adds this medicinal pair into a wide range of formula variants for the treatment of pathoconditions that require yang-subduing spirit-quieting, astringing and checking, and hardness-softening bind-dissipating actions.

Long Yan He (龍眼核 / Semen Longan/Longan Seed)

In classical literature on pharmacopoeia, it is described as follows: "Treats mounting qi (疝氣 shàn qì) [taken orally] and sores and lichen applied topically, and also stanches bleeding from incised wounds" and "For the treatment of foxy smell [armpit odor], grind six **Long Yan He** and 27 pepper kernels together, and apply [topically] when perspiration presents."

In contemporary texts, it is described as having a slightly bitter and astringent flavor and balanced nature; entering the liver, spleen, and urinary bladder channels; and having qi-moving bind-dissipating, dampness-drying diarrhea-checking, blood-stanching, and pain-relieving actions.

Taken orally, it is commonly prescribed for the treatment of stomach pain and mounting qi (hernia) pain (i.e., in combination with **Li Zhe He** and **Xiao Hui Xiang**); and applied topically it can treat bleeding from wounds, burns, arm pit odor, scabs and lichen, and damp sores. It is also possible to crush the entire fruit, including the **shell** (殼 ké), **flesh** (肉 ròu), **pit** (核 hé), and **seed** (子 zi), for decoction.

*For more details, refer to **The Seeds** profile.

Lu Jiao (鹿角) – refer to **Lu Rong**

Lu Jiao Shuang (鹿角霜) – refer to **Lu Rong**

Lu Lu Tong (路路通/Fructus Liquidamberis/Sweetgum Fruit/aka Feng Qiu, Feng Guo)

In classical literature on pharmacopoeia, it is described as follows: "Frees the twelve channels" and "Repels miasma and eliminates scourge (辟瘴却瘟 pì zhàng què wēn), brightens the eyes, eliminates dampness, soothes hypertonicity of the sinew network vessels (筋絡拘攣 jīn luò jū luán), whole body impediment pain, limb and lumbar pain, and the smell of its smoke upon burning will cure all."

In contemporary texts, it is described as having a bitter flavor and balanced nature; entering the liver and kidney channels; and having wind-expelling network vessel-freeing and water-disinhibiting dampness-eliminating actions.

It is traditionally prescribed for the treatment of impediment pain in the limbs and hypertonicity of the extremities, water swelling (edema), distention and fullness, scant breast milk and menstrual block, and welling- and flat-abscesses, scab, lichen, and eczema (damp papules).

Dr. Lee further classifies **Lu Lu Tong**, **Ci Ji Li** (calms and courses the liver and dispels wind and brightens the eyes), and **Zao Jiao Ci** (quickens the blood and disperses swelling and expels pus and frees milk) as pore conductor medicinals with their capacity to regulate—*opening* and *closing* (開闔 kāi hé)—of the pores and promote dermal circulation. Thus, he also adds this medicinal combination into formula variants for exterior wind-heat (or wind-heat-damp) and blood desiccation pattern with exterior wind-heat (or with exterior wind-heat-damp) skin pathoconditions presenting with pruritic papules and maculopapular and vesicular eruptions (e.g., dyshidrotic eczema (pompholyx), palmoplantar pustulosis (PPP), wind papules (urticaria), acute stage atopic dermatitis).

*For more details, refer to **The Eye Brighteners** and **The Itch Relievers** profiles.

Lu Rong (鹿茸/Cornu Cervi Pantotrichum/Deer Antler)

In classical literature on pharmacopoeia, it is described as follows: "Sweet [in flavor], warm [in nature], and pure yang" and "Engenders essence and supplements marrow, nourishes blood and assists yang, and strengthens the sinews and fortifies bone. Treats lumbar and kidney vacuity cold, aching and pain in the extremities, dizzy head and eye blackening (眼黑 yǎn hēi) [spots in visual field], flooding and vaginal discharge and seminal emission, and all [types of] vacuity-detriment taxation damage. Suitable for patients with a fine sunken pulse and debilitation of the ministerial fire."

In contemporary texts, it is described as having a sweet and salty flavor and warm nature; entering the kidney and liver channels; and having yang-invigorating, blood essence-supplementing, sinew- and bone-strengthening, thoroughfare and controlling vessel-harmonizing, and toxin- and sore-expressing actions.

Lu Rong is the whole cartilaginous antler in a pre-calcified stage, with hair that looks and feels like velvet. It contains many growth factors (e.g., NT-3, NGF, IGF) and has been experimentally and clinically proven to increase hormone levels (e.g., testosterone, luteinizing hormone), stimulate adrenal cortical function, and promote hematopoiesis.

In his clinical practice, Dr. Lee prescribes either **Cu Lu Rong** or **Xi Lu Rong** depending on the pathocondition and presenting signs, symptoms, and pattern.

Cu Lu Rong (粗鹿茸/Coarse-Haired Deer Antler)

This is a type of **Lu Rong** that is fully developed, but *not* yet completely calcified (hormone level production low), for which Dr. Lee identifies as **Cu Lu Rong**, with the "coarse" (粗 cū) antler hairs describing its texture and appearance. This medicinal is less expensive than **Xi Lu Rong** and requires larger doses (typically, 8 qian/3x/day) to achieve efficacy, thus Dr. Lee administers this medicinal in decocting piece form rather than powder.

Cu Lu Rong is *inferior* to **Xi Lu Rong** at increasing hormone levels and promoting hematopoiesis, but *superior* to **Lu Jiao** at quickening the blood and transforming stasis. This medicinal has been experimentally and clinically proven to inhibit tumor vasculature from generating hormones and thus functioning to inhibit tumor angiogenesis and tumerogenesis.

Dr. Lee typically prescribes **Cu Lu Rong** for cancer patients at high risk of bone metastasis or with existing metastasis, and for bone cancers, spinal cord tumors, and fractures that fail to heal properly (i.e., delayed union, nonunion).

Xi Lu Rong (細鹿茸/Fine-Haired Deer Antler)

This is a premium quality **Lu Rong** (reaching 60% to 70% growth at peak hormone production levels) offering superior medicinal efficacy, for which Dr. Lee identifies as **Xi Lu Rong**, with the "fine" (細 xì) velvet sheen of the antler describing its texture and appearance. This medicinal is a precious natural resource, very expensive, and typically only requires small doses (typically, 5 fen/3x/day) to achieve efficacy, thus Dr. Lee administers this medicinal in pulverized powder form rather than decocting pieces.

Xi Lu Rong offers superior efficacy for severe cases of thrombocytopenia (low platelet count), whether it is caused by *impaired platelet production* resulting from bone marrow failure (e.g., aplastic anemia), bone marrow suppression (e.g., chemotherapy, radiotherapy, immunotherapy), infection (e.g., cytomegalovirus (CMV), Epstein-Barr virus (EBV), hepatitis C virus (HCV), HIV), and malignancy (e.g., leukemia, lymphoma, myelodysplastic syndrome); *increased platelet turnover* resulting from immune thrombocytopenia (ITP) and other autoimmune diseases (e.g., systemic lupus erythematosus (SLE), rheumatoid arthritis (RA)), drug-induced drug side effects (e.g., heparin, quinine, sulfa drugs, NSAIDS, anticonvulsants), pregnancy, and infection; or *redistribution and dilution* (e.g., liver disease, splenomegaly, gestational, post-transfusion).

Lu Jiao (鹿角/Cervi Cornu/Mature Deer Antler)

Lu Jiao is the completely calcified antler whose coarse hairs have shed and it contains high calcium phosphate content.

In classical literature on pharmacopoeia, it is described as follows: "Salty [in flavor] and warm [in nature]. …dissipates heat and moves blood, disperses swelling and repels evil…."

In contemporary texts, it is described as having a salty flavor and a warm nature; entering the liver and kidney channels; and having blood-quickening stasis transforming actions. Traditionally, it is prescribed for the treatment of all types of vacuity taxation and offers exceptional efficacy for flat-abscesses and cold-type pus sores.

Lu Jiao can be processed into **Lu Jiao Shuang (Cervi Cornu Degelatinatum/degelatinated deer antler)**, which Dr. Lee uses in powder form combined with **Fu Zi** and **Gan Jiang** for the treatment of chronic (dry) skin ulcerations (e.g., diabetic ulcers).

Lu Jiao can also be processed into **Lu Jiao Jiao (Cervi Cornus Gelatinum/deer antler glue)** combined with **Gui Ban Jiao (tortoise plastron glue)** to make Gui Lu Er Xian Jiao (Tortoise Shell and Deerhorn Two Immortals Glue), which Dr. Lee typically includes in formulas treating pathoconditions such as true origin vacuity detriment, extreme exhaustion of essence, extreme exhaustion of bone (e.g., osteoporosis), emaciation and shortage of qi, and dim vision (e.g., presbyopia). **Lu Jiao Jiao** can also be administered in small doses and eaten like candy (soft and chewy) as a method of regulating the constitution for the elderly.

Ma Huang (麻黃/Herba Ephedrae/Ephedra Stem)

In classical literature on pharmacopoeia, it is described as follows: "Enters Tai Yang [channel] along with hand Shao Yin [and] Yang Ming [channels], and is a lung domain (家 jiā) chief medicinal" and "Promotes sweating and resolves flesh, and dispels cold evil at the construction [level] and wind-heat at the defense [level]. It regulates blood vessels, frees the nine orifices, and opens the pores; treats wind strike and cold damage, headache and warm malaria, cough and counterflow qi ascent, phlegm wheezing and panting, red and black macule toxin, toxic wind papules (measles) impediment (毒風疹痹 dú fēng zhěn bì), skin insensitivity, sore red swollen eyes, and water swelling and wind swelling."

In contemporary texts, it is described as having an acrid and slightly bitter flavor and a warm nature; entering the lung and urinary bladder channels; and having sweating-promoting exterior-resolving, lung-diffusing panting-calming, water-disinhibiting swelling-dispersing, nasal orifice-freeing, papule-outthrusting, and itch-relieving actions. However, this medicinal takes on an even broader role in Dr. Lee's pharmacopoeia.

Dr. Lee interprets **Ma Huang**'s action of opening the pores (開竅 kāi qiào) broadly to mean it can "open up" and transport other medicinals across all membranes of the body at the cellular level, which makes it an effective systemic channel conductor for treating all types of diseases (e.g., dermatology, rheumatology, cardiology, neurology). And he also interprets **Ma Huang**'s action of "opening the nine orifices" as innervating the nervous system (i.e., CNS, PNS, ANS), prompting its application for neurological disorders of the brain and nervous system.

Of course, Dr. Lee utilizes the revered bronchodilation action of **Ma Huang** for the treatment of respiratory tract pathoconditions (e.g., sinusitis, bronchitis, COPD, pneumonia) as well. He also commonly pairs this medicinal with **Di Long** for pathoconditions affecting the respiratory and vasomotor centers in the brainstem (e.g., cerebrovascular accident (CVA), trauma, microbial infection, enduring illness) and for the treatment of wind-cold-damp impediment.

As for dosage, it depends on the individual's constitution and the particular season. Typically, I would start out with a small dose of anywhere from 5 fen to 1.5 qian, incrementally increasing in 5 fen doses up until the patient notices difficulty sleeping, and then, adjusting the dose back down a bit to where sleep is unaffected. A typical dose would be 1.5 qian to 3 qian.

Mang Xiao (芒硝/Mirabilitum/Glauber's Salt)

The primary constituent of this medicinal is sodium sulfate decahydrate (Na2SO4 ·10H2O). However, depending on availability and physician preference, **Mang Xiao** may be substituted with **Epsom salt** (aka **Magnesium Sulfate**). In the past, a distinction was made establishing different grades of processed crude mirabilite based on the level of purity, with **Po Xiao (朴消)** classified as having the most *impurities*, **Mang Xiao** as a *purer* form, and **Xuan Ming Fen (玄明粉)** as the *purest* form. Nowadays, there is no such distinction made, and if *less refined* medicinals are used, it is standard practice to denote these medicinals as **Po Xiao** in the prescription.

In classical literature on pharmacopoeia, it is described as follows: "**Po Xiao** settles at the bottom, the crystals are coarse, and turbid and heavy in substance. **Mang Xiao** and **Ya Xiao (牙消)** form [float] on the top, the crystals are refined, and clear and light in substance…, "**Mang Xiao** is salty [in flavor] and cold [in nature], can eliminate abiding grime, transform accumulations and disperse phlegm, and abate all [types of] heat," and "Acridity can moisten dryness, saltiness can soften hardness, bitterness can precipitate diarrhea, and great cold can eliminate heat…. [It] can flush away triple burner and gastrointestinal repletion heat, and remove the old and institute the new…."

In contemporary texts, it is described as having a salty, bitter flavor and a cold nature; entering the stomach and large intestine channels; and having heat-draining stool-freeing, dryness-moistening hardness-softening, and fire-clearing swelling-dispersing actions.

This medicinal has the action of inhibiting the large intestine's capacity to absorb water and thus promotes the excretion of large amounts of water. It must be prescribed prudently in small doses to prevent excessive watery diarrhea that may lead to malabsorption. Dr. Lee only prescribes this medicinal in cases where large doses (5–7 qian) of **Da Huang** have already been administered for a period of time without efficacy to promote defecation and maintain 2–3 stools per day.

Mi Meng Hua (密蒙花/Flos Buddlejae/Pale Butterfly Bush Flower)

In classical literature on pharmacopoeia, it is described as follows: "Treats clear-eye blindness [glaucoma] (青盲 qīng máng) and floating screens [corneal opacities] (浮翳 fú yì), red and dry eyes and copious eye discharge and tearing, and disperses red vessels in the eyes, and bran and legumes (麩豆 fū dòu) and gan qi (疳氣 gān qì) attacking the eyes in children."

In contemporary texts, it is described as having a sweet flavor and slightly cold nature; entering the liver channel; and having liver-clearing eye-brightening and blood-cooling screen-abating actions.

Mi Meng Hua is an essential ophthalmological medicinal traditionally prescribed for blood vacuity liver heat pattern and liver channel repletion heat pattern pathoconditions of the eyes that present with sore, red, swollen and itchy eyes, copious tearing and eye discharge, red vessels in the eyes, clouded vision, and aversion to light (e.g., acute and chronic conjunctivitis, uveitis, retinitis, clouded vision, night blindness, eye screen (目中翳障 mù zhōng yì zhàng), wind ulceration of the eyelid rim (風弦赤爛 fēng xián chì làn), gan accumulation (疳積 gān jī) in children).

Dr. Lee commonly pairs this medicinal with **Qian Li Guang** (clears heat and resolves toxin, abates screens and brightens eyes, and kills worms and relieves itch), utilizing their function as eye orifice conductors for the treatment of all types of heat—exterior wind-heat, residual heat, liver channel repletion heat, liver channel vacuity heat, blood stasis heat, blood desiccation with heat, and yin vacuity heat—pattern ophthalmological pathoconditions presenting with sore, red, swollen and itchy eyes (e.g., acute and chronic conjunctivitis, uveitis, retinitis, ocular hypertension).

*For more details, refer to **The Eye Brighteners** profile.

Mo Yao (沒藥/Myrrha/Myrrh)

In classical literature on pharmacopoeia, it is described as follows: "Enters the twelve channels" and "Dissipates qi bind, frees stagnant blood, disperses swelling, stabilizes pain, and engenders flesh. Supplements heart and gallbladder vacuity and liver blood insufficiency. Treats incised wound and club injuries, malign sores and hemorrhoids, nebulous eye screen (雲翳 yún yì) and red eye, postpartum qi and blood pain, and breaks accumulations and aborts the fetus."

In contemporary texts, it is described as having a bitter and acrid flavor and balanced nature; entering the heart, liver, and spleen channels; and having blood-quickening pain-relieving and swelling-dispersing flesh engendering actions.

It has been experimentally and clinically proven to have inhibitory affects on pathogenic mycoses (fungi); and the resins of these medicinals have been proven in laboratory experiments to have a hypolipidemic effect on male rabbits with hypercholesterolemia, and also in the prevention of plaque formation.

*For more details, refer to the **Ru Xiang and Mo Yao** medicinal pair profile.

Mu Dan Pi (牡丹皮/Cortex Moutan/Tree Peony Root Bark)

In classical literature on pharmacopoeia, it is described as follows: "**Mu Dan Pi** is cold [in nature], breaks blood and frees channels, and [treats] heat in the blood aspect and steaming bone without sweating," "[It] is acrid and sweet [in flavor] and slightly cold [in nature] and enters the hand and foot Shao Yin and Jue Yin [channels]," and "Drains latent heat in the blood and harmonizes and cools the blood, thus engenders the blood, breaks blood accumulations, frees the channels and vessels, and is an essential medicinal for blood ejection and spontaneous external bleeding. Treats wind strike [stroke] and five taxations, and fright epilepsy and tugging and slackening [clonic spasm]. Eliminates vexation heat, treats welling-abscesses and sores, aborts the fetus and placenta, and abates steaming bone without sweating."

In contemporary texts, it is described as having a bitter and acrid flavor and slightly cold nature; entering the heart, liver, and kidney channels; and having heat-clearing blood-cooling and blood-quickening stasis-dissipating actions. It is recognized as among the best medicinals for eliminating yin aspect latent heat and treating steaming bone blood aspect pathoconditions.

Dr. Lee pairs this medicinal together with **Di Gu Pi** (a steaming bone qi aspect medicinal) in the formula Di Gu Pi Yin and with **Sheng Di Huang** in Zhi Bo Di Huang Tang. It is also one the medicinals in Gui Zhi Fu Ling Wan, which is included in Po Xiao

Dang Bao Tang. Additionally, Dr. Lee commonly adds **Mu Dan Pi** into Ru Mo Si Wu Tang, forming a medicinal pair with **Chi Shao** to inhibit tumor angiogenesis; adds the medicinal pair **Mu Dan Pi** and **Shan Zhi Zi** into formulas to treat acute inflammation of vasculature walls (e.g., vasculitis, arteritis); and adds the medicinal pair **Mu Dan Pi** and **Sheng Di Huang** into formulas to treat chronic inflammation of vasculature walls (e.g., vasculitis, arteritis).

Mu Li (牡蠣/Concha Ostreae/Oyster Shell)

In classical literature on pharmacopoeia, it is described as follows: "Salty [in flavor], thus softens hardness and transforms phlegm and disperses scrofula and nodes and old blood and conglomeration-mounting (瘕疝 jiǎ shàn). Astringent [in flavor], thus contracts desertion (脫 tuō) and treats seminal emission and flooding and vaginal discharge, suppresses cough and constrains sweat, and secures the small and large intestines. Slightly cold [in nature], thus [it] clears heat and supplements water [for the] treatment of vacuity taxation and vexation heat, warm malaria and red dysentery; and [it] serves as a liver and kidney blood aspect medicinal."

In contemporary texts, it is described as having a salty and astringent flavor and slightly cold nature; entering the liver and kidney channels; and having liver-calming yang-subduing, hardness-softening bind-dissipating, and astringing and securing actions.

Mu Li is a commonly prescribed medicinal for checking vacuity sweating and transforming phlegm and softening hardness. It contains 80 to 95% calcium carbonate (CaCO3), calcium phosphate (Ca3(PO4)2), and calcium sulfate (CaSO4), along with small amounts of magnesium (Mg), aluminum (Al), silicon (Si), iron oxide (Fe3O4), and organic matter. The calcium salts in **Mu Li** contain antacid properties and mild sedative (fright-settling) and anti-inflammatory actions. This medicinal has been experimentally and clinically proven to offer efficacy for the treatment of gastric and duodenal ulcers and boosting the immune system. Traditionally, **Duan Long Gu** is ground into powder for use as a topical application in the treatment of damp sores with discharge (i.e., transudation, exudation) that fail to heal over a prolonged period of time.

Despite the fact that **Duan Mu Li (煅牡蠣/Calcined Oyster Shell)** offers superior astringing efficacy for topical application, it also causes more *intense* skin and tissue irritation (e.g., stinging pain) lasting for up to an hour after topical application. Based on clinical experience,

Dr. Lee believes **Sheng Mu Li (生牡蠣/Crude Oyster Shell)** provides adequate astringing efficacy with only *mild*, *if any*, skin irritation, thus he only prescribes the crude form for both internal and external administration.

*For more details, refer to the **Long Gu and Mu Li** medicinal pair profile.

Niu Xi (牛膝/Radix Achyranthis Bidentatae/Oxknee Root/aka **Huai Niu Xi)**

Dr. Lee uses **Huai Niu Xi (懷牛膝)** (*Achyranthes bidentata* Bl.) in his pharmacopoeia, which has superior liver- and kidney-supplementing and sinew-soothing bone-fortifying actions compared to **Chuan Niu Xi (川牛膝)** (*Cyathula officinalis* Kuan), which has superior blood-quickening stasis-dissipating and joint-perfusing actions.

In classical literature on pharmacopoeia, it is described as follows: "A foot Jue Yin channel and Shao Yin channel medicinal [that] conducts all other medicinals downwards. Steamed with wine it is sweet and sour [in flavor] and warm [in nature], boosts the liver and kidneys and strengthens sinews and bones, and treats pain in the lumbus, knees and bones, wilting of the legs and hypertonicity of the sinews (筋攣 jīn luán), yin wilt [impotence] and incontinence, enduring malaria and dysentery, and scant qi during injury. Used raw it dissipates evil blood, breaks accumulations and binds, and treats all [types of] pain in the heart [region] and abdomen, stranguric urination (淋痛 lín tòng) and bloody urine, menstrual block and difficult delivery, throat impediment and toothache, welling-abscess, swellings and evil sores, and incised wounds and fractures. Removes bamboo and wood [splinters]."

In contemporary texts, it is described as having a bitter, sweet, and sour flavor and balanced nature; entering the liver and kidney channels; and having blood-quickening channel-freeing, liver- and kidney-supplementing, sinew- and bone-strengthening, water-disinhibiting strangury-freeing, and fire (blood)-conducting downward actions. **Niu Xi** is recognized as an essential channel conductor directing other medicinals to the lumbus and lower limbs.

Dr. Lee includes the medicinal pair **Niu Xi** and **Du Zhong** (supplements the liver and kidney, strengthens sinews and bones, conducts medicinals downward to the lumbus and lower limbs, and quiets the fetus) in the Yu Sheng formulas You Gui Yin, Tong Jing

Fang, Paralysis Formula #1, Paralysis Formula #3, and Zuo Gui Yin. Dr. Lee also includes the medicinal combination that forms San Miao Wan—**Niu Xi**, **Huang Bo**, and **Cang Zhu**—in the formulas You Gui Yin and Zhi Bo Di Huang Tang.

Po Xiao (朴消) – refer to **Mang Xiao**

Qian Li Guang (千里光/Herba Senecionis Scandens/Ragwort)

In classical literature on pharmacopoeia, it is described as follows: "Treats unclear vision, eliminates red-thread [bloodshot eyes] (紅絲 hóng sī) and white obstruction [cataract] (內障 nèi zhàng), and tearing on exposure to wind" and "Brightens the eyes and eliminates stars obstruction (星障 xīng zhàng)…."

In contemporary texts, it is described as having a bitter flavor and cold nature; entering the lung and liver channels; and having heat-clearing toxin resolving, screen-abating eye-brightening, and worm-killing itch-relieving actions. Traditionally, this medicinal is prescribed for the treatment of all types of acute infections and inflammation involving the eyes, skin, and respiratory, digestive, and genitourinary systems.

Dr. Lee commonly pairs this medicinal with **Mi Meng Hua** (clears heat and resolves toxin, abates screens and brightens eyes, and kills worms and relieves itch), utilizing their function as eye orifice conductors for the treatment of all types of heat—exterior wind-heat, residual heat, liver channel repletion heat, liver channel vacuity heat, blood stasis heat, blood desiccation with heat, and yin vacuity heat—pattern ophthalmological pathoconditions presenting with sore, red, swollen and itchy eyes (e.g., acute and chronic conjunctivitis, uveitis, retinitis, ocular hypertension).

*For more details, refer to **The Eye Brighteners** profile.

Qing Hao (青蒿/Herba Artemisiae Annuae/Sweet Wormwood)

In classical literature on pharmacopoeia, it is described as follows: "[**Qing Hao**] is bitter [in flavor] and cold [in nature]," "Obtains Spring wood Shao Yang the earliest, thus enters Shao Yang and Jue Yin blood aspect," "Treats steaming bone taxation heat, childbirth taxation vacuity heat, wind toxin heat jaundice, enduring malaria and enduring diarrhea, scabies and malign sores, demonic qi and cadaverous infixation (鬼氣戶疰 guǐ qì hù zhù), and supplements the center and brightens the eyes," and "Treats malaria heat (fever) and [aversion to] cold."

In contemporary texts, it is described as having a bitter and acrid flavor and cold nature; entering the liver, gallbladder, and kidney channels; and having yin vacuity heat-clearing, steaming bone-eliminating, summerheat-resolving, and malaria-interrupting actions.

Qing Hao contains the active constituent artemisinin, which can inhibit the development of and directly kill malaria parasites. And because of its fragrant qi and flavor, unlike other cold bitter medicinals, it does *not* damage the spleen and stomach.

Dr. Lee includes this medicinal in combination with **Di Gu Pi** and **Zhi Mu** in Hyperactive Immune Formula and commonly adds the combination of **Qing Hao**, **Di Gu Pi**, and **Zhi Mu** into formula variants for the treatment of all types of pathoconditions presenting with symptoms such as intermittent fever, enduring heat, enduring cough, and yin vacuity dryness.

Qiu Yin (蚯蚓) – refer to **Di Long**

Quan Xie (全蠍/Buthus Martensi/Scorpion/aka **Xie)**

In classical literature on pharmacopoeia, it is described as follows: "Green-blue is associated with wood, thus [**Quan Xie**] treats all [types of] wind with shaking and dizzy vision, fright epilepsy and pulling, deviated eyes and mouth, malarial wind sores, deafness, vaginal discharge, and hernia, and Jue Yin wind and wood diseases."

In contemporary texts, it is described as having an acrid flavor, balanced nature, and toxicity; entering the liver channel; and having wind-extinguishing tetany-checking, toxin-attacking bind-dispersing, and network vessel-freeing pain-relieving actions.

Traditionally, it is commonly paired with **Wu Gong** for the treatment of pathoconditions involving spasm and convulsion (e.g., acute and chronic fright wind, tetanus, wind striking the channels and network vessels with deviated eyes and mouth). It is also combined with **Wu Gong** and **Bai Jiang Can** for the treatment of neuropathic pain (e.g., trigeminal neuralgia) and intractable headache (e.g., migraine, cluster headache).

*For more details, refer to **The Three Insects** profile.

Ren Dong Teng (忍冬藤/Caulis Lonicerae/Honeysuckle Stem)

In classical literature on pharmacopoeia, it is described as follows: "Sweet and bitter flavor and slightly cold nature," "Enters the heart and lung channels," and "Governs heat-toxin, blood dysentery, and water dysentery."

Traditionally this medicinal is prescribed for its heat-clearing toxin-resolving and network vessel-freeing actions. In Dr. Lee's pharmacopoeia it is an essential medicinal for inhibiting the synthesis of blood urea nitrogen (BUN) and serum creatinine (Cr) for the treatment of pathological conditions that result from hypoperfusion of blood through functionally normal kidneys (prerenal), structural damage to the renal parenchyma (intrinsic renal), and urinary tract obstruction (postrenal).

Dr. Lee commonly prescribes **Ren Dong Teng** paired with **Ding Shu Xiu**, adding them into Wu Ling San (Nephritis Formula), Chai Ling Tang, or other formula variants based on presenting signs, symptoms, and pattern identification.

Ren Shen (人參/Radix Ginseng/Ginseng Root)

In classical literature on pharmacopoeia, it is described as follows: "**Ren Shen** is sweet [in flavor] and balanced [in nature], greatly supplements original qi, checks thirst and engenders fluid, and regulates construction and nourishes defense."

In contemporary texts, it is described as having a sweet and slightly bitter flavor and mildly warm nature; entering the heart, lung, and spleen channels; and having great original qi-supplementing vacuity desertion-stemming, spleen-supplementing lung-boosting, liquid-engendering, and spirit-quieting actions.

Ren Shen is an expensive medicinal and the process of decoction diminishes potency, thus Dr. Lee typically administers it as a pulverized powder to minimize cost and maximize efficacy. This powder is either added directly into a formula after the decoction has cooled or taken separately. Since Dr. Lee prescribes **Ren Shen** in pulverized powder form, it is omitted from Yu Sheng formula composition listings, which are decocting pieces only. This medicinal is often paired with **Chuan Qi (powder)** to form **Ren Shen/Chuan Qi Powder**, one of the pillars of Dr. Lee's therapeutic approaches.

Dr. Lee explains in a more modern biomedical perspective: "As an adaptogenic medicinal, **Ren Shen** has the capacity to regulate cell metabolism throughout the entire body, down-regulating and up-regulating whenever it is necessary, and offers exceptional efficacy in repairing and maintaining physiological function of spinal nerves."

*For more details, refer to the **Ren Shen/Chuan Qi Powder** profile.

Ren Shen/Chuan Qi Powder (人參/川七粉)

This medicinal pair forms one of the pillars of Dr. Lee's therapeutic approaches. These two medicinals have qi-boosting fluid-engendering, origin-supporting desertion-stemming, blood-quickening stasis-transforming, and blood-stanching actions that exemplify the TCM classical theory of qi is the commander of blood and blood is the mother of qi (氣為血之帥、血為氣之母 qì wèi xuè zhī shuài, xiě wéi qì zhī mǔ).

Together, they can be prescribed for the treatment of a wide spectrum of pathoconditions that involve compromised vasculature leading to insufficient blood perfusion, excessive blood loss or hemorrhage, and chronic diseases in which taxation and desertion present. Specific pathoconditions include cardiovascular disease (e.g., coronary heart disease (CHD), aortic aneurysm, peripheral artery disease (PAD), deep vein thrombosis (DVT)), cerebrovascular disease (e.g., stroke, transient ischemic attack (TIA), vascular dementia), autoimmune disorders (e.g., systemic lupus erythematosus (SLE), dermatomyositis), gynecological disorders (e.g., menorrhagia, hypermenorrhagia, spotting), and end-stage cancer patients among others.

For severe blood stasis, **Dan Shen** decocting pieces are commonly prescribed along with this medicinal pair to further enhance the blood-quickening stasis-transforming actions and complement the pair with blood-cooling actions. The administration of medicinals with blood-quickening stasis-transforming actions in chronic pathoconditions is based on the TCM classical theory of enduring illness results in stasis.

The pulverized powder of these medicinals are mixed together and placed in zip lock packets with a typical dosage of 7g/3x/day (a total of 21 g/day).

Rou Gui (肉桂/Cortex Cinnamoni Cassiae/Cinnamon Bark/aka Yu Gui)

In classical literature on pharmacopoeia, it is described as follows: "Acrid and sweet [in flavor] and great heat [in nature] and thick qi pure yang," "Enters the blood aspect of the liver and kidney [channels]," and "Supplements insufficiency of the life gate ministerial fire and boosts yang to disperse yin. Treats intractable cold and deep cold, can promote sweating, free the blood vessels, and perfuses and conducts the hundred medicinals. Eliminates construction and defense wind-cold, exterior vacuity spontaneous sweating, cold pain in the abdomen, and cough and counterflow qi bind…."

In contemporary texts, it is described as having an acrid and sweet flavor and hot nature; entering the spleen, kidney, heart, and liver channels; and having fire-supplementing yang-assisting, cold-dissipating pain-relieving, and channel-warming vessel-freeing actions.

The majority of formulas Dr. Lee prescribes are variants of classical formulas derived from *Treatise on Cold Damage and Miscellaneous Diseases* (**傷寒雜病論** *Shang Han Za Bing Lun*) (which was subsequently compiled into two books called *On Cold Damage* (**傷寒論** *Shang Han Lun*) and *Essential Prescriptions of the Golden Coffer* (**金匱要略方論** *Jin Gui Yao Lue Fang Lun*)). In this text, the instructions to "remove the skin" (i.e., scrape away the thin layers of fungal growth on the surface of the bark) from **Gui Zhi** suggests that the bark (**Rou Gui**) with its higher volatile oil content was in fact used instead of the twig (**Gui Zhi**). Also, due to logistical considerations during the Eastern Han Dynasty (25-220 CE), it would have been much more viable to transport the relatively lighter bark (**Rou Gui**) up to northern China, where Zhang Zhong-Jing wrote his TCM classic, from southern China (or Vietnam), where the cinnamon tree (*Cinnamomum cassia* Presl.) grows.

And from a practical perspective, it is also much simpler to decoct the entire formula composition together, instead of adding the medicinals containing volatile oils towards the end of decoction to mitigate the extent of evaporation. Since **Rou Gui** contains a much higher volatile oil content than **Gui Zhi**, a higher potency of the bioactive constituents in these volatile oils will be retained during decoction. Thus, Dr. Lee predominantly prescribes **Rou Gui** in place of **Gui Zhi** even in exterior-resolving formulas such as Gui Zhi Tang, and with the exception of **Chai Ling Tang**, the only other time he prescribes **Gui Zhi** is for its function as an upper extremity channel-conducting medicinal. Amidst this dynamic, **Rou Gui**'s actions can be interpreted as encompassing those of **Gui Zhi** (e.g., exterior-resolving, spleen-fortifying, pain-relieving, antimicrobial), while also containing vasodilation actions that more effectively promote blood circulation.

*For more details, refer to **The Three Great Yang-Supplementers** profile.

Ru Xiang (乳香/Olibanum/Frankincense)

In classical literature on pharmacopoeia, it is described as follows: "Disperses welling-abscesses, flat-abscesses, and all toxins; internally expresses and safeguards the heart; quickens the blood, stabilizes pain, and extends sinews; and treats female difficult delivery and fractures" and "Fragrant [odor] penetrates and enters the heart [region], bitter [flavor] and warm [nature] supplement the kidney, [and] acrid [flavor] and warm [nature] free the twelve channels, [**Ru Xiang**] can dispel wind and extend sinews, quicken the blood and regulate qi, internally express and safeguard the heart, [and] engender flesh and relieve pain."

In contemporary texts, it is described as having a warm nature and acrid and bitter flavor, entering the liver, heart, and spleen channels; and having blood-quickening qi-moving, swelling-dispersing flesh-engendering, and pain-relieving actions. It is recognized as an external medicine and traumatology essential medicinal.

*For more details, refer to the **Ru Xiang and Mo Yao** medicinal pair profile.

Ru Xiang and Mo Yao

This is one of Dr. Lee's commonly prescribed medicinal pairs for the treatment of static blood pattern pathoconditions presenting in internal medicine (e.g., gynecology, ophthalmology, oncology), external medicine (e.g., dermatology), and traumatology (e.g., sprains, knocks and falls, pulling of the sinews and bone fractures).

In classical literature on pharmacopoeia, this medicinal pair is described as follows: "**Ru Xiang** quickens the blood, **Mo Yao** dissipates the blood, [and] both can relieve pain, disperse swelling and engender flesh, thus these two medicinals are often prescribed together" and "**Ru Xiang and Mo Yao** prescribed together are an essential organ- and viscera-perfusing and channel-freeing medicinal [pair] that can be prescribed for the treatment of all types of stomach, rib-side, abdomen, limb, and joint pain. The pair also treats abdominal pain during menstruation, postpartum static blood pain, and menstruation at irregular intervals [menstrual irregularities]. The capacity for freeing qi and quickening the blood makes the pair effective in the treatment of wind-cold-damp impediment, generalized numbness, paralysis [paresis] of the limbs, and all types of swollen and painful sores or hard sores without pain. For external application, pulverize [the decocting pieces] into powder and apply on sores to resolve toxin and disperse swelling and engender flesh and relieve pain. Despite having freeing actions, the pair will not damage qi and blood; indeed, it is a superb medicinal [pair]."

In contemporary texts, this medicinal pair is described as having similar mutually accentuating actions and indications, with **Ru Xiang** having more pronounced qi-moving sinew-extending actions and **Mo Yao** having more pronounced blood-dissipating stasis-transforming actions.

Ru Xiang and Mo Yao improve the elasticity and functional patency of the vasculature, specifically the tunica intima (innermost layer of arteries and veins), which is made up of one layer of endothelial cells and supported by an internal elastic lamina. These endothelial cells are in direct contact with the blood flow and influence the secretion of inflammatory and clotting factors. Thus, **Ru Xiang and Mo Yao** provide exceptional anti-inflammatory actions and mild blood-stanching actions, with the overall effect of accelerating the healing process. **Ru Xiang and Mo Yao** serve as the principal medicinals in Yu Sheng formulas such as Ru Mo Si Wu Tang, Xian Fang Huo Ming Yin, Diao Fen Gao (Suspension Powder Paste), and Huo Luo Dan.

San Qi (三七) – refer to **Chuan Qi**

Sang Bai Pi (桑白皮/Cortex Mori Albae Radicis/Mulberry Root Bark)

In classical literature on pharmacopoeia, it is described as follows: "Sweet and acrid [in flavor] and cold [in nature]," "Drains lung fire, disinhibits urine and stool, dissipates static blood, precipitates qi and moves water, and suppresses cough and clears phlegm. It treats lung heat panting and fullness, spitting of blood and heat thirst, and water swelling and cranium distention. Made into string it can [be used for] sewing incised wounds," and "Drains fire evil in the lung, but not lung qi. Fire and original qi are incompatible, and once fire is eliminated then qi will be calm."

In contemporary texts, it is described as having a sweet flavor and cold nature; entering the lung channel; and having lung-draining panting-calming and water-disinhibiting swelling-dispersing actions.

Dr. Lee describes this medicinal as having the capacity to "clean up the metabolic waste that clogs cell membranes throughout the entire body." Metabolic waste build-up may derive from normal metabolic processes or from inflammatory responses to disease, which may inhibit (or further exacerbate) the normal function of cellular mechanisms, disrupt homeostasis, and lead to heat pattern pathoconditions such as diabetes. For this reason, **Sang Bai Pi** is an essential medicinal for the treatment of diabetes and it is also prescribed for other heat pattern pathoconditions of the respiratory tract (e.g., acute bronchitis, emphysema) and skin (e.g., atopic dermatitis).

Sha Yuan Ji Li (沙苑蒺藜/Semen Astragali Complanati/Flattened Milkvetch Seed/aka Sha Yuan Zi)

This medicinal is processed in-house in Dr. Lee's own medicinal processing and decoction facility. Raw **Sha Yuan Ji Li** is stir-fried on low flame until faint crackling sounds can be heard, an aromatic scent arises, and the seeds turn a dark yellow to light brown color. The purpose for processing in this way is to crack open the seed coat, thus allowing the bioactive constituents to be easily extracted upon decoction.

In classical literature on pharmacopoeia, it is described as follows: "Supplements the kidney, treats lumbar pain and seminal discharge and vacuity detriment and taxation" and "**Sha Yuan Ji Li** [is a] kidney-supplementing essence-astringing medicinal. …[it] nourishes the liver and brightens the eyes and moistens the pupils, supplements the kidney and secures essence, strengthens yang [increases male libido] for bearing seeds [promotes fertility], [it's] neither harsh nor dry, checks dribble after voiding, and is a balanced and moderate moistening medicinal."

In contemporary texts, it is described as having a sweet flavor and warm nature; entering the liver and kidney channels; and having kidney-supplementing essence-securing and liver-nourishing eye-brightening actions. It is traditionally prescribed for the treatment of liver and kidney insufficiency, aching lumbus and knees, hemorrhoids and fistulas, clouded vision, seminal emission and premature ejaculation, enuresis, bloody urine (hematuria), and vaginal discharge.

Dr. Lee includes the medicinal pair **Sha Yuan Ji Li** and **Tu Si Zi** (supplements the kidney and secures essence, nourishes the liver and brightens the eyes, checks diarrhea, and quiets the fetus) in Atopic Dermatitis Formula and Blood Desiccation Formula; and commonly adds the pair into formula variants for their balanced and moderate liver and kidney yin-nourishing actions. Together, these medicinals offer superior capacity for retaining moisture (cellular hydration) and maintaining cell metabolic activity.

Sha Yuan Zi (沙苑子) – refer to **Sha Yuan Ji Li**

Shan Qi (山七) – refer to **Chuan Qi**

Shan Yao (山藥/Rhizoma Dioscoreae/Chinese Yam/aka **Huai Shan)**

In classical literature on pharmacopoeia, it is described as follows: "**Shan Yao** fortifies the spleen and supplements vacuity and enriches essence and secures the kidney, and treats all types of vacuity and the hundred injuries (百損 bǎi sǔn) and five taxations (五勞 wǔ láo) and seven damages (七傷 qī shāng). Its qi is light and nature moderate and not suitable for single medicinal prescription. Thus, for supplementing the spleen and lung, [**Ren**] **Shen** and [**Bai**] **Zhu** must be included as chief medicinals; for supplementing the kidney water, [**Shan**] **Zhu** [**Yu**] and [**Shou**] **Di** [**Huang**] must be included as sovereign medicinals; for astringing turbid vaginal discharge, **Po Gu** [**Zhi**] must be ground together; and for securing emissions and diarrhea, rely on **Tu Si** [**Zi**] for mutual assistance" and "Enters the spleen and lung channels, supplements their insufficiencies, clears their vacuity heat, secures the intestines and stomach, moistens the skin and [body] hair, transforms phlegm-drool, and checks diarrhea and dysentery. Lung is the mother of kidney, thus [**Shan Yao**] also boosts the kidney and strengthens yin and treats vacuity-detriment taxation damage. The spleen is the son of the heart, thus [**Shan Yao**] can boost heart qi and treat forgetfulness and seminal emission. Crush raw and topically apply on welling-abscesses and sores and [it] disperses swelling and hardness."

In contemporary texts, it is described as having a sweet flavor and balanced nature; entering the spleen, lung, and kidney channels; and having qi-boosting yin-nourishing, spleen, lung, and kidney-supplementing, and essence-securing vaginal discharge-checking actions.

Shan Yao contains a broad spectrum of amino acids, proteins, hormones, steroids, vitamins, and trace minerals that can provide exceptional efficacy when administered as processed decocting pieces or simply eaten as medicinal food (藥膳 yào shàn).

Dr. Lee includes **Shan Yao** in a wide range of Yu Sheng formulas for its moderating action (Jian Ling Tang and Yu Sheng Wan), its spleen, lung and kidney-supplementing actions (Mai Men Dong Tang and Asthma Formula), and its kidney-supplementing and yin-enriching actions (You Gui Yin and Zuo Gui Yin).

Shan Zha (山楂/Fructus Crataegi/Hawthorn Fruit/aka Xian Zha)

In classical literature on pharmacopoeia, it is described as follows: "Sour, sweet, and salty [in flavor] and warm [in nature]," "Shan Zha is sour and sweet [in flavor], grinds and disperses meat-type food, treats mounting (疝 shàn) and moves stasis, and disperses bloating and fortifies the stomach," and "Fortifies the spleen and moves qi, dissipates stasis and transforms phlegm, disperses food and grinds accumulations, effuses infantile pox, and relieves infant's-pillow [postpartum abdominal] pain."

In contemporary texts, it is described as having a sour and sweet flavor and a slightly warm nature; entering the spleen, stomach, and liver channels; and having food-dispersing accumulation-transforming actions and qi-moving stasis-dispersing actions.

Shan Zha is an essential medicinal for promoting digestion of greasy, rich and meat-type food accumulation and stagnation; and its **seed (pit)** (核 hé) is also prescribed in combination with **Li Zhi He** and **Ju He** for the treatment of stomach pain and mounting qi (hernia) pain.

Dr. Lee commonly adds the medicinal pair **Shan Zha** and **Ji Nei Jin** into formulas (e.g., heat-clearing toxin-resolving, yin-nourishing blood-supplementing, blood-quickening stasis-transforming, yin-enriching yang-subduing) that may impair digestion and cause sloppy stools in some patients. This medicinal pair is also added into formula variants for the treatment of hyperlipidemia and hypertrigliceridemia. Additionally, Dr. Lee adds **Shan Zha** into formula variants for the treatment of static blood pattern pathoconditions, such as postpartum infant's-pillow pain (postpartum abdominal pain) and coronary artery spasm.

*For more details, refer to **The Seeds** profile.

She Tui (蛇蛻/Periostracum Serpentis/Snake Slough/aka **She Pi)**

In classical literature on pharmacopoeia, it is described as follows: "Miraculous in nature (性靈 xìng líng) can repel evil, thus [it] treats ghosts and goblins (鬼魅 guǐ mèi) and gu toxin (蠱毒 gǔ dú). Scurrying in nature (竄性 cuàn xìng) excels at dispelling wind, thus [it] treats fright epilepsy and wind malaria, and double tongue (重舌 chóng shé) and throat wind. Toxic in nature kills insects, thus [it] treats scab, lichen, and malign sores, and swollen clove sores and hemorrhoids and fistulas. It is skin so [its] nature excels at sloughing, thus [it] treats skin sores, difficult delivery and eye screen."

In contemporary texts, it is described as having a sweet and salty flavor and balanced nature; entering the liver channel; and having wind-dispelling, swelling-dispersing, worm-killing, fright-stabilizing, and screen-abating actions.

Dr. Lee classifies **She Tui** as an exterior membrane conductor (i.e., eyes, skin) based on its innate substance as slough (shed epithelial tissue) and its inherent capacity to *peel off* the agglutinated protein build-up on the membranous surfaces of the eyes. This is an example of the classical TCM treatment method of resembling forms treat respective body parts and resembling organs treat respective organs (以形治形、以臟治臟 yǐ xíng zhì xíng, yǐ zàng zhì zàng).

Dr. Lee typically prescribes the medicinal pair **She Tui** and **Chan Tui** (courses wind and dissipates heat, outthrusts papules and relieves itch, brightens the eyes and abates screens, and checks fright) for the treatment of ophthalmological pathoconditions such as lens opacities (e.g., cataract) and corneal opacities (e.g., eye screen (目翳 mù yì), scarring), and for dermatological pathoconditions presenting with intense pruritis.

*For more details, refer to **The Eye Brighteners** and **The Itch Relievers** profiles.

Sheng Di Huang (生地黃/Radix Rehmanniae/Rehmannia Root/aka **Gan Di Huang)**

Clarification is warranted for the confusing parallel nomenclature used to describe the **Rehmannia Root (Di Huang)** throughout history. To clarify this ambiguity, contemporary texts make the clear distinction of **Xian Di Huang** (鮮 xiān = fresh) as opposed to **Sheng Di Huang** (生 shēng = raw), a term that is now used synonymously in reference to **Gan Di Huang** (乾 gān = dried). **Gan Di Huang** is the term used at Dr. Lee's clinic for this medicinal; however, since most readers may be more familiar with the term **Sheng Di Huang**, it is referred to as such for the purpose of this text.

In classical literature on pharmacopoeia, it is described as follows: "Sweet and bitter [in flavor] and cold [in nature] and sinks yin and downbears," "Enters the hand and foot Shao Yin and Jue Yin and hand Tai Yang channels," and "Enriches yin, abates yang, and engenders and cools blood. It treats blood vacuity heat effusion, taxation damage cough, wilting and impediment fright palpitations, blood ejection and bloody urine, blood dizziness and flooding, heat and pain on the underside of the foot, and sinew expiration from fractures and falls. It replenishes the bone marrow, generates flesh, disinhibits stool and urine, regulates menstruation, and quiets the fetus. It can also kill worms and treats acute pain in the heart [region] and abdomen."

In contemporary texts, it is described as having a sweet and bitter flavor and cold nature; entering the heart, liver, and lung channels; and having heat-clearing blood-cooling and yin-nourishing liquid-engendering actions.

Xian Di Huang (鮮地黃/Fresh Rehmannia Root)

It has a sweet and bitter flavor and a cold nature; enters the heart, liver and lung channels; and has heat-clearing blood-cooling and yin-nourishing liquid-engendering actions. Due to the cost concerns of shipping and storage, Dr. Lee does *not* keep **Xian Di Huang** in his dispensary and uses **Sheng Di Huang** instead. In cases where the heat-abating action of **Xian Di Huang** is preferred, Dr. Lee will typically pair **Sheng Di Huang** with **Huang Bo**.

Shu Di Huang (熟地黃/Cooked Rehmannia Root)

It has a sweet flavor and a slightly warm nature; enters the liver and kidney channels; and has blood-supplementing yin-enriching and essence-boosting marrow-replenishing actions. The traditional processing method—involving steeping **Sheng Di Huang** in yellow wine mixed with **Sha Ren (砂仁)** and steaming and sun-drying repeatedly a total of nine times—is extremely time-consuming, labor-intensive and expensive, and thus seldom implemented anymore. The modern method of processing **Shu Di Huang** results in inferior quality that differs in nature and property compared to its predecessor.

Taking these factors into consideration, in cases where the blood-supplementing yin-enriching and essence-boosting marrow-replenishing actions of **Shu Di Huang** are preferred, Dr. Lee typically pairs **Sheng Di Huang** with medicinals such as **Fu Zi** (frees the twelve channels), **Rou Gui** (enters the liver and kidney blood aspect and supplements life gate ministerial fire), **Ma Huang** (frees the nine orifices), and **Shi Chang Pu (石菖蒲)** (opens heart hole [passage] and disinhibits the nine orifices).

However, Dr. Lee *does* keep traditionally processed **Shu Di Huang** in his dispensary for inclusion in Du Huo Ji Sheng Tang, which is typically prescribed for impediment pattern (痹症 bì zhèng) pathoconditions such as postpartum blood vacuity engendering wind, pulling of the extremities, hypertonicity of the sinews and vessels, intermittent convulsions, and hemiparesis.

Sheng Jiang (生薑/Rhizoma Zingiberis Recens/Fresh Ginger)

In classical literature on pharmacopoeia, it is described as follows: "Moves yang aspect, thus dispels cold and effuses the exterior; diffuses lung qi, thus resolves depression and regulates the center; and opens the appetite, thus eliminates phlegm and allows food to go down. Treats cold damage headache, wind damage nasal congestion, cough and counterflow and retching, chest congestion and phlegm blockage, and cold pain and damp diarrhea. Disperses water qi, moves blood impediment, frees spirit light (神明 shén míng), eliminates foulness, rescues sudden collapse, treats foxy smell (armpit odor), rub on frozen ears (chilblain), kills Ban Xia, Nan Xing, fungus and plants, and wild beast toxins, and repels mist and dew mountain forest miasmic qi (山嵐瘴氣 shān lán zhàng qì). Crush to extract the juice and decoct with Oxhide Glue (黃明膠 huáng míng jiāo) and apply on wind-damp impediment pain."

In contemporary texts, it is described as having an acrid flavor and warm nature; entering the lung, spleen, and stomach channels; having sweat-promoting (-effusing) exterior-resolving, center-warming vomiting-checking, lung-warming phlegm-transforming, and cough-suppressing actions.

Sheng Jiang is recognized as a sage medicinal for people suffering from retching and vomiting and is traditionally prescribed for the treatment of externally contracted wind-cold, stomach cold vomiting, and cold-phlegm cough.

Dr. Lee includes **Sheng Jiang** in his Yu Sheng versions of Ge Gen Tang, Mai Men Dong Tang, Xiao Chai Hu Tang, Chai Ling Tang, Da Qing Long Tang (Major Green-Blue Dragon Decoction), and Gui Zhi Jia Long Gu Mu Li Tang. However, he will replace **Sheng Jiang** with **Gan Jiang** in Yu Sheng versions of Gui Qi Jian Zhong Tang and Xiang Sha Liu Jun Zi Tang. Exceptions to this rule would be Xiang Sha Liu Jun Zi Tang including **Sheng Jiang** for the treatment of morning sickness during the first trimester of pregnancy and **Gan Jiang** replacing **Sheng Jiang** in Ge Gen Tang for the treatment of crick in the neck (落枕 lào zhěn) and painful stiff nape (頭項強痛 tóu xiàng qiáng tòng).

Sheng Long Gu (Crude Dragon Bone) – refer to **Long Gu**

Sheng Mu Li (Crude Oyster Shell) – refer to **Mu Li**

Sheng Shi Gao (Crude Gypsum) – refer to **Shi Gao**

Shi Gao (石膏/Gypsum Fibrosum/Gypsum)

Gypsum is a soft sulfate mineral composed of calcium sulfate dehydrate ($CaSO_4 \cdot 2H_2O$). It is heavy in substance and requires the prescription of relatively large doses in order to achieve therapeutic efficacy.

In classical literature on pharmacopoeia, it is described as follows: "A great cold foot Yang Ming channel medicinal, the color white enters the lung, and also enters the triple burner" and "Cold [in nature] clears heat and downbears fire, acrid [in flavor] promotes sweating and resolves the flesh, and sweet [in flavor] moderates the spleen and boosts qi and engenders liquid and allays thirst. [**Shi Gao**] treats cold damage binding depression (鬱結 yù jié) in the absence of sweating, Yang Ming headache, heat effusion and aversion to cold, late afternoon tidal heat, vigorous heat of the flesh, turbid reddish urine, great thirst with fluid intake, summerheat strike (中暑 zhòng shǔ) and spontaneous sweating, and parched tongue and toothache. Also, [since] stomach governs the flesh and the lung governs skin and hair, [it] is an essential medicinal for [treating] macular (斑 bān) and papular (疹

zhěn) eruptions. However, when used in small amounts, actions will not become apparent."

In contemporary texts, it is described as having an acrid and sweet flavor and extremely cold nature; entering the liver and stomach channels; and having heat-clearing fire-draining, vexation-eliminating thirst-allaying, astringing, and flesh-engendering actions. **Shi Gao** is recognized as an essential medicinal for clearing and draining qi aspect repletion heat of the lung and stomach channels.

Sheng Shi Gao (生石膏/Crude Gypsum) is traditionally prescribed for oral intake and **Duan Shi Gao (煅石膏/Calcined Gypsum)** for topical application. Despite the fact that **Duan Shi Gao** offers superior astringing efficacy for topical application in the treatment of external medicine pathoconditions, it also causes more *intense* skin and tissue irritation (e.g., stinging pain) that may last up to an hour after application. Based on clinical experience, Dr. Lee believes **Sheng Shi Gao** still provides adequate astringing efficacy with *mild*, *if any*, skin irritation, thus he only prescribes the crude form for both internal and external administration.

Sheng Shi Gao is by far Dr. Lee's most commonly prescribed medicinal for the treatment of interior repletion heat pattern and exterior damp-heat pattern pathoconditions. Dr. Lee includes this medicinal in the orally administered heat-draining, lung-diffusing panting-calming, and cough-suppressing formulas Ma Xing Shi Gan Tang and Da Qing Long Tang; the external medicine formulas Xian Fang Huo Ming Yin and Seborrheic Dermatitis Formula; and also in the topically applied formulas Shuang Shen Fen (Body Soothing Powder) and Lu Fu Gan Shi Fen (Antler Aconite Ginger Gypsum Powder).

Typically, Dr. Lee prescribes a base minimum oral dose of 1 liang up to a maximum of 4 liang depending on the extent of heat.

Shu Di Huang (熟地黃) – refer to **Sheng Di Huang**

The Eye Brighteners (明目藥)

Dr. Lee commonly adds pairs or combinations of **Qian Li Guang**, **Mi Meng Hua**, **She Tui**, **Chan Tui**, **Ci Ji Li**, and **Zao Jiao Ci** into formula variants for the treatment of ophthalmological disorders.

Qian Li Guang and **Mi Meng Hua** can be classified as eye orifice conductor medicinals, which are prescribed for the treatment of all types of heat—exterior wind-heat, residual heat, liver channel repletion heat, liver channel vacuity heat, blood stasis heat, blood desiccation with heat, and yin vacuity heat—pattern ophthalmological pathoconditions presenting with sore, red, swollen and itchy eyes (e.g., acute and chronic conjunctivitis, uveitis, retinitis, ocular hypertension).

She Tui and **Chan Tui** can be classified as exterior membrane conductor (i.e., eyes, skin) medicinals, which are prescribed specifically for the treatment of lens opacities (e.g., cataract) and corneal opacities (e.g., eye screen (目翳 mù yì), scarring), with their capacity to *peel off* the agglutinated protein build-up on the membranous surfaces of the eyes.

Ci Ji Li and **Zao Jiao Ci** are typically prescribed for the treatment of exterior wind-heat or wind-heat-damp pattern ophthalmological pathoconditions affecting the lacrimal drainage system (e.g., dacryocystitis, dacryoadenitis, epidemic keratoconjunctivitis ("pinkeye")).

The Four Lings (四苓)

This medicinal combination derives from Si Ling Tang (四苓湯)—**Fu Ling**, **Ze Xie**, **Zhu Ling**, and **Bai Zhu**—recorded in the *Teachings of Dan Xi* (丹溪心法 *Dan Xi Xin Fa*). However, Dr. Lee usually substitutes **Cang Zhu** in place of **Bai Zhu** for its spleen-fortifying dampness-drying and antimicrobial actions, which are ideal for Taiwan's humid subtropical climate.

Fu Ling, **Ze Xie**, and **Zhu Ling** all have similar flavor and nature (sweet, bland, and balanced); enter the kidney and urinary bladder channels; and share the complementary actions of disinhibiting water, percolating dampness, fortifying the spleen, and discharging heat. **Cang Zhu** has an acrid and bitter flavor and warm nature; enters the spleen and stomach channels; and has spleen-fortifying dampness-drying, wind-damp-dispelling sweat-promoting, and antimicrobial actions. The combination of these medicinals fortifies the spleen, disinhibits water, and percolates dampness for the treatment of water-damp collecting internally, inhibited urination, diarrhea, swelling (edema), and bloody urine.

These medicinals form one of the pillars of Dr. Lee's therapeutic approaches administered for a broad scope of pathoconditions involving water amassment or water-rheum collecting internally, which causes obstruction or stagnation and leads to the disruption of physiological mechanisms and pathological disorders. The resulting homeostatic imbalance may manifest in pathoconditions such as generalized edema, ascites, pericardial effusion, pleural effusion, and increased intracranial pressure (ICP) (e.g., traumatic injury, hemorrhage, tumor, herniation, heart failure, obstruction of cerebrospinal fluid).

Dr. Lee typically includes these medicinals in Wu Ling San (Calculi Formula), Wu Ling San (Nephritis Formula), and Chai Ling Tang or adds them into a formula variant based on presenting signs, symptoms, and pattern identification. For pathoconditions such as diarrhea, ascites, and ICP, Dr. Lee commonly includes **Da Huang** to enhance the draining precipitation action and adds **Ren Shen** as a counterbalance that aides the reabsorption of nutrients and electrolytes.

Depending on the specific pathocondition, Dr. Lee may prescribe large doses (up to 8 qian–1 liang each) of **The Four Lings** (especially **Fu Ling** and **Ze Xie**) to ensure an adequate level of water disinhibition is achieved.

The Itch Relievers (止癢藥)

Dr. Lee commonly prescribes pairs or combinations of **Ci Ji Li**, **Zao Jiao Ci**, **Lu Lu Tong**, **She Tui**, and **Chan Tui** for the treatment of all types of skin pathoconditions that result from inflammatory responses and the build-up of metabolic waste that block pores and disrupt normal epidermal homeostasis (i.e., epidermopoiesis and its regulation). This may present clinically in manifestations such as pruritis, erythema, macules, papules, scaling, lichenification, pustules, furuncles, abscesses, wheals, and plaques.

Ci Ji Li, **Zao Jiao Ci**, and **Lu Lu Tong** can be classified as pore conductor medicinals with their capacity to regulate—*opening* and *closing* (開闔 kāi hé)—of the pores and promote dermal circulation. This medicinal combination can be added into formula variants for the treatment of all types of acute (e.g., exterior wind-heat, exterior wind-damp-heat patterns) and chronic (e.g., blood desiccation pattern with exterior wind-heat or exterior wind-heat-damp) dermatological pathoconditions.

She Tui and **Chan Tui** can be classified as exterior membrane conductor (i.e., eyes, skin) medicinals with their capacity of promoting epidermal cell proliferation. This medicinal pair can be added into formula variants for the treatment of both acute (e.g., exterior wind-heat, damp-heat patterns) and chronic (e.g., vacuity heat, yang vacuity, blood desiccation patterns) dermatological pathoconditions.

However, due to their lightness in substance, high cost, tendency for patient aversion, and the fact that renewal of the dermis occurs naturally—*peeling off* on its own, Dr. Lee rarely prescribes this medicinal pair for skin pathoconditions unless the case is particularly severe or recalcitrant (e.g., eczema, atopic dermatitis, psoriasis).

The Seeds (種子)

Dr. Lee commonly prescribes pairs or combinations of **Long Yan He (Longan Seed)**, **Li Zhe He (Litchi Seed)**, **Ju He (Tangerine Seed)**, and **Shan Zha He (Hawthorn Berry Seed)** for pathoconditions of the male genitourinary system (e.g., benign prostatic hyperplasia (BPH), scrotal dermatitis, epididymitis, hydrocele, erectile dysfunction (ED), infertility, prostate cancer).

These medicinals share the common traits of entering the liver channel, have qi-moving bind-dissipating actions, and serve as channel conductors for their likeness of the gonads in both external appearance and physiological function. This is an example of the classical TCM treatment method of "resembling forms supplement respective body parts and resembling organs supplement respective organs (以形補形、以臟補臟 yǐ xíng bǔ xíng, yǐ zàng bǔ zàng)."

Dr. Lee's choice of these particular seeds (pits) is simply based on the fact that these fruits are grown locally, inexpensive and easily accessible. The seeds (pits) of many other fruits contain either identical or similar bioactive constituents and can be readily prescribed in place of those mentioned above for effective results. Prior to decoction, the seeds (pits) must be crushed to facilitate extraction of their bioactive constituents during decoction.

Note: The term seed (種子 zhǒng zǐ) and pit (果核 guǒ hé) are used interchangeably here. Many seed medicinals also have a pit and are thus designated as such in their names. For example, **Long Yan He (龍眼核/Longan Seed)** also has a pit (核 hé), but it is commonly translated as a seed, since the seed is indeed enclosed within the pit. To clarify, a seed is an ovule containing an embryo, while a pit is the part of the fruit that protects the seed until growth time.

The Three Great Yang-Supplementers (三大補陽)

The medicinal combination of **Gan Jiang**, **Fu Zi**, and **Rou Gui** comprise one of the pillars of Dr. Lee's therapeutic approaches. These great spleen and kidney yang-supplementing medicinals are prescribed for the post-acute and chronic stages that present with yang vacuity and cold stasis pattern. They are also prescribed following surgery, radiotherapy, and the administration of chemotherapeutic agents—*suppress* bone marrow function, thus *inhibiting* hematopoiesis—and corticosteroids—*suppress* the hypothalamic-pituitary-adrenal (HPA) axis, thus *decreasing* corticotropin-releasing hormone (CRH), adrenocorticotropic hormone (ACTH), and endogenous cortisol)—which result in yang vacuity and cold stasis pattern.

Additionally, Dr. Lee may prescribe this medicinal combination when the therapeutic regimen has reached a point where marginal or no significant improvement is being made. In this instance, the treatment method of returning and reinforcing yang is applied to "boost" the metabolism and immune system, giving the body the strength and capacity to bolster right qi and win the struggle between right and evil.

These great yang-supplementing medicinals boost the metabolism and immune system by innervating the central nervous system (CNS), peripheral nervous system (PNS), and autonomic nervous system (ANS) and by engaging a cascade of endocrine and hormonal factors. And when **Ren Shen**, **Huang Qi**, and **Lu Rong** are prescribed together with **The Three Great Yang-Supplementers** in a formula, this combination stimulates the body's capacity for self-repair, regeneration (e.g., nerves, skin, tissue, bone), and hematopoiesis.

An initial dose of 2–3 qian for each medicinal will be prescribed, increasing incrementally up to 5–8 qian each. Once the combined dose reaches 10–12 qian, then 3–5 qian of either one or a combination of **The Three Yellows** (**Huang Qin**, **Huang Bo**, and **Huang Lian**) are added to counteract excessive heat and mitigate the potential adverse effects.

The Three Insects (三蟲)

This term refers to the combination of **Quan Xie**, **Wu Gong**, and **Bai Jiang Can**. These arthropods have evolutionary ancestry dating back nearly 500 million years and are composed of relatively smaller, more basic fundamental amino acid and protein archetypes, offering exceptional efficacy at regulating the transmission of neurotransmitters across chemical synapses.

These three medicinals all enter the liver channel and share common actions of extinguishing wind and checking tetany, with

Quan Xie and **Wu Gong** attacking toxins, dissipating binds, and freeing the network vessels and relieving pain, and **Bai Jiang Can** dispelling wind and relieving pain and transforming phlegm and dissipating binds.

Dr. Lee typically adds **The Three Insects** into formula variants for the treatment of neuropathic pain (e.g., trigeminal neuralgia) and intractable headache (e.g., migraine, cluster headache).

The Three Yellows (三黃)

This term refers to the combination of **Huang Qin**, **Huang Bo**, and **Huang Lian**. The heat-clearing toxin-resolving (antimicrobial and anti-inflammatory) actions of these medicinals make them among the most important and commonly used medicinals in Dr. Lee's pharmacopoeia, comprising one of the pillars of Dr. Lee's therapeutic approaches. They provide exceptional efficacy for the treatment of all kinds of infections and inflammation (e.g., nasal, upper respiratory tract, gastrointestinal, hepatic, renal, autoimmune), and are also added into Yu Sheng formula variants to counteract the great heat of **The Three Great Yang-Supplementers—Gan Jiang**, **Fu Zi**, and **Rou Gui**.

Classical literature on pharmacopoeia differentiates the specific actions of these three medicinals as follows: "…**Huang Lian** drains heart fire and middle burner fire, **Huang Qin** drains upper burner fire, **Huang Bo** drains lower burner fire…." Dr. Lee also acknowledges these differentiations, using **Huang Lian** for the gastrointestinal tract, **Huang Qin** for the upper respiratory tract, and **Huang Bo** for the kidneys and genitourinary tract. However, from his clinical experience, these specific distinctions are *not* vital to achieve efficacy, and when evil qi (i.e., microbial infection) is being treated, the combination of **The Three Yellows** provides effective broad-spectrum antimicrobial action.

Tian Ma (天麻/Rhizoma Gastrodiae Elatae/Gastrodia Rhizome)

In classical literature on pharmacopoeia, it is described as follows: "Acrid [in flavor] and warm [in nature]," "Enters the liver channel qi aspect," and "Boosts qi and strengthens yin, frees the blood vessels, strengthens the sinews, and courses phlegm qi. Treats all types of wind dizziness and shaking, dizzy head and eye blackening [spots in visual field], speech not complying (語言不逐 yǔ yán bù zhú), wind-damp insensitive impediment (頑痹 wán bì) [paralysis of the extremities], and infantile fright epilepsy."

In contemporary texts, it is described as having a sweet flavor and balanced nature; entering the liver channel; and having wind-extinguishing tetany-checking, liver yang uprising-repressing, wind-dispelling, and network vessel-freeing actions.

Tian Ma shares many common properties with **The Three Insects**, thus Dr. Lee typically administers this medicinal either along with them or in combination with **Chuan Xiong**, **Chai Hu**, **Ban Xia**, and **Ge Gen** for the treatment of dizziness, vertigo (e.g., Meniere disease, benign paroxysmal positional vertigo (BPPV), idiopathic), and intractable headache (e.g., migraine, cluster headache). Dr. Lee also prescribes this medicinal for the treatment of neurogenic hypertension caused by brainstem dysfunction.

Depending on the severity of the patient's signs and symptoms, Dr. Lee may prescribe a dose of 3 qian up to 1 liang.

Tian Xiong (天雄) – refer to **Fu Zi**

Tu Si Zi (菟絲子/Semen Cuscutae Chinensis/Cuscuta)

This medicinal is processed in-house in Dr. Lee's own medicinal processing and decoction facility. Raw **Tu Si Zi** is mix-fried over a low flame until faint crackling sounds can be heard and an aromatic scent arises. At this time, these seeds will be dark yellow to light brown in color. The purpose for processing in this way is to crack open the seed coat, thus allowing the constituents to be easily extracted upon decoction.

In classical literature on pharmacopoeia, it is described as follows: "Sweet and acrid [in flavor] and harmonious and balanced [in nature] and condenses qi of right yang (凝正陽之氣 níng zhèng yáng zhī qì)," "Enters the three yin [channels] of the foot," and "Strengthens yin and boosts essence, warms without drying, and does not reinforce ministerial fire. Treats the five taxations and seven damages, seminal cold and dribbling, and bitterness of mouth with dryness and thirst. Dispels wind and brightens the eyes, supplements defense qi, aides the sinews and vessels, boosts qi and bodily strength, and fattens and fortifies the body."

In contemporary texts, it is described as having a sweet flavor and a warm nature; entering the liver, kidney and spleen channels; and having kidney-supplementing essence-securing, liver-nourishing eye-brightening, diarrhea-checking, and fetus-quieting actions.

Dr. Lee includes the medicinal pair **Tu Si Zi** and **Sha Yuan Ji Li** (supplements the kidney and secures essence and nourishes the liver and brightens the eyes) in Atopic Dermatitis Formula and Blood Desiccation Formula; and commonly adds the pair into formula variants for their balanced and moderate liver and kidney yin-nourishing actions. Together, these medicinals offer superior capacity for retaining moisture (cellular hydration) and maintaining cell metabolic activity.

Wu Gong (蜈蚣/Scolopendra Subspinipes/Centipede)

In classical literature on pharmacopoeia, it is described as follows: "Mobile and able to dissipate, [it] treats umbilical wind clenched jaw, fright epilepsy and scrofula, snake concretions and nail sores, and kills worms and aborts the fetus."

In contemporary texts, it is described as having an acrid flavor, a warm, mobile and penetrating nature able to reach the interior and exterior, and toxicity; entering the liver channel; and having wind-extinguishing tetany-checking, toxin-attacking bind-dissipating, and network vessel-freeing pain-relieving actions. Traditionally, it is commonly paired with **Quan Xie** for the treatment of pathoconditions presenting with spasm and convulsion, such as acute and chronic fright wind, tetanus, and wind striking the channels and network vessels with deviated eyes and mouth.

Dr. Lee combines this medicinal with **Quan Xie** and **Bai Jiang Can** for the treatment of neuropathic pain (e.g., trigeminal neuralgia) and intractable headache (e.g., migraine, cluster headache). Due to its high market price, Dr. Lee typically only prescribes it in cases where the pain is "unbearable."

*For more details, refer to **The Three Insects** profile.

Xi Lu Rong (細鹿茸) – refer to **Lu Rong**

Xian Di Huang (鮮地黃) – refer to **Sheng Di Huang**

Xian Zha (仙楂) – refer to **Shan Zha**

Xie (蠍) – refer to **Quan Xie**

Xiong Huang (雄黃/Realgar)

In classical literature on pharmacopoeia, it is described as follows: "Acrid [in flavor] and warm [in nature] with toxicity and obtains qi of right yang," "Enters the liver channel qi aspect," and "Tracks (down) the liver (搜肝 sōu gān) and strengthens the spleen, dissipates great wind of the hundred joints (百節大風 bǎi jié dà fēng), kills hundred toxin, and repels ghosts and goblins. Treats fright epilepsy and phlegm-drool, headache and dizziness, summerheat malaria and afflux dysentery (澼痢 pì lì), and diarrhea and accumulations and gatherings. [It] can also transform blood into water, dry dampness and kill worms, and treat taxation gan (勞疳 láo gān), sores and boils, and snake bite."

In contemporary texts, it is described as having an acrid flavor, warm nature, and toxicity; entering the heart, liver and stomach channels; and having toxin-resolving worm-killing, dampness-drying, and wind-dispelling actions.

This medicinal contains the toxic constituent arsenic sulfide (As2S2). To mitigate the potential for harmful side effects and ensure safety, a time-consuming and rigorous traditional water grind (water-refining) processing method must be performed (calcination is strictly prohibited!). This processed pulverized powder form of **Xiong Huang** is then used for clinical application. It is experimentally and clinically proven to contain potent and effective toxin-resolving, worm-killing (i.e., antimicrobial), and anticancer actions (i.e., suppresses cell differentiation, induces apoptosis, inhibits tumor growth and angiogenesis).

Administered orally, this medicinal can only be prescribed in minuscule doses and added within a well-balanced formula composition due to the potential risk of adverse effects if taken in excessive dosages (e.g., suppression of hematopoiesis). **Xiong Huang** powder is included in the Yu Sheng formula compositions of Bao An Wan Ling Dan, Sai Ji (Vaginal Suppository), Xi Ji (Vaginal Wash/Douche), Shuang Shen Fen, and Medicated Thread (Yao Xian). Dr. Lee also uses this medicinal as an external application for the treatment of herpes zoster skin rash.

Xu Duan (續斷/Radix Dipsaci/Teasal Root)

In classical literature on pharmacopoeia, it is described as follows: "An essential medicinal for supplementing and joining the blood vessels" and "Bitterness and warmth supplement the kidney and acridity and warmth supplement the liver. [**Xu Duan**] perfuses blood vessels and rectifies the sinews and bones, thus supplements insufficiency during injury, relaxes the uterus, reduces urination, and breaks static blood. [It] treats lumbar pain and fetal spotting, flooding and vaginal discharge and seminal emission, intestinal wind and blood dysentery, and welling-abscesses, hemorrhoids, and toxin swelling. [It] treats incised wounds, breaks, and knocks and falls, relieves pain and engenders flesh, and is considered a first-class medicinal for women's medicine and external medicine."

In contemporary texts, it is described as having a bitter, sweet, and acrid flavor and slightly warm nature; entering the liver and kidney channels; and having liver- and kidney-supplementing, sinew- and bone-strengthening, blood-stanching, and fetus-quieting actions for the treatment of injuries and mending breakages.

Dr. Lee commonly includes **Xu Duan** paired or in combination with other medicinals containing similar properties in his formulas as follows: **Du Zhong** (serves as a channel conductor directing medicinals downwards to the lumbar and lower limbs, supplements the liver and kidney, and quiets the fetus) in Dang Gui San; **Gu Sui Bu** (enters the kidney channel, quickens the blood and transforms stasis, breaks blood, and treats injury and mends breakages) in Diao Fen (Suspension Powder); and **Gu Sui Bu** and **Niu Xi** (quickens the blood and dissipates stasis, supplements the liver and kidney, and frees the channels (menstruation) and relieves pain) in Tong Jing Fang. Additionally, Dr. Lee commonly adds the medicinal pair **Xu Duan** and **Gu Sui Bu** into formula variants for the treatment of skeletal bone, marrow, and tooth pathoconditions, such as fractures, osteoporosis, and periodontitis; and this pair also serves as a conductor that targets hard tissue—eliminating stasis and engendering the new—for the treatment of both malignant and benign tumors.

Yin Xing Ye (銀杏葉/Folium Ginkgo/Ginkgo Leaf/aka Bai Guo Ye)

This medicinal is the leaf of *Ginkgo biloba* L. and its seed is **Bai Guo**. In classical literature on pharmacopoeia, it is described as follows: "Grind into powder, knead into dough, make into cake, roast and eat cooked, [it] checks diarrhea and dysentery."

In contemporary texts, it is described as having a bitter, sweet and astringent flavor, balanced nature, and mild toxicity; entering the heart, lung, and spleen channels; and having blood-quickening heart-nourishing and lung-constraining intestine-astringing actions.

Traditionally, it is prescribed for the treatment of chest impediment heart pain, panting with phlegm cough, diarrhea and dysentery, and white vaginal discharge. Experimental animal studies have shown that the flavonols (i.e., quercetin, kaempferol, and isorhamnetin) and biflavonols in **Yin Xing Ye** have the capacity to dilate coronary blood vessels, increase coronary blood flow, lower serum cholesterol, and inhibit platelet aggregation. Dr. Lee explains that one of its main physiological mechanisms involves increasing exchanges across blood vessel membranes.

This is a commonly prescribed medicinal in Dr. Lee's pharmacopoeia and is prescribed for the treatment of such conditions as coronary artery disease (CAD), angina pectoris, hyperlipidemia, atherosclerosis, hypertension, cerebral vasospasm, and aneurysms. It is also an essential medicinal in (Yu Sheng) Bu Yang Huan Wu Tang, which is typically prescribed for sequelae of cerebrovascular accident (CVA), Parkinson's disease (PD), Alzheimer's disease (AD), and other cerebrovascular, cardiovascular and neurodegenerative pathoconditions.

Yu Gui (玉桂) – refer to **Rou Gui**

Zao Jiao Ci (皂角刺/Spina Gleditsiae/Chinese Honeylocust Spine)

In classical literature on pharmacopoeia, it is described as follows: "Acrid [in flavor] and warm [in nature]. [**Zao Jiao Ci**] tracks (down) wind and kills worms, just like **Zao Jia (皂筴)** [**Zao Jiao**], but it is sharp [and] can reach the affected site [to] break and disperse welling- and flat-abscesses for the treatment of welling-abscess toxin, begrudging milk [excess of breast milk] (妒乳 dù rǔ), pestilential wind [leprosy] (癘風 lì fēng) and malign sores, and retention of the placenta. [It is] contraindicated for welling- and flat-abscesses that have already ruptured [and] for pregnant women" and "[**Zao**] **Jiao Ci** opens the orifices for all welling- and flat-abscesses that have not yet ruptured; and for those that have already ruptured, [it] can conduct medicinals to the sore, thus is an essential medicinal for all types of malign sores and lichen and pestilential wind [leprosy]."

In contemporary texts, it is described as having an acrid flavor and warm nature; entering the liver and stomach channels; and having blood-quickening swelling-dispersing and pus-expelling milk-freeing actions.

Traditionally, **Zao Jiao Ci** is prescribed in the early stage of swelling and toxin of welling-abscesses and sores, for pus formation that fails to rupture, and for breast milk stoppage. It can also be applied topically for the treatment of sores and lichen. The medicinal combination of **Zao Jiao Ci**, **Ci Ji Li**, and **Chan Tui** can be prescribed to promote the dispersion and rupture of welling-abscesses and sores and relieve itching.

Dr. Lee commonly adds the medicinal pair **Zao Jiao Ci** and **Ci Ji Li** (calms and courses the liver and dispels wind and brightens the eyes) into formula variants for the treatment of exterior wind-heat or wind-heat-damp pattern ophthalmological pathoconditions affecting the lacrimal drainage system (e.g., dacryocystitis, dacryoadenitis, epidemic keratoconjunctivitis ("pinkeye")) and damp-heat pattern dermatological pathoconditions (e.g., lipomas, flat warts).

Dr. Lee classifies **Zao Jiao Ci**, **Ci Ji Li**, and **Lu Lu Tong** (expels wind and frees the network vessels and disinhibits water and eliminates dampness) as pore conductor medicinals with their capacity to regulate—*opening* and *closing* (開闔 kāi hé)—of the pores and promote dermal circulation. Thus, he adds this medicinal combination into formula variants for the treatment of exterior wind-heat (or wind-heat-damp) and blood desiccation pattern with exterior wind-heat (or with exterior wind-heat-damp) skin pathoconditions presenting with pruritic papules and maculopapular and vesicular eruptions (e.g., dyshidrotic eczema (pompholyx), palmoplantar pustulosis (PPP), wind papules (urticaria), atopic dermatitis).

Dr. Lee explains that blood-quickening stasis-transforming medicinals, such as **Dang Gui**, **Chuan Xiong**, **Ru Xiang**, **Mo Yao**, promote an increase of angiogenic proteins, the precursors necessary for angiogenesis, while the medicinal pair **Zao Jiao Ci** and **Ci Ji Li** has the capacity to open up pathways in the granulation tissue and collagen deposition formed during the wound healing process. The prescription of these mutually complementary medicinals reestablishes patent vasculature and perfusion at the site of the fibrous tissue (i.e., scar) formation, restores the natural skin coloration, and shrinks the size of the scar, thus improving the cosmetic appearance of both hypertrophic and keloid scars.

*For more details, refer to **The Eye Brighteners** and **The Itch Relievers** profiles.

Ze Xie (澤瀉/Rhizoma Alismatis Orientalitis/Alisma)

In classical literature on pharmacopoeia, it is described as follows: "Enters the urinary bladder [channel], disinhibits urine, drains fire evil in the kidney channel, and specializes in disinhibiting dampness and moving water."

In contemporary texts, it is described as having a sweet and bland flavor and cold nature; entering the kidney and urinary bladder channels; and having water-disinhibiting dampness-percolating and heat-discharging actions. It is experimentally proven to increase urine output along with the excretion of urea and chloride, lower blood pressure, and lower blood sugar levels.

As a general rule, if large doses of this medicinal are prescribed (≥ 8 qian), Dr. Lee will include a comparable dose of **Fu Ling** to enhance water-disinhibiting actions.

*For more details, refer to **The Four Lings** profile.

Zhu Ling (豬苓/Sclerotium Polyporus Umbellati/Polyporus)

In classical literature on pharmacopoeia, it is described as follows: "Bitter [in flavor] drains stagnation, bland [in flavor] disinhibits the orifices, and sweet [in flavor] assists yang. Enters the urinary bladder kidney channel, upbears thus can downbear, opens the interstices and promotes sweating, disinhibits urine and moves water, and has similar actions as **Fu Ling** except that it does not supplement…."

In contemporary texts, it is described as having a sweet and bland flavor and a balanced nature; entering the kidney and urinary bladder channels; and having water-disinhibiting dampness-percolating actions. **Zhu Ling** has a stronger water-disinhibiting action compared to **Fu Ling**, but not as strong of a supplementing action. The physiological mechanism of its urine-disinhibiting (diuretic) action primarily involves inhibiting the absorption of water and electrolytes (specifically potassium (K^+), sodium (Na^+), and chlorine (Cl^-)) in the renal tubules of the nephron.

*For more details, refer to **The Four Lings** profile.

DR. LEE'S FORMULAS

This section introduces the formulas Dr. Lee commonly prescribes and includes details about the dose and action of each medicinal, the composite action of each formula, and the types of pathoconditions for which each formula is typically administered. Many of these formulas are variants on Han dynasty classical formulas from the *Treatise on Cold Damage and Miscellaneous Diseases* (傷寒雜病論 *Shang Han Za Bing Lun*), some are variants on more contemporary classic formulas from the Tang, Song, Ming, and Qing dynasties, and others are original formulas designed by Dr. Lee. Additionally, other formulas that Dr. Lee mentions as alternatively effective therapeutic options in the text are also listed for reference, but with only the compositions provided.

Throughout the text, the name "(Yu Sheng)" may be included in front of a formula's name to distinguish that it is a Dr. Lee variant on an existing formula or his own unique composition. Even when not included, it is still implied that all of the formulas Dr. Lee prescribes are indeed (Yu Sheng) formulas. The term Yu Sheng simply refers to Yu Sheng Chinese Medicine Clinic of which Dr. Lee is the founder, director, and chief physician.

The following formulas are set compositions designed to treat the extensive scope of pathoconditions that Dr. Lee commonly incurs in his clinical practice. The medicinals comprising the formulas are either purchased already processed or processed in-house, and then pre-weighed and pre-packaged into semiporous decocting packets (not yet sealed) for convenient storage and administration. Upon prescription, Dr. Lee will subsequently make modifications to these formulas by adding medicinals based on each individual patient's signs, symptoms, and pattern identification. The packets are then sealed and ready for administration and decoction. This is not an exhaustive listing: when special cases present, Dr. Lee will compose formulas specifically designed for a particular case.

As time evolves, social and environmental factors impact the manifestation of maladies in the human body, mind, and spirit. Dr. Lee continues to search for the best approaches to provide the most effective treatment in our modern world.

*__Disclaimer__: The formula compositions and medicinal doses provided in Dr. Lee's commonly prescribed formulas listed below and throughout this entire three-volume series are *for reference purposes only* and are *not* intended for indiscriminate administration by other individuals or parties. Prescription of these formulas should only be administered by a licensed traditional Chinese medicine (TCM) physician or practitioner who has carefully evaluated the patient's history, signs, and symptoms, and conducted pattern identification as the basis for determining treatment. Licensed TCM practitioners must be aware that these formula compositions and medicinal doses are *for reference purposes only* and solely intended for administration by Dr. Lee in his own clinical practice.

An Zhong San (安中散)
Gui Zhi, Yan Hu Suo, Mu Li, Xiao Hui Xiang, Sha Ren, Gan Cao, Liang Jiang

Asthma Formula (氣喘方/Qi Chuan Fang)

Ma Huang	1.5 qian
Dan Shen, Cang Zhu, Fu Ling, Gan Cao	3 qian each
Mu Xiang, Sha Ren, Wu Wei Zi	3 qian each
Chen Pi, Ban Xia, Xing Ren, Bai Guo	4 qian each
Shan Yao, Rou Gui	5 qian each

This original Yu Sheng formula contains the qi-boosting spleen-fortifying and qi-moving phlegm-transforming actions of **Xiang Sha Liu Jun Zi Tang** adding Ma Huang, Wu Wei Zi, Xing Ren, Bai Guo, Shan Yao, and Rou Gui. Ma Huang promotes sweating and resolves the exterior; Wu Wei Zi constrains the lung and stabilizes panting; Xing Ren suppresses cough and calms panting; Bai Guo constrains the lung and dispels phlegm; Shan Yao supplements the spleen, lung, and kidneys and nourishes yin; and Rou Gui supplements fire and assists yang for the treatment of vacuity asthma debilitation of the life gate fire. Dr. Lee will also add Ren Shen (powder), which enters the lung and spleen channels, greatly supplements original qi, and supplements the spleen and boosts the lung. As its name indicates, this formula is designed for the treatment of asthma, and specifically for the spleen yang vacuity pattern type that presents with panting (asthma) and shortness of breath (dyspnea).

Spleen yang vacuity pattern presents in the early stages of this pathocondition, when it can be more readily managed and often even cured. If this pathocondition progresses to the more severe, chronic stage of kidney yang vacuity pattern, Dr. Lee typically prescribes **You Gui Yin** variant. For acute flare-ups, heat-clearing toxin-resolving, lung-depurating phlegm-transforming, and cough-suppressing panting-calming medicinals will be added to the formula; or the original formula will be substituted with a heat-clearing, cough-suppressing, and panting-calming formula variant (e.g., **Ma Xing Gan Shi Tang**, **Da Qing Long Tang**) until the flare-up subsides.

Athlete's Foot/Pompholyx Infusion (香港腳/汗皰疹泡藥)
Xiong Huang, Da Huang, Ru Xiang, Hua Shi, Gan Shi, and Qing Fen

Atopic Dermatitis Formula (異位性皮膚炎方/Yi Wei Xing Pi Fu Yan Fang)

Ma Huang	1.5 qian
Dan Shen, Cang Zhu, Fu Ling, Gan Cao	3 qian each
Chen Pi, Ban Xia, Mu Xiang, Sha Ren	3 qian each
Xing Ren, Bai Guo, Wu Wei Zi, Shan Yao	3 qian each
Dang Gui, He Shou Wu, Tu Si Zi, Sha Yuan Zi	5 qian each

This is an Yu Sheng original compound formula derived from **Asthma Formula (Qi Chuan Fang)** (subtracting Rou Gui) and **Blood Desiccation Formula (Xue Ku Fang)** (subtracting Ci Ji Li). **Asthma Formula** supplements the spleen, lung, and kidneys, nourishes yin, resolves the exterior, opens the pores, and dispels phlegm; and **Blood Desiccation Formula** nourishes blood, enriches yin, and dispels wind. As its name indicates, Dr. Lee administers this formula for the treatment of atopic dermatitis and specifically spleen yang vacuity pattern type.

Depending on the patient's presenting signs, symptoms and pattern, the following medicinals are commonly added: for severe pruritis—Shi Gao, Lu Lu Tong, and Hua Shi; for flare-ups with excessive suppuration—Bai Xian Pi, Huang Qin, Yi Yi Ren; and for chronic persistent cases with erythematous lesions (in body creases or generalized), cracking, suppuration, pruritis, and agitation—the medicinal doses in **Blood Desiccation Formula** will be increased with small amounts of The Three Great Yang-Supplementers (Gan Jiang, Fu Zi, and Rou Gui) added to supplement kidney and spleen vacuity and return and reinforce yang.

Ba Xian Chang Shou Wan (八仙長壽丸)

Sheng Di Huang, Shan Zhu Yu, Huai Shan, Fu Ling, Mu Dan Pi, Ze Xie, Mai Men Dong, Wu Wei Zi

Ba Zheng San (八正散)

Mu Tong, Qu Mai, Che Qian Zi, Bian Xu, Hua Shi, Gan Cao, Da Huang, Zhi Zi, Deng Xin Cao

Bai He Gu Jin Tang (百合固金湯)

Bai He, Sheng Di Huang, Shu Di Huang, Yuan Shen	3 qian each
Jie Geng, Gan Cao, Mai Men Dong	3 qian each
Dang Gui, Chi Shao, Cang Zhu	3 qian each

Bai Hu Tang (白虎湯)

Zhi Mu, Shi Gao, Gan Cao, Jing Mi

Ban Xia Hou Po Tang (半夏厚朴湯)

Ban Xia, Hou Po, Fu Ling, Sheng Jiang, Gan Su Ye

Ban Xia Tian Ma Bai Zhu San (半夏天麻白朮散)

Dang Gui	2 qian
Ban Xia, Bai Zhu, Fu Ling, Cang Zhu	3 qian each
Ze Xie, Chen Pi, Shen Qu	3 qian each
Mai Ya, Gan Jiang, Huang Bo	3 qian each
Fu Zi, Tian Ma	5 qian each
Huang Qi	1 liang

The Yu Sheng version is virtually the same as the original formula except for the addition of Dang Gui and Fu Zi, and the fact that Ren

Shen (powder) is either taken separately or added into the formula after decoction. Dang Gui supplements and quickens the blood and Fu Zi returns yang and stems counterflow, supplements fire and reinforces yang, and dissipates cold and relieves pain. These additions complement this foot Tai Yin spleen channel formula's overall spleen and stomach-supplementing, phlegm-damp transforming, and wind-stabilizing actions. The classical TCM pathomechanisms of this formula are explained as follows: "Phlegm reversal [refers to] phlegm-damp reverse flow ascending. Phlegm counterflow leads to upper body repletion, causing headache, dizzy head, and black [spots] in front of the eyes [visual field]."

This is among Dr. Lee's most commonly prescribed formulas, administered for a wide range of pathoconditions including Meniere disease, benign paroxysmal positional vertigo (BPPV), psychosomatic symptoms (e.g., abdominal distention, malaise, and fatigue), migraine and cluster headaches, traumatic brain injury resulting in increased intracranial pressure, and benign brain tumors. It is also one of the commonly prescribed formulas in Dr. Lee's cancer treatment protocol, specifically administered for malignant brain tumors.

Bao An Wan Ling Dan (保安萬靈丹/Safeguard Unlimited Efficacy Elixir)

Tian Ma, Chuan Xiong, Chuan Wu, Wu Cao	1 liang each
Fang Feng, Jing Jie, Ma Huang, Xi Xin	1 liang each
Qiang Huo, He Shou Wu, Dang Gui	1 liang each
Shi Hu, Quan Xie, Gan Cao	1 liang each
Cang Zhu	8 liang
Xiong Huang	6 qian

Dr. Lee uses the *Orthodox Manual of External Medicine* (外科正宗 *Wai Ke Zheng Zong*) version of this formula and commonly abbreviates the name, calling it simply **Wan Ling Dan**. This is a pill specially prepared for Dr. Lee by an outsourced medicinal processing facility. It is composed of medicinals that dispel wind, eliminate dampness, dissipate cold, extinguish wind, quicken the blood, supplement the blood, check tetany, free the network vessels, open the orifices, resolve toxin, dissipate binds, and relieve pain. Xiong Huang is among the principal medicinals in this composition with its antimicrobial and anticancer actions (e.g., suppresses cell differentiation, induces apoptosis, and inhibits tumor growth and angiogenesis).

As its name implies, this formula has been traditionally administered for the treatment of a broad spectrum of pathoconditions including welling- and flat-abscesses, deep pus sores, clove toxin, mouth-level nape flat abscess, jowl effusion, damp phlegm streaming sore, bone flat-abscesses, crane's-knee wind, wind-cold-damp impediment, paralysis, tetanus, and migraine headaches.

Dr. Lee prescribes this formula for various types of acute, chronic, and intractable pathoconditions including innominate toxin-swelling, benign tumors, and paralysis resulting from parasitic infection. It also constitutes one of the pillars of Dr. Lee's cancer treatment protocol, prescribed as a part of the regimen for all types of solid tumors (e.g., carcinoma, sarcoma) and hematological cancers (i.e., leukemia, lymphoma, myeloma). Combined with other formulas, **Wan Ling Dan** has the capacity to induce partial or complete remission and lower the chances of recurrence and metastasis.

Blood Desiccation Formula (血枯方/Xue Ku Fang)

Cang Zhu, Ci Ji Li	4 qian each
Dang Gui, He Shou Wu, Tu Si Zi, Sha Yuan Zi	8 qian each

The term blood desiccation first appears in the *The Yellow Emperor's Inner Canon* (黃帝內經 *Huang Di Nei Jing*) and refers to this pathocondition as blood vacuity following hemorrhage. Indeed, Dr. Lee's adaptation of this term covers a much broader scope of applications. This Yu Sheng original formula has similar actions and clinical applications as **Dang Gui Yin Zi** containing the essential medicinals Dang Gui, He Shou Wu, and Ci Ji Li. However, it replaces Shao Yao, Chuan Xiong, and Sheng Di Huang with large doses of Dang Gui and He Shou Wu; subtracts Fang Feng, Jing Jie, and Huang Qi; and adds Sha Yuan Zi, Tu Si Zi, and Cang Zhu.

Sha Yuan Zi and Tu Si Zi both supplement the kidney, secure essence, and nourish the liver; and Cang Zhu dispels wind-damp and dries dampness and fortifies the spleen to counteract the potential for digestion impairment and loose stools resulting from the blood-nourishing yin-enriching medicinals. These additions complement this formula's overall actions of nourishing the blood, moistening dryness, dispelling wind, and relieving itch for the treatment of yin vacuity, blood vacuity, and blood desiccation patterns. For the treatment of skin pathoconditions, the relatively hardier Ma Huang is added to resolve the exterior instead of Fang Feng and Jing Jie (their volatile oils readily vaporize upon decoction and thus require large doses to achieve efficacy); and if itch presents, add Ci Ji Li, Zao Jiao Ci, and Lu Lu Tong.

Dr. Lee typically prescribes this formula for wind-dryness presenting as dry, itchy skin, and possibly mild redness (e.g., pruritis, erythema, urticaria, eczema, atopic dermatitis), liver blood vacuity (e.g., late stage hepatic cirrhosis with darkened skin and compromised hematopoiesis), and endometrial hypoperfusion (e.g., causing infertility and miscarriage).

Bu Yang Huan Wu Tang (補陽還五湯)

Dang Gui, Chuan Xiong, Chi Shao	4 qian each
Dan Shen, Yin Xing Ye	4 qian each
Huang Qi	2 liang

The Yu Sheng version is based on the original formula, but only contains 2 liang of Huang Qi as opposed to 4 liang; excludes Di Long, Tao Ren, and Hong Hua; and adds Yin Xing Ye and Dan Shen. Though not listed above, Ren Shen *is* included in this composition just as in the original formula, except in pulverized powder form, and is often paired with Chuan Qi (aka Ren Shen/Chuan Qi Powder). This medicinal pair serves to complement the qi-supplementing action of Huang Qi and the blood-quickening action of Dan Shen. Dr. Lee has chosen a relatively smaller dose of Huang Qi for this composition, because starting out with an excessive dose may result in the rupture of compromised blood vessels or a sudden increase in intracranial pressure in patients with arteriosclerosis, atheroclerosis, hematoma, or adhesions in the subarachnoid space of the meninges.

Yin Xing Ye is an essential medicinal in this formula and Dr. Lee utilizes its capacity of increasing exchanges across blood vessel membranes (e.g., promotes lymphatic circulation) and phlegm-transforming actions to reduce blood viscosity and eliminate plaque for patients with cerebrovascular accident (CVA) (stroke) sequelae, transient ischemic attack (TIA) sequelae, Parkinson's disease (PD), Alzheimer's disease (AD), and other cerebrovascular and neurodegenerative pathoconditions. Tao Ren, Hong Hua, and Di Long are excluded, because unlike stroke patients in the 18th and 19th centuries when this formula was designed, modern biomedicine has already intervened during the acute stage to accelerate reperfusion with drugs and surgical decompression. This intervention obviates the need for these potent blood-quickening stasis-dispelling and network vessel-freeing medicinals.

Nowadays, the primary role of TCM is to treat the neurological sequelae and prevent subsequent attacks. This requires the administration of dual supplementation of blood and qi, blood-quickening, and phlegm-transforming medicinals to reduce blood viscosity, maintain plaque-free vasculature, and prevent the development of emboli or thrombi. Prescribed for the treatment of neurodegenerative diseases (e.g., AD, PD, Huntington's disease), this formula slows down the rate of degeneration, enhances quality of life, and extends life expectancy.

Bu Zhong Yi Qi Tang (補中益氣湯)

Huang Qi	1 liang
Dang Gui	2 qian
Dan Shen, Cang Zhu, Chen Pi	3 qian each
Gan Cao, Sheng Ma, Chai Hu	3 qian each

The Yu Sheng version is similar to the original formula except that Dan Shen replaces Ren Shen for its blood-quickening stasis-dispelling action, and Cang Zhu replaces Bai Zhu for its spleen-fortifying dampness-drying action, which aids digestion and is more suitable for Taiwan's humid subtropical climate. However, depending on the presenting signs, symptoms, and pattern, Dr. Lee may also add Ren Shen (powder) (or Ren Shen/Chuan Qi Powder).

Dr. Lee prescribes this qi-boosting, yang-upbearing fall-raising, and spleen-supplementing stomach-regulating formula for pathoconditions such as anal prolapse, uterine prolapse, gastroptosis, nephroptosis, inguinal hernia, anal fissures, hemorrhoids, myasthenia gravis (qi-vacuity type), leukorrhea (qi-vacuity type), and proteinuria (intrinsic renal disease) in pediatric patients. Additionally, this formula's exceptional efficacy at promoting tissue repair and mucous membrane healing makes it an essential formula for patients with post-surgical wounds and cancer patients who have undergone (or are currently receiving) radiotherapy or chemotherapy.

Chai Ling Tang (柴苓湯)

Huang Qin, Fu Ling, Zhu Ling, Ze Xie	3 qian each
Cang Zhu, Yuan Hu Suo, Mu Xiang, Gui Zhi	3 qian each
Dan Shen, Ban Xia, Gan Cao, Sheng Jiang	5 qian each
Da Zao	3 pieces
Chai Hu	6 qian

The Yu Sheng version is similar to the original formula with the addition of Yuan Hu Suo, Mu Xiang, and Dan Shen, and the replacement of Bai Zhu with Cang Zhu; Ren Shen pulverized powder is used instead of decocting pieces; and unlike other Yu Sheng formulas, Gui Zhi *is* included (instead of Rou Gui) for its yang-assisting qi-transforming actions. Yan Hu Suo and Mu Xiang relax smooth muscle and thus relieve pain.

This is a compound formula that includes elements of **Xiao Chai Hu Tang (小柴胡湯)** and **Wu Ling San (Calculi Formula) (五苓散) (結石方)** and functions to eliminate heat, disinhibit water, and transform phlegm for the treatment of symptoms and patterns involving water amassment collecting above and below the diaphragm, amassed phlegm and collecting rheum, cold damage with residual Shao Yang heat, chest and rib-side distention and impediment, difficult urination, and vomiting and diarrhea upon drinking water.

Dr. Lee typically prescribes this formula for pathoconditions that manifest as ascites, portal hypertension, pleural effusion, pleuritis, pericardial effusion, cerebral edema, and increased intracranial pressure, such as in chronic liver disease (e.g., hepatitis, cirrhosis, fulminant hepatitis, hepatorenal syndrome (HRS), hepatocellular carcinoma), encephalitis, trauma, and radiotherapy. It is also one of the commonly prescribed formulas in Dr. Lee's cancer treatment protocol, specifically administered for Shao Yang cancers, which are identified as membranous tissue cancers manifesting in organs such as the liver, kidney, and lung.

Chai Ping Tang (柴平湯)

Chai Hu, Ren Shen, Ban Xia, Huang Qin, Gan Cao, Chen Pi, Hou Po, Cang Zhu, Sheng Jiang, Da Zao

Chong He Tang (冲和湯)

Ren Shen, Chen Pi, Huang Qi, Bai Zhu, Dang Gui, Bai Zhi, Fu Ling, Chuan Xiong, Zao Jiao Ci, Ru Xiang, Mo Yao, Jin Yin Hua, Gan Cao

Chou Feng Tang (抽風湯/Tugging Wind Formula)

Fang Feng, Yuan Ming Fen, Chai Hu, Da Huang, Huang Qin, Che Qian Zi, Jie Geng, Xi Xin

Da Huang Zhe Chong Wan (大黄哲蟲丸)

Da Huang, Huang Qin, Gan Cao, Tao Ren, Xing Ren, Bai Shao, Shou Di Huang, Gan Qi, Meng Chong, Shui Zhi, Qi Cao, Tu Bie Chong, Mi (Honey)

Da Qing Long Tang (大青龍湯/Major Green-Blue Dragon)

Ma Huang	2 qian
Xing Ren, Cang Zhu	4 qian each
Rou Gui, Sheng Jiang, Gan Cao	3 qian each
Sheng Shi Gao	1 liang
Da Zao	5 pieces

The Yu Sheng version is virtually identical to the original formula, which is a derivative of **Ma Huang Tang** that includes large doses of Ma Huang and Gan Cao and adds Sheng Shi Gao, Sheng Jiang, and Da Zao. However, as is the case in many of Dr. Lee's formulas, Rou Gui replaces Gui Zhi, and Cang Zhu is added due to considerations for Taiwan's humid subtropical climate. Its name, **Major Green-Blue Dragon**, refers to the fact that after taking this formula, sweat flows and evil abates as if a dragon rose up to the skies and brought rain pouring down, thus resulting in the immediate elimination of depressed heat.

This formula is traditionally prescribed for the treatment of external contraction wind-cold exterior repletion with interior heat pattern, presenting in pathoconditions such as the common cold, influenza, bronchitis, measles papules, wind papules, urticaria, and itchy skin. Similarly, Dr. Lee prescribes this formula for the treatment of Tai Yang cold damage with vexation and agitation from interior heat;

however, for external medicine (i.e., dermatology) manifestations he may also consider prescribing formula variants such as **Yue Bi Tang**, **Gui Zhi Ma Huang Ge Ban Tang**, or **Ma Xing Gan Shi Tang** instead.

Dang Gui Liu Huang Tang (當歸六黃湯)

Dang Gui, Sheng Di Huang, Shu Di Huang, Huang Qin, Huang Lian, Huang Bo, Huang Qi

Dang Gui San (當歸散)

Dang Gui, Chuan Xiong, Sheng Bai Shao	3 qian each
Sheng Di Huang, Chao Bai Zhu, Xu Duan	3 qian each
Du Zhong, Gan Cao	3 qian each
Shan Yao, Ai Cao	5 qian each
Huang Qin	2 qian

The Yu Sheng version is composed of the same essential medicinals as the original formula— Dang Gui, Chuan Xiong, Sheng Bai Shao, Chao Bai Zhu, and Huang Qin—along with the addition of Shan Yao, Ai Ye, Sheng Di Huang, Xu Duan, Du Zhong, and Gan Cao.

Sheng Di Huang clears heat and cools the blood and nourishes yin and engenders liquid; Xu Duan quickens the blood and stanches bleeding and supplements the liver and kidney and quiets the fetus; Du Zhong serves as a channel conductor directing medicinals downwards to the lumbus and lower limbs and supplements the liver and kidney and quiets the fetus; Ai Ye warms the channels and stanches bleeding, dissipates cold and regulates menstruation, and quiets the fetus; Shan Yao boosts qi and nourishes yin, supplements the spleen, lung, and kidney, and secures essence and checks vaginal discharge; and Gan Cao supplements the center and harmonizes the nature of medicinals. These additions enhance and complement the blood-nourishing blood-harmonizing, blood quickening stasis-moving, liver-emolliating construction aspect harmonizing, heat-clearing blood-cooling, and spleen-fortifying dampness-drying actions of this formula's essential medicinals.

This blood-nourishing fetus-quieting formula promotes a healthy pregnancy and treats all types of prenatal and postpartum pathoconditions. It is traditionally prescribed for women with a history of habitual abortion and/or premature labor, stirring fetus, scant blood with heat, heat vexation and thirst, hysteria, and aching lumbus and abdominal pain. This is Dr. Lee's first-line formula for a broad spectrum of obstetric pathoconditions such as the prevention of spontaneous abortions due to poor implantation of the blastocyst embryo during the first two weeks of pregnancy, absence of cervical mucus, ovulation disorders (e.g., anovulation, oligoovulation), thin endometrial lining, absence of cervical mucus, morning sickness, preeclampsia, and gestational diabetes; and also postpartum pathoconditions (e.g., "baby blues" (depression), perineal pain, uterine infection, mastitis).

Dang Gui Shao Yao San (當歸芍藥散)
Dang Gui, Shao Yao, Chuan Xiong, Fu Ling, Ze Xie, Bai Zhu

Dang Gui Si Ni Jia Wu Zhu Yu Sheng Jiang Tang (當歸四逆加吳茱萸生薑湯)
Dang Gui, Gui Zhi, Bai Shao, Xi Xin, Gan Cao, Tong Cao, Da Zao, Wu Zhu Yu, Sheng Jiang

Dang Gui Yin Zi (當歸飲子)
Dang Gui, Bai Shao, Chuan Xiong, Sheng Di Huang, Bai Ji Li, Fang Feng, Jing Jie, He Shou Wu, Huang Qi, Gan Cao, Sheng Jiang

Di Dang Tang (抵擋湯)

Tao Ren	1 g
Meng Chong	2 g
Shui Zhi	2 g
Da Huang	3 g

Note: This formula is administered as a pulverized medicinal powder.

Di Gu Pi Yin (地骨皮飲)

Dang Gui, Chuan Xiong, Chi Shao	3 qian each
Sheng Di Huang, Gan Cao, Huang Qin	3 qian each
Cang Zhu	4 qian
Di Gu Pi, Mu Dan Pi	5 qian each

The Yu Sheng version is based on the *On Blood Pathoconditions* (血症論 *Xue Zheng Lun*) formula. It is composed of a **Si Wu Tang** variant

(Dang Gui, Chuan Xiong, Chi Shao, Sheng Di Huang) adding Di Gu Pi, Mu Dan Pi, Huang Qin, and Cang Zhu. **Si Wu Tang** supplements and quickens the blood; Di Gu Pi nourishes yin, cools the blood, downbears latent heat in the lung, and supplements right qi; Mu Dan Pi drains latent heat in the blood and harmonizes, cools, and engenders blood; Huang Qin clears heat and dries dampness and drains fire and resolves toxin; and Cang Zhu fortifies the spleen and dries dampness to counteract the digestion impairment and loose stools some patients experience when administered blood-nourishing yin-enriching medicinals.

The blood-nourishing yin-enriching and heat-clearing blood-cooling actions of this formula are traditionally prescribed for the treatment of fire effulgence due to yin-vacuity, steaming bone taxation heat, heat entering the blood chamber, antepartum heat, and alternating tidal heat. Similarly, Dr. Lee typically prescribes this formula for yin-vacuity blood heat with stasis heat (or Shao Yang heat) pattern and steaming bone taxation heat (fever) pattern that manifests in pathoconditions such as autoimmune diseases, leukemia, lymphoma, idiopathic thrombocytopenic purpura (ITP), menopausal transition symptoms, sweating of the five hearts, dengue fever, tuberculosis, and vasculitis.

Di Long San (地龍散)

Rou Gui, Di Long, Huang Bo, Gan Cao, Qiang Huo, Su Mu, Ma Huang, Tao Ren, Dang Gui, Du Huo

Di Tan Tang (滌痰湯)

Ban Xia, Tian Nan Xing, Ju Hong, Zhi Shi, Fu Ling, Ren Shen, Shi Chang Pu, Zhu Ru, Gan Cao, Sheng Jiang, Da Zao

Diao Fen Gao (吊粉膏/Suspension Powder Paste)

Da Huang, Huang Bo	1 part
Ru Xiang, Mo Yao	1 part
Xu Duan, Gu Sui Bu	1 part
Chuan Wu, Cao Wu	1 part
Rice Wine	

These medicinals are pulverized into medicinal powder and then mixed with rice wine (27% alcohol) to form a medicinal paste (藥膏 yào gāo) that is applied topically in the acute stage of inflammation.

This is the stage presenting with heat, pain, redness (or purplish), and swelling in traumatic injuries (e.g., sprains, subluxation, fractures). It comprises equal parts of heat-dispersing inflammation-resolving; blood-quickening stasis-transforming and swelling-dispersing flesh-engendering; sinew- and bone-strengthening and injury-treating breakage-mending; and anesthetic and pain-relieving medicinals.

This medicinal paste is spread on fine burlap cloth, covered with gauze, and then sufficiently wrapped with bandage and secured with tubular elastic net dressing (wrapped just tight enough to secure the cloth in place without adversely affecting circulation). For best efficacy, it is recommended that the medicinal paste be left on for 6 to 8 hours; however, in the rare case of mild allergic reaction (e.g., patient feels itchiness, tingling, and discomfort), it should be removed ahead of the recommended time.

Du Huo Ji Sheng Tang (獨活寄生湯)

Shu Di Huang	8 qian
Ren Shen, Gan Jiang, Fu Zi, Qin Jiao, Xu Duan	5 qian each
Gu Sui Bu, Gui Ban, Bie Jia, Du Zhong	5 qian each
Niu Xi, Chen Pi, Du Huo, Wu Jia Pi	5 qian each
Fu Ling, Chao Shao Yao, Chao Bai Zhu	4 qian each
Dang Gui, Chuan Xiong, Rou Gui, Huang Qin	3 qian each
Fang Feng, Xi Xin, Gan Cao	3 qian each
Dang Shen, Huang Qi, Sang Ji Sheng	1 liang each

Er Chen Tang (二陳湯)

Huang Qin	3 qian
Chen Pi, Ban Xia, Fu Ling, Gan Cao	4 qian each

The Yu Sheng version is similar to the original except for the subtraction of Sheng Jiang and Wu Mei and the addition of Huang Qin, whose heat-clearing dampness-drying actions are acclimated for Taiwan's humid subtropical climate, complementing this formula's overall dampness-drying phlegm-harmonizing and qi-normalizing center-harmonizing actions. The derivatives of **Er Chen Tang—Wen Dan Tang** and **Ban Xia Tian Ma Bai Zhu San**—are frequently prescribed for a broad scope of pathoconditions ranging from external contraction (common cold), psychosomatic symptoms (e.g., abdominal distention, malaise, and fatigue) to infertility, glaucoma and brain tumors.

Er Miao San (二妙散)
Huang Bo, Cang Zhu, Sheng Jiang Zhi (Raw Ginger Juice)

Fang Feng Tong Sheng San (防風通聖散)
Fang Feng, Jing Jie, Lian Qiao, Ma Huang, Bo He, Chuan Xiong, Dang Gui, Bai Shao, Bai Zhu, Shan Zhi Zi, Da Huang, Mang Xiao, Huang Qin, Shi Gao, Jie Geng, Gan Cao, Shi Gao, Sheng Jiang, Cong Bai

Feng Shi Fang (風濕方)

Ma Huang	1.5 qian
Rou Gui, Chi Shao, Gan Cao, Gan Jiang	3 qian each
Fu Zi, Huang Qin, Huang Bo, Fu Ling	3 qian each
Zhu Ling, Ze Xie, Cang Zhu, Sheng Shi Gao	3 qian each
Jin Yin Hua, Wu Wei Zi, Yin Yang Huo	3 qian each
Da Zao	5 pieces

This Yu Sheng original formula was designed by Dr. Lee early on in his clinical practice and was specifically administered for patients with rheumatic disorders (e.g., osteoarthritis (OA), rheumatoid arthritis (RA)) either currently receiving or having recently received administration of immunosuppressants (e.g., corticosteroids).

In years past, Western medical doctors in Taiwan indiscriminately prescribed systemic corticosteroids for the treatment of all types of inflammatory pain, including rheumatic disorders, without any consideration given to the deleterious side effects. This practice has been largely superseded by a more responsible approach that has in part been driven by the advent of new drugs and drug combinations.

Attuned to the pulse of our ever-evolving modern environment, nowadays, Dr. Lee typically prescribes **(Yu Sheng) Hyperactive Immune Formula** for these types of pathoconditions instead.

Fu Yuan Huo Xue Tang (復原活血湯)
Da Huang, Chai Hu, Dang Gui, Tao Ren, Hong Hua, Chuan Shan Jia, Gua Lou Gen, Gan Cao

Gan Jiang Ren Shen Ban Xia Wan (乾薑人参半下丸)

Gan Jiang, Ren Shen, Ban Xia, Sheng Jiang

Gan Lu Yin (甘露飲)

Sheng Di Huang, Shu Di Huang, Tian Men Dong, Mai Men Dong, Shi Hu, Yin Chen, Huang Qin, Zhi Ke, Pi Pa Ye, Gan Cao

Gan Mai Da Zao Tang (甘麥大棗湯)

Gan Cao, Xiao Mai, Da Zao

Gan Mai Da Zao Tang Combining Ban Xia Hou Po Tang (甘麥大棗湯合併半夏厚朴湯)

Ban Xia, Hou Po, Zi Su Zi, Fu Ling	4 qian
Gan Cao	5 qian
Da Zao	10 pieces
Fu Xiao Mai	1 liang

This is a compound formula with a composition almost identical to the original formulas except for the subtraction of Sheng Jiang. **Gan Mai Da Zao Tang** has center-harmonizing spirit-quieting and tension-relaxing agitation-calming actions, and is traditionally prescribed for the treatment of visceral agitation. **Ban Xia Hou Po Tang** has qi-moving counterflow-downbearing and stagnation-dissipating phlegm-transforming actions, and is traditionally prescribed for the treatment of seven-affect binding depression (七情鬱結 qī qíng yù jié) (e.g., anxiety, depression, and hypomania), insomnia, palpitations, gastrointestinal neurosis, vocal cord nodules and polyps, plum-pit qi, and menopausal transition symptoms.

Since the actions and indications of these two formulas are complementary, Dr. Lee has combined them for the treatment of a broad spectrum of mood, psychosomatic, and neuropsychiatric disorders (e.g., mild cases of Tourette syndrome) including those mentioned above. For patients presenting with phlegm reversal and ascending counterflow symptoms (e.g., abdominal distention, headache, malaise, fatigue), Dr. Lee will prescribe this compound formula in combination with **Ban Xia Tian Ma Bai Zhu San**. And for relatively mild pathoconditions, he may prescribe one of these simple formulas on its own.

Ge Gen Qin Lian Tang (葛根芩連湯)/aka **Ge Gen Huang Qin Huang Lian Tang (葛根黃芩黃連湯)**

Ge Gen, Huang Qin, Huang Lian, Gan Cao

Ge Gen Tang (葛根湯)

Ma Huang	1.5 liang
Huang Qin, Cang Zhu	3 qian each
Ge Gen, Chi Shao, Gan Cao, Rou Gui, Sheng Jiang	5 qian each
Da Zao	5 pieces

The Yu Sheng version is very similar to the original formula, which is a derivative of **Gui Zhi Tang**. But as in Dr. Lee's other formulas, Rou Gui replaces Gui Zhi and Chi Shao replaces Bai Shao, and Cang Zhu and Huang Qin are added due to considerations for Taiwan's humid subtropical climate. This formula promotes sweating and resolves the exterior and upbears liquid and courses the channels.

Dr. Lee commonly prescribes variants of this formula for external contraction with Yang Ming headache and body ache, heat effusion (fever) without sweating, aversion to cold, stretched stiffness of the nape and back (項背強几几 xiàng bèi qiáng shū shū), crick in the neck, and sinusitis. This formula is also prescribed for patients with acute stage facial palsy (caused by trauma or tumor), Bell's palsy (caused by a virus such as herpes simplex), or trigeminal neuralgia, who have *not* been prescribed corticosteroids.

The inclusion of Huang Qin and Cang Zhu in the Yu Sheng version of this formula also makes it easily modified into **Ge Gen Huang Qin Huang Lian Tang** (by adding Huang Lian) for the treatment of heat evil entering the interior causing diarrhea or dysentery (gastroenteritis) and exterior evil that has not yet resolved.

Ge Xia Zhu Yu Tang (膈下逐瘀湯)

Wu Ling Zhi, Dang Gui, Chuan Xiong, Tao Ren, Mu Dan Pi, Chi Shao, Wu Yao, Yan Hu Suo, Gan Cao, Xiang Fu, Hong Hua, Zhi Ke

Gui Lu Er Xian Jiao (龜鹿二仙膠)

Lu Jiao, Gui Ban, Ren Shen, Gou Qi Zi

Gui Ma Ge Ban Tang (桂麻各半湯) – refer to **Gui Zhi Ma Huang Ge Ban Tang (桂枝麻黃各半湯)**

Gui Pi Tang (歸脾湯)

Ren Shen, Huang Qi, Bai Zhu, Fu Ling, Dang Gui, Suan Zao Ren, Gui Yuan Rou, Yuan Zhi, Mu Xiang, Gan Cao, Sheng Jiang, Da Zao

Gui Qi Jian Zhong Tang (歸耆建中湯)

Dang Gui	2 qian
Gan Jiang, Huang Qin, Cang Zhu	3 qian each
Rou Gui, Chi Shao, Gan Cao, Fu Zi	5 qian each
Da Zao	5 pieces
Huang Qi	1 liang

This formula is derived from **Xiao Jian Zhong Tang** adding Dang Gui and Huang Qi. The Yu Sheng version of this formula is similar to the original version, but includes large doses of Huang Qi; replaces Bai Shao with Chi Shao, Sheng Jiang with Gan Jiang, and Gui Pi with large doses of Rou Gui (superior quality and efficacy); and adds Cang Zhu, Da Zao, and a large dose of Fu Zi. Huang Qin is also added for its heat-clearing dampness-drying and fire-draining toxin-resolving actions that counteract the great heat medicinals of Gan Jiang, Rou Gui, and Fu Zi. Huang Qi functions as a channel conductor for the upper limbs and Rou Gui as a channel conductor for the four extremities (the limbs).

The additions to the Yu Sheng version of this formula enhance its qi-supplementing center-fortifying, tension-relaxing interior-harmonizing, and blood supplementing actions, while also equipping it with the capacity to treat vacuity cold pathoconditions of the upper body.

Dr. Lee commonly prescribes this formula for cold impediment of the Tai Yang small intestine channel, neuropathy, frozen shoulder, and Raynaud disease (and phenomenon); and for skin pathoconditions (e.g., non-erupting papules (acne), menopausal pruritis).

Gui Zhi Fu Ling Wan (桂枝茯苓丸)

Rou Gui, Fu Ling	4 qian each

Mu Dan Pi, Chi Shao, Tao Ren	4 qian each
Gan Cao, Cang Zhu	3 qian each

Gui Zhi Jia Long Gu Mu Li Tang (桂枝加龍骨牡蠣湯)

Cang Zhu	4 qian
Rou Gui, Chi Shao, Gan Cao, Sheng Jiang	5 qian each
Sheng Long Gu, Sheng Mu Li, Shan Yao, Dang Shen	5 qian each
Da Zao	5 pieces

The Yu Sheng version contains all of the essential medicinals of the original formula with the exception of Rou Gui replacing Gui Zhi and the addition of Dang Shen, Shan Yao, and Cang Zhu. The qi-boosting spleen-fortifying and essence-securing dampness-drying actions of these additional medicinals complement this formula's overall action of neutrally supplementing yin and yang, subduing and settling, and securing essence and containing urine.

This formula is traditionally prescribed for pathoconditions such as vacuity taxation with dual yin and yang vacuity, dreaming with seminal emission, hypertonicity of the lesser abdomen, lower burner vacuity cold, stirring palpitations below the umbilicus resulting from urinary incontinence, and hysteria.

In addition to these pathoconditions, Dr. Lee also prescribes this formula for the treatment of juvenile acne, stress-related hair loss (e.g., alopecia areata, hair shedding (telogen effluvium), hair pulling disorder (trichotillomania)), and children with hyperactivity or impulsivity (e.g., attention deficit hyperactivity disorder (ADHD)). Early on in Dr. Lee's clinical practice, he would prescribe this formula for obstetrics pathoconditions, but in recent years he typically prescribes **Dang Gui San** variants instead.

Gui Zhi Ma Huang Ge Ban Tang (桂枝麻黃各半湯)
Gui Zhi, Ma Huang, Shao Yao, Sheng Jiang, Xing Ren, Gan Cao, Da Zao

Gui Zhi Ren Shen Tang (桂枝人參湯)
Gui Zhi, Gan Cao, Bai Zhu, Ren Shen, Gan Jiang

Gui Zhi Tang (桂枝湯) – refer to **Yang Dan Tang (陽但湯)**

Hei Xi Dan (黑錫丹)

Hei Xi, Liu Huang, Chen Xiang, Fu Zi, Hu Lu Ba, Yang Qi Shi, Xiao Hui Xiang, Bu Gu Zhi, Rou Dou Kou, Chuan Lian Zi, Mu Xiang, Rou Gui

Huan Shao Dan (還少丹)

Shu Di Huang, Shan Yao, Niu Xi, Gou Qi, Shan Zhu Rou, Fu Ling, Du Zhong, Yuan Zhi, Wu Wei Zi, Chu Shi, Xiao Hui Xiang, Ba Ji Tian, Rou Cong Rong, Shi Chang Pu

Huang Lian Jie Du Tang (黃連解毒湯)

Huang Lian, Huang Qin, Huang Bo, Zhi Zi	3 qian each
Cang Zhu	4 qian
Gan Cao	5 qian

The Yu Sheng version is virtually the same as the original formula except for the addition of Cang Zhu and Gan Cao. Cang Zhu fortifies the spleen and dries dampness and Gan Cao supplements the center and harmonizes the nature of medicinals—a pair that combines to promote digestion and protect the stomach from the bitter flavor and cold nature of the essential medicinals. The essential medicinals of this formula are The Three Yellows (Huang Qin, Huang Bo, and Huang Lian), which Dr. Lee commonly utilizes for their heat-clearing toxin-resolving (antimicrobial and anti-inflammatory) actions.

This is a commonly administered formula for triple burner heat toxin congestion. Huang Lian drains heart fire and middle burner fire; Huang Qin drains upper burner fire; Huang Bo drains lower burner fire; and Zhi Zi frees and drains heat in all three burners, abducting heat downward where the heat evil is excreted in the urine. These medicinals contain powerful heat-clearing toxin-resolving (antimicrobial and anti-inflammatory) actions, and when combined together into one formula provide exceptional efficacy for the treatment of all types of infections and inflammation throughout the body (e.g., upper respiratory, gastrointestinal, hepatic, renal, genitourinary, autoimmune disorders).

It is important to note here that long-term administration (≥ 3 months) of Zhi Zi may cause transient grayish yellow skin pigmentation in some patients. In cases where long-term administration is necessary, Dr. Lee will either subtract Zhi Zi or prescribe another formula, such as the heat-clearing toxin-resolving and yin vacuity-heat clearing yin-enriching **Hyperactive Immune Formula**, instead.

Huang Long Tang (黃龍湯)

Da Huang, Mang Xiao, Zhi Shi, Hou Po, Gan Cao, Ren Shen, Dang Gui, Sheng Jiang, Da Zao, Jie Geng

Huang Qin Tang (黃芩湯)

Huang Qin, Bai Shao, Gan Cao, Da Zao

Hui Yang Sheng Xian Tang (回陽升陷湯)

Huang Qi, Gan Jiang, Dang Gui, Gui Zhi, Gan Cao

Huo Luo Dan (活絡丹/Network-Quickening Elixir)

Dang Gui, Ru Xiang, Mo Yao	5 jin each
Dan Shen, Di Long, Chuan Wu	5 jin each
Wu Cao, Tian Nan Xing, Ma Huang	5 jin each

The Yu Sheng version is identical to the original formula, which is also known as **Xiao Huo Luo Dan (小活絡丹/Minor Network-Quickening Elixir)**, except for the addition of Dang Gui, Dan Shen, and Ma Huang. Dang Gui supplements and quickens the blood; Dan Shen quickens the blood and dispels stasis; and Ma Huang "opens up" and transports medicinals across all membranes. These additions complement and further enhance this formula's overall wind-dispelling dampness-dispersing, blood-quickening stasis-dispelling, and network vessel-freeing pain-relieving actions.

This formula is traditionally prescribed for the treatment of wind-cold-damp evil invading the channels and network vessels, contraction and pain of the sinews and vessels, inhibited bending and stretching of the joints, and wandering aches and pain; insensitivity of the limbs following stroke and phlegm-damp dead blood in the channels and network vessels; and knocks and falls (traumatic injury) and stasis obstruction in the channels and network vessels causing pain.

Dr. Lee utilizes this pill's blood-quickening stasis-dispelling and channel- and network vessel-freeing actions for its exceptional efficacy in relieving pain, particularly for wind-damp impediment and traumatic injuries involving the lumbus and lower limbs. This pill is produced and processed in-house, using a strictly controlled fermentation method and oven-roast process that safely ensures elimination of the potential for toxicity.

Hyperactive Immune Formula (免疫過抗方/Mian Yi Guo Kang Fang)

Huang Lian, Huang Qin, Huang Bo, Cang Zhu	5 qian each
Qing Hao, Zhi Mu, Di Gu Pi	5 qian each

This formula was designed relatively later in Dr. Lee's clinical practice primarily for the treatment of connective tissue diseases, degenerative disorders, and systemic inflammation in patients who are *not* being administered immunosuppressants (e.g., systemic corticosteroids, high dose methotrexate (MTX)) or those who *have* been administered immunosuppressants for $\leq$ 1 week.

It is composed of the essential medicinals from **(Yu Sheng) Huang Lian Jie Du Tang** (Huang Lian, Huang Qin, Huang Bo, and Cang Zhu) along with the additions of Qing Hao, Zhi Mu, and Di Gu Pi. These medicinals combine to form a potent combination of heat-clearing toxin-resolving (anti-inflammatory), vacuity heat-clearing steaming bone-eliminating, yin-enriching dryness-moistening, and blood-cooling fire-draining actions.

As mentioned in the **Feng Shi Fang** profile, the changing practice of Western medicine in Taiwan has seen a trend away from indiscriminate administration of systemic corticosteroids. In response, Dr. Lee now commonly prescribes this formula for treating patients with a broad scope of pathoconditions presenting with acute stage inflammation and chronic autoimmune and degenerative diseases (e.g., osteoarthritis (OA), rheumatoid arthritis (RA), ankylosing spondylitis (AS), systemic lupus erythematosus (SLE), polymyositis, dermatomyositis, scleroderma, multiple sclerosis (MS), Behcet's disease (BD), Sjogren's syndrome (SS), immune thrombocytopenic purpura (ITP), inflammatory bowel disease (IBS), vasculitis).

In addition to applying eight-principle and six-channel pattern identification methods, inflammatory indices (e.g., erythrocyte sedimentation rate (ESR), antinuclear antibody (ANA), rheumatoid factor (RF)) are invaluable diagnostic tools for determining the severity of inflammation and gauging clinical efficacy. This formula provides reliable and lasting effectiveness in resolving inflammation and relieving symptoms (i.e., treat the tip). Once the inflammation is under control, the patient can proceed on to other supplementing and nourishing TCM formulas in the process of bringing the pathocondition into complete remission (i.e., treat the root).

Jia Wei Er Miao San (加味二妙散)

Cang Zhu, Huang Bo, Gui Ban, Bi Xie, Zhi Mu

Jia Wei Xiao Chai Hu Tang (加味小柴胡湯)

Chai Hu, Huang Qin, Zhi Mu, Dang Shen, Bie Jia, Ban Xia, Chang Shan, Cao Guo, Gan Cao, Jiu Qu, Sheng Jiang, Da Zao

Jian Ling Tang (健瓴湯)

Ci Shi	3 qian
Bo Zi Ren	4 qian
Niu Xi, Chi Shao, Sheng Long Gu	5 qian each
Sheng Mu Li, Sheng Di Huang, Shan Yao	5 qian each
Dai Zhe Shi	8 qian

The Yu Sheng version is virtually the same as the original formula with the exception of Chi Shao replacing Bai Shao and the addition of Ci Shi. As in many Yu Sheng formulas, Chi Shao is selected for its superior blood-quickening stasis-dispelling actions. The primary constituents of this spirit-quieting by heavy settling formula are Dai Zhe Shi—enters the blood aspect of the liver and heart channels, eliminates heat, calms the liver and subdues yang, and downbears counterflow by heavy settling; Ci Shi—enters the liver and kidney channels, governs the lung and kidney, settles fright and quiets the spirit, and calms the liver and subdues yang; Sheng Long Gu—enters the heart, liver, and kidney channels, subdues yang, and quiets the spirit; and Sheng Mu Li—calms the liver and subdues yang, softens hardness and dissipates binds, and astringes and secures.

Dr. Lee typically reserves this formula for only the most severe cases of ascendant hyperactivity of yang, manifesting in pathoconditions such as hyperglycemia (diabetes), hypertension, hyperthyroidism, insomnia, schizophrenia, and Tourette syndrome. This includes cases in which Western medicine drug therapy has been administered without efficacy, or with initial efficacy, but is no longer able to effectively control the pathocondition.

Jin Suo Gu Jing Wan (金鎖固精丸)
Sha Yuan Zi, Qian Shi, Lian Xu, Long Gu, Mu Li, Lian Zi Fen

Jing Fang Bai Du San (荊防敗毒散)
Jing Jie, Fang Feng, Chai Hu, Fu Ling, Jie Geng, Chuan Xiong, Qiang Huo, Du Huo, Zhi Ke, Gan Cao, Sheng Jiang

Ju He Wan (橘核丸)
Ju He, Hai Zao, Kun Bu, Hai Dai, Chuan Lian Zi, Tao Ren, Ho Po, Yu Zhi Zi, Zhi Shi, Yan Hu Suo, Gui Xin, Mu Xiang

Li Zhong Tang (理中湯/Center-Rectifying Decoction/aka **Ren Shen Tang**)
Bai Zhu, Ren Shen, Gan Jiang, Gan Cao

Liang Ge San (涼膈散)

Lian Qiao, Huang Qin, Bo He Ye	3 qian each
Zhu Ye, Shan Zhi Zi, Gan Cao	3 qian each
Da Huang, Mang Xiao	1 qian each
Cang Zhu	4 qian

Ling Gui Zhu Gan Tang (苓桂朮甘湯)
Fu Ling, Gui Zhi, Bai Zhu, Gan Cao

Liu Jun Zi Tang (六君子湯)
Ren Shen, Gan Cao, Fu Ling, Bai Zhu, Chen Pi, Ban Xia, Sheng Jiang, Da Zao

Liu Wei Di Huang Wan (六味地黃丸)
Shu Di Huang, Shan Zhu Yu, Shan Yao, Ze Xie, Fu Ling, Mu Dan Pi

Long Dan Xie Gan Tang (龍膽瀉肝湯)

Long Dan Cao, Huang Qin, Zhi Zi, Dang Gui	3 qian each
Sheng Di Huang, Mu Tong, Chai Hu, Che Qian Zi	3 qian each
Cang Zhu, Ze Xie	4 qian
Sheng Gan Cao	5 qian

The Yu Sheng version is identical to the original except for the addition of Cang Zhu, with its wind-damp dispelling actions further enhancing this formula's potent overall liver-clearing dampness-disinhibiting actions, as it drains liver and gallbladder repletion fire and clears lower burner damp-heat.

Traditionally, this formula is prescribed for liver and gallbladder repletion fire flaming upward pattern pathoconditions presenting with rib-side pain (e.g., herpes zoster) and headache (e.g., acute hepatitis, acute cholecystitis), red eyes (e.g., acute conjunctivitis, keratitis) and bitter taste in mouth, and deafness and swelling of the ear (e.g., otitis media, sinusitis); and liver channel damp-heat pouring downward pattern presenting with urinary dribbling and strangury-turbidity (e.g., urinary tract infection, enlarged prostate), pudendal itch, genital swelling (e.g., acute epididymitis), and vaginal discharge (e.g., vaginitis). In addition to these pathoconditions, Dr. Lee also administers this formula for pain wind (gout and pseudogout).

Ma Huang Fu Zi Xi Xin Tang (麻黃附子細辛湯)
Ma Huang, Fu Zi, Xi Xin

Ma Huang Jia Zhu Tang (麻黃加朮湯)
Ma Huang, Gui Zhi, Gan Cao, Xing Ren, Bai Zhu

Ma Huang Lian Yao Chi Xiao Dou Tang (麻黃連軺赤芍豆湯)
Ma Huang, Lian Yao (aka Lian Qiao Gen), Xing Ren, Chi Xiao Dou, Da Zao, Zi Bai Pi, Sheng Jiang, Gan Cao

Ma Huang Tang (麻黃湯)
Ma Huang, Gui Zhi, Gan Cao, Xing Ren

Ma Xing Gan Shi Tang (麻杏甘石湯)

Ma Huang	1.5 qian
Cang Zhu	3 qian
Xing Ren	4 qian
Gan Cao	5 qian
Shi Gao	1 liang

The Yu Sheng version is identical to the original formula except for the addition of Cang Zhu, which is included for its wind-damp dispelling dampness-drying actions. This formula's heat-draining, lung-diffusing panting-calming, and cough-suppressing actions are traditionally administered for the treatment of externally contracted wind-cold and exuberant lung heat, failure to resolve generalized heat (fever), and panting counterflow and rapid breathing.

Dr. Lee typically prescribes this formula for the treatment of the common cold (exterior wind-heat external contraction), acute bronchitis, and pneumonia. Additionally, Dr. Lee may also add Yi Yi Ren to form a variant of **Ma Xing Yi Gan Tang** for the treatment of wind-damp exterior pattern external medicine (dermatological) pathoconditions (e.g., eczema, urticaria, seborrheic dermatitis).

Ma Xing Yi Gan Tang (麻杏薏甘湯)/aka **Ma Huang Xing Ren Yi Yi Ren Gan Cao Tang (麻黃杏仁薏苡甘草湯)**

Ma Huang, Gan Cao, Yi Yi Ren, Xing Ren

Mai Men Dong Tang (麥門冬湯)

Ma Huang	1.5 qian
Xing Ren, Cang Zhu	4 qian each
Mai Men Dong, Xuan Shen, Ban Xia	5 qian each
Gan Cao, Shan Yao, Sheng Jiang	5 qian each
Da Zao	5 pieces

The Yu Sheng version is the same as the original formula except for the subtraction of Jing Mi; Ren Shen pulverized powder is used instead of decocting pieces; and the addition of Ma Huang, Xing Ren, Cang Zhu, Xuan Shen, Shan Yao, and Sheng Jiang. As in **Jia Wei Mai Men Dong Tang**, the qi-boosting yin-enriching, spleen- and lung-supplementing, and kidney-supplementing essence-securing actions of Shan Yao replaces Jing Mi. Xuan Shen's heat-clearing blood-cooling and yin-enriching toxin-resolving actions complement Mai Men Dong (nourishes yin, engenders liquid, and moistens the lung) and Ren Shen (supplements the spleen, boosts the lung, and engenders liquid). Ma Huang suppresses cough and counterflow qi and opens the nine orifices; Xing Ren downbears and drains lung qi and suppresses cough and calms panting; and Cang Zhu has the action of drying dampness and fortifying the spleen.

Mai Men Dong Tang is traditionally prescribed to clear heat, nourish the lung and stomach, downbear counterflow, and precipitate qi for the treatment of lung yin vacuity, lung wilting, upflaming vacuity fire, and qi counterflow panting and coughing. These types of pathoconditions typically result from microbial infections (i.e., bacteria, virus, fungus) damaging the mucous membranes of the respiratory tract (e.g., larynx, trachea, bronchi) and inhibiting the secretion of epithelial lining fluid (ELF). In health, this fluid maintains epithelial moisture, traps particulate material and pathogens moving through the airway, and transports mucous (e.g., metabolic waste, pus, phlegm-rheum) upwards through the trachea towards the mouth, where it is either coughed out or swallowed.

This formula functions to promote healing of these mucous membranes and serves to restore normal regulation of fluid secretion in the respiratory tract. Dr. Lee classifies these types of pathoconditions as yin vacuity cough (陰虛發咳 yīn xū fā ké) (aka dryness cough) in the lung and kidney channels, and he will also prescribe this formula for side effects resulting from radiotherapy (e.g., head and neck cancers) such as dry mouth and throat and skin redness, blistering and peeling.

Paralysis Formula Series (截癱方系)

These three formulas were specially designed early on in Dr. Lee's clinical practice for the treatment of paresis and paralysis, which correlates with wilting pattern (痿證 wěi zhèng) in TCM classical pathologic terminology, resulting from traumatic injury (including iatrogenic), microbial infection, and degenerative diseases of autoimmune and hereditary etiology.

Each formula in this series has a specific function throughout the various stages of the pathocondition. Since the determination of treatment is based on signs, symptoms, and pattern identification, in addition to the selections in this **Paralysis Formula** series, Dr. Lee may also prescribe other formulas for the treatment of paresis, paralysis, and neuropathies. For instance, in cases involving paralysis induced by viral infection, if the patient has not yet been administered corticosteroids and it is still in the acute stage (approximately < 3 to 4 days), Dr. Lee will approach this as an external contraction wind-heat pattern, prescribing a formula such as **Ge Gen Tang** variant with its cool acrid exterior resolution actions combined with other medicinals such as Di Long that free the orifices.

The typical protocol is as follows:
Paralysis Formula #1 (Di Long San Variant) (截癱一號方) (地龍散加方)—acute stage (approximately ≤ 1 week following the onset of symptoms, *unless* corticosteroids have already been administered) with static blood and metabolic waste (e.g., hyaline degeneration, inflammatory factors) congesting the vasculature, channels, and network vessels that can be identified as collection of static blood pattern; **Paralysis Formula #2 (Shi Quan Da Bu Tang Variant) (截癱二號方) (十全大補湯加方)**—post-acute and chronic stage (approximately ≥ 1 week) with enduring symptoms that can be identified as dual qi and blood vacuity pattern, and specifically for cases involving cervical and thoracic spine injuries; and **Paralysis Formula #3 (You Gui Yin Variant) (截癱三號方) (右歸飲加方)**—post-acute and chronic stages (approximately ≥ 1 week) with enduring symptoms that can be identified as kidney yang vacuity pattern, and specifically for cases involving lumbar spine injuries.

Formula Paralysis #1 (Di Long San Variant)
(截癱一號方) (地龍散加方)

Ma Huang, Hong Hua	1.5 qian each
Tao Ren, Gan Cao, Gan Jiang, Rou Gui	3 qian each
Di Long, Dang Gui, Huang Bo	3 qian each
Du Zhong	4 qian
Wei Ling Xian, Niu Xi, Fu Zi	5 qian each

The Yu Sheng version is composed of the original formula's essential medicinals—Di Long, Tao Ren, Rou Gui, Huang Bo, Gan Cao, Ma Huang, and Dang Gui—along with the addition of Hong Hua, Niu Xi, Wei Ling Xian, Gan Jiang, Fu Zi, and Du Zhong. Hong Hua, Niu Xi, and Wei Ling Xian enhance the formula's blood-quickening stasis-dispelling, blood-supplementing blood-breaking, and channel-freeing actions. Wei Ling Xian is a Tai Yang urinary bladder channel medicinal that perfuses the twelve channels and network vessels; and Du Zhong and Niu Xi are channel conductors directing medicinals into the lumbar spine and lower limbs. Fu Zi and Gan Jiang combine with Rou Gui to form one of the pillars of Dr. Lee's treatment approaches—The Three Great Yang-Supplementers—that boost the metabolism by innervating the central nervous system (CNS) and peripheral nervous system (PNS), repairing damaged cells, rejuvenating weakened cells, and promoting tissue regeneration. Ma Huang "opens up" and transports other medicinals across all membranes of the body down to the cellular level, thus making it an effective channel-conductor, while its action of opening the nine orifices innervates the nervous system (i.e., CNS, PNS, ANS). Di Long is a Tai Yang urinary bladder channel medicinal that extinguishes wind, clears heat and disinhibits urine, and frees the channels and quickens the network vessels; Huang Bo clears heat and resolves toxin, abates heat and dries dampness, drains fire and eliminates steam in the lower burner, and counteracts the heat of The Three Great Yang-Supplementers; and Gan Cao supplements the center and harmonizes the nature of medicinals.

The original formula is traditionally prescribed for the treatment of knocks and falls, pain in the cervical, thoracic, and lumbar spine, pain in the arms, accumulations and gatherings in the abdomen, and blood stasis and static blood pain.

As mentioned in the **Paralysis Formula Series** introduction, Dr. Lee typically administers this formula during the acute stage (approximately ≤ 1 week following the onset of symptoms, *unless* corticosteroids have already been administered) with static blood and metabolic waste (e.g., hyaline degeneration, inflammatory factors) congesting the vasculature, channels, and network vessels that can be identified as collection of static blood pattern.

Paralysis Formula #2 (Shi Quan Da Bu Tang Variant)
(截癱二號方) (十全大補湯加方)

Da Huang	5 fen
Ma Huang	1.5 qian
Dan Shen, Chao Bai Zhu, Fu Ling, Gan Cao	3 qian each
Dang Gui, Chuan Xiong, Chi Shao	3 qian each
Sheng Di Huang, Huang Qi, Rou Gui	3 qian each
Di Long, Niu Xi, Huang Qin, Gan Jiang	3 qian each
Fu Zi	5 qian

This formula is composed of **(Yu Sheng) Shi Quan Da Bu Tang** with Chao Bai Zhu replacing Cang Zhu for its emphasis on supplementing qi and fortifying the spleen, along with the addition of Da Huang, Ma Huang, Di Long, and Niu Xi. Da Huang drains precipitation and damp heat, quickens the blood and transforms stasis, and disperses accumulation to effectively lower intracranial pressure, relieve tension in the diaphragm, and promote lysis of hyaline degeneration and the removal of metabolic waste that obstructs neurotransmitters. Ma Huang "opens up" and transports other medicinals across all membranes of the body down to the cellular level, thus making it an effective channel-conductor, and its action of opening the nine orifices innervates the nervous system (i.e., CNS, PNS, ANS). Di Long is a Tai Yang urinary bladder channel medicinal that extinguishes wind, clears heat and disinhibits urine, and frees the channels and quickens the network vessels. Niu Xi quickens the blood and frees the channels, supplements the liver and kidney, strengthens the sinews and bones, conducts fire (blood) downward, and serves as a channel conductor directing medicinals into the lumbar spine and lower limbs.

The addition of the precipitation-draining, water-disinhibiting, accumulation-dispersing, blood-quickening stasis-transforming, and wind-extinguishing channel-freeing network vessel-quickening medicinals complements and enhances the blood-quickening blood-supplementing, qi-boosting spleen-fortifying, and kidney yang-supplementing actions of **Shi Quan Da Bu Tang**.

As mentioned in the **Paralysis Formula Series** introduction, Dr. Lee typically administers this formula during the post-acute and chronic stage (approximately ≥ 1 week) with enduring symptoms that can be identified as dual qi and blood vacuity pattern, and specifically for cases involving cervical and thoracic spine injuries.

Paralysis Formula #3 (You Gui Yin Variant)
(截癱三號方) (右歸飲加方)

Da Huang	5 fen
Ma Huang	1.5 qian
Fu Ling, Dang Gui	2 qian each
Gou Qi Zi, Niu Xi, Du Zhong, Huang Bo	3 qian each

Di Long, Gan Jiang, Rou Gui	3 qian each
Sheng Di Huang, Shan Zhu Yu, Shan Yao, Tu Si Zi	4 qian each
Fu Zi	5 qian

This formula is derived from **(Yu Sheng) You Gui Yin** subtracting Cang Zhu and adding Di Long, Da Huang, and Ma Huang, just as in the **Paralysis #2 Formula (Shi Quan Da Bu Tang Variant)** above. Ma Huang "opens up" and transports other medicinals across all membranes of the body down to the cellular level, thus making it an effective channel-conductor, and its action of opening the nine orifices innervates the nervous system (i.e., CNS, PNS, ANS). Di Long is a Tai Yang urinary bladder channel medicinal that extinguishes wind, clears heat and disinhibits urine, and frees the channels and quickens the network vessels. Da Huang drains precipitation and damp heat, quickens the blood and transforms stasis, and disperses accumulation to effectively lower intracranial pressure, relieve tension in the diaphragm, and promote lysis of hyaline degeneration and the removal of metabolic waste that obstructs neurotransmitters.

The addition of the precipitation-draining, water-disinhibiting, accumulation-dispersing, blood-quickening stasis-transforming, and wind-extinguishing channel-freeing network vessel-quickening medicinals complements and enhances the overall kidney yang-warming and -supplementing, blood-quickening stasis-dissipating, sinew- and bone-strengthening, and dampness-eliminating pain-relieving actions of this formula.

As mentioned in the **Paralysis Formula Series** introduction, Dr. Lee typically administers this formula during the post-acute and chronic stage (approximately ≥ 1 week) with enduring symptoms that can be identified as kidney yang vacuity pattern, and specifically for cases involving lumbar spine injuries.

Ping Wei San (平胃散)

Chen Pi, Hou Po, Cang Zhu, Gan Cao, Sheng Jiang, Da Zao

Po Xiao Dang Bao Tang (朴硝盪胞湯)

Da Huang, Mang Xiao	1 qian each
Rou Gui, Fu Ling, Mu Dan Pi, Chi Shao	3 qian each

Tao Ren, Dang Shen, Gan Cao	3 qian each
Niu Xi, Dang Gui, Hou Po, Xi Xin	3 qian each
Jie Geng, Huang Qin, Qing Pi, Shui Zhi	3 qian each
Cang Zhu	4 qian
Gan Jiang, Fu Zi	5 qian each
Meng Chong	20 pieces

The Yu Sheng version is virtually identical to the original formula with the exception of Dang Shen replacing Ren Shen and the addition of Huang Qin, Cang Zhu, and Gan Jiang. Meng Chong, Shui Zhi, Hou Po, Da Huang, and Mang Xiao are among the essential medicinals combining to provide an effective formula for treating female infertility with its draining-precipitation, stasis-dispelling accumulation-breaking, phlegm-transforming accumulation-dispersing, qi-moving downwards, and channel-freeing actions. Po Xiao is a lesser refined grade of mirabilite and generally not used for medicinal purposes anymore, instead being replaced by the more refined form called Mang Xiao.

As its name indicates—**Dang Bao (盪胞)** means to "flush the uterus." This formula functions to "flush away" the residual metabolic waste (e.g., pus, cellular matter, blood clots) that may stagnate on the uterine lining and fallopian tube junctions (i.e, uterotubal junction) as a result of inflammation, adhesions, polyps, endometrial hyperplasia, endometriosis, and leiomyomas. This formula also elicits uterine contractions, which sends a definitive feedback signal to the hypothalamus and pituitary gland so that the body clearly recognizes it should recalibrate normal hormone regulation and continue the regeneration process once again (e.g., a pathophysiological phenomenon occurring in some women whom have already given birth or have had a spontaneous abortion, either knowingly or unknowingly).

Dr. Lee administers this formula specifically as a first-line treatment for female infertility—defined as *absence* of a live birth despite ≥ 1 years of efforts with a male partner (primary infertility), during which they have *not* used contraceptives; or in women who *have* consummated a live birth previously, but are subsequently *unable* to despite ≥ 1 years of efforts (secondary infertility), during which they have *not* used contraceptives.

The treatment regimen involves administration of this formula for 1 week starting a few days before menstruation, with the couple subsequently proceeding in an attempt at natural insemination over a 6-month period. In approximately 70% of these cases, this approach will lead to pregnancy within that 6-month period. If this treatment does *not* result in pregnancy, then Dr. Lee will advise the couple to undergo further evaluation (e.g., ultrasound to determine the thickness of the endometrial lining, scrotal ultrasound) and testing (e.g., postcoital test (PCT), semen analysis to determine the presence of anti-sperm antibodies) prior to conducting further pattern identification and proceeding with other therapeutic approaches.

Qi Bao Mei Ran Dan (七寶美髯丸)
He Shou Wu, Fu Ling, Niu Xi, Dang Gui, Gou Qi Zi, Tu Si Zi, Po Gu Zhi

Qi Chuan Fang (氣喘方) refer to **Asthma Formula**

Qi Fu Tang (耆附湯)
Huang Qi, Fu Zi, Sheng Jiang

Qian Zheng San (牽正散)
Bai Fu Zi, Bai Jiang Can, Quan Xie

Qin Jiao Bie Jia San (秦艽鱉甲散)
Di Gu Pi, Chai Hu, Qin Jiao, Zhi Mu, Dang Gui, Bie Jia, Qing Hao, Wu Mei

Qin Lian Si Wu Tang (芩連四物湯)
Dang Gui, Chuan Xiong, Chi Shao, Gan Di Huang, Huang Qin, Huang Lian

Qing Shang Fang Feng Tang (清上防風湯)
Fang Feng, Lian Qiao, Bai Zhi, Jie Geng, Huang Qin, Chuan Xiong, Huang Lian, Jing Jie, Shan Zhi Zi, Zhi Ke, Bo He, Gan Cao

Qing Wei San (清胃散)

Huang Lian, Sheng Ma, Dang Gui	3 qian each
Sheng Di Huang, Mu Dan Pi	3 qian each

Qing Xin Lian Zi Yin (清心蓮子飲)
Huang Qin, Mai Men Dong, Di Gu Pi, Che Qian Zi, Chai Hu, Gan Cao, Lian Zi, Fu Ling Huang Qi, Dang Shen

Qing Yan Li Ge San (清咽利膈散)
Jin Yin Hua, Fang Feng, Jing Jie, Bo He, Jie Geng, Huang Qin, Huang Lian, Shan Zhi Zi, Lian Qiao, Xuan Shen, Da Huang, Mang Xiao, Niu Bang Zi, Gan Cao

Qing Zao Jiu Fei Tang (清燥救肺湯)
Sang Ye, Shi Gao, Gan Cao, Ren Shen, Hua Ma Ren, E Jiao, Mai Men Dong, Xing Ren, Pi Pa Ye

Ren Shen Bai Du San (人參敗毒散)
Ren Shen, Qiang Huo, Du Huo, Chai Hu, Qian Hu, Chuan Xiong, Zhi Ke, Jie Geng, Fu Ling, Gan Cao, Sheng Jiang, Bo He

Ren Shen Yang Rong Tang (人參養榮湯)
Ren Shen, Bai Zhu, Huang Qi, Gan Cao, Chen Pi, Rou Gui, Dang Gui, Shu Di Huang, Wu Wei Zi, Fu Ling, Yuan Zhi, Bai Shao, Da Zao, Sheng Jiang

Ru Mo Si Wu Tang (乳沒四物湯)

Dang Gui, Chuan Xiong, Chi Shao	3 qian each
Sheng Di Huang, Ru Xiang, Mo Yao	3 qian each
Cang Zhu, Gan Cao, Tao Ren	3 qian each
Hong Hua	1.5 qian

This Yu Sheng formula is a variant of **Tao Hong Si Wu Tang** with Sheng Di Huang replacing Shu Di Huang, Chi Shao replacing Bai Shao, and adding Cang Zhu and Gan Cao. Sheng Di Huang supplements yin and cools the blood; Chi Shao cools the blood and expels stasis; Tao Ren quickens the blood and dispels stasis; and Hong Hua quickens the blood, dispels stasis, and frees the channels (menstruation). The addition of the medicinal pair Ru Xiang (quickens the blood and moves qi, disperses swelling and engenders flesh, and relieves pain) and Mo Yao (dissipates the blood and transforms stasis, disperses swelling and engenders flesh, and relieves pain) complements **Tao Hong Si Wu Tang**'s blood-nourishing blood-quickening, network vessel-freeing channel (menstruation)-regulating, and stasis-dispelling pain-relieving actions

This is a commonly prescribed formula for gynecological pathoconditions presenting with blood stasis and concretions, conglomerations, accumulations, and gatherings (e.g., uterine fibroids (leiomyomas), endometrial hyperplasia, ovarian cysts, menstrual irregularities). Dr. Lee prescribes this formula for treating a broad spectrum of pathoconditions involving blockage of the flow of blood both inside the vessels (e.g., thrombus, embolus) and outside in the interstitium (e.g., hemorrhage) where it is capable of promoting absorption of blood and stanching bleeding. And it is also one of the main formulas prescribed in Dr. Lee's cancer treatment protocol, specifically administered for malignant (or benign) tumors of the smooth muscle (soft tissue) (e.g., carcinomas, fibromas, leiomyosarcomas, hamartomas) involving the breast, urinary bladder, uterus, gastrointestinal tract, and respiratory tract.

Sai Ji (塞劑/Vaginal Suppository)

She Chuang Zi	1 g
Xiong Huang, Liu Huang, Da Huang	0.3 g each

Sai Ji is a vaginal suppository prescribed for various types of vaginal infections including bacterial vaginosis (i.e., *Gardnerella vaginalis*), yeast (candidiasis), parasites (trichomoniasis), and sexually transmitted diseases (STDs) (e.g., genital herpes, gonorrhea, Chlamydia) that present with itching, irritation, and watery or viscous vaginal discharge.

This formula is typically prescribed as part of a therapeutic regimen that includes decocted formulas taken orally such as **Long Dan Xie Gan Tang**, **Jin Suo Gu Jing Wan**, or **Bu Zhong Yi Qi Tang**.

San Bi Tang (三痹湯)

Ren Shen, Huang Qi, Fu Ling, Gan Cao, Dang Gui, Chuan Xiong, Bai Shao, Sheng Di Huang, Du Zhong, Niu Xi, Xu Duan, Gui Xin, Xi Xin, Qin Jiao, Du Huo, Fang Feng

San Ceng Hui Xiang Wan (三層茴香丸)

Ba Jiao Hui Xiang, Chuan Lian Zi, Mu Xiang, Fu Ling, Bei Sha Shen, Bi Ba, Bin Lang, Fu Zi

San Miao Wan (三妙丸)

Huang Bo, Cang Zhu, Niu Xi

San Zhong Kui Jian Tang (散腫潰堅湯)
Huang Qin, Zhi Mu, Huang Bo, Long Dan Cao, Tian Hua Fen, Jie Geng, Kun Bu, Chai Hu, Sheng Ma, Lian Qiao, Gan Cao, San Leng, E Zhu, Ge Gen, Dang Gui, Shao Yao, Huang Lian

Seborrheic Dermatitis Formula (脂漏方/Zhi Lou Fang)

Ma Huang	1.5 qian
Huang Qin	3 qian
Xing Ren, Cang Zhu	4 qian
Gan Cao, Jin Yin Hua	5 qian each
Lu Lu Tong	10 pieces
Shi Gao, Yi Yi Ren	1 liang each

This Yu Sheng original formula is composed of **(Yu Sheng) Ma Xing Yi Gan Tang** adding Huang Qin, Jin Yin Hua, and Lu Lu Tong. Huang Qin clears heat and resolves toxin, dries dampness, and drains fire; Jin Yin Hua clears heat and resolves toxin, courses wind and dissipates heat, disperses welling-abscess and swelling, and is an essential medicinal for the treatment of all types of yang pattern swollen welling-abscesses and clove sores (carbuncles, furuncles, boils); and Lu Lu Tong dispels wind, eliminates dampness, and resolves toxin for the treatment of wind-damp streaming sores, welling-abscesses, scab, and lichen.

As the name indicates, this Yu Sheng formula is designed for the treatment of seborrheic dermatitis, and specifically for the acute and post-acute stages that can be identified as exterior wind-heat or exterior wind-heat-damp pattern. Seborrheic dermatitis correlates with the classical TCM pathologic terms wandering wind of the face (面游風 miàn yóu fēng) and white scaling wind (白屑風 bái xiè fēng).

She Gan Ma Huang Tang (射干麻黃湯)

Ma Huang	2 qian
She Gan, Zi Wan, Kuan Dong Hua	3 qian each
Wu Wei Zi, Xi Xin, Sheng Jiang, Gan Cao	3 qian each
Ban Xia, Xing Ren, Chen Pi, Fu Ling	4 qian each
Hong Zao	3 pieces

Shen Fu Tang (參附湯)
Fu Zi, Gan Cao, Gan Jiang, Ren Shen

Shen Ling Bai Zhu San (參苓白朮散)
Bian Dou, Ren Shen, Bai Zhu, Fu Ling, Gan Cao, Shan Yao, Lian Zi, Yi Yi Ren, Jie Geng, Sha Ren, Da Zao

Shen Qi Wan (腎氣丸)

Sheng Di Huang, Shan Zhu Yu	4 qian each
Shan Yao, Cang Zhu, Du Zhong	4 qian each
Fu Ling, Ze Xie, Mu Dan Pi, Huang Bo	2 qian each
Niu Xi, Fu Zi, Rou Gui	5 qian each
Gan Cao, Gan Jiang	3 qian each

Sheng Yang Yi Wei Tang (升陽益胃湯)
Huang Qi, Ban Xia, Ren Shen, Gan Cao, Du Huo, Fang Feng, Bai Shao, Qiang Huo, Ju Pi, Fu Ling, Chai Hu, Ze Xie, Bai Zhu, Huang Lian, Sheng Jiang, Da Zao

Sheng Yu Tang (聖愈湯)

Dang Gui, Chuan Xiong, Chi Shao	3 qian each
Sheng Di Huang, Cang Zhu	3 qian each
Dan Shen	5 qian
Huang Qi	1.5 liang

The Yu Sheng version is similar to the original formula except that Sheng Di Huang replaces Shu Di Huang and Dan Shen replaces Ren Shen, and Chi Shao and Cang Zhu are added. Due to the time-consuming and costly method of traditional processing, the Shu Di Huang on the market today is either very expensive or uses modern processing methods resulting in inferior quality; thus, Dr. Lee typically substitutes it with Sheng Di Huang, which has yin-enriching, blood-nourishing, and blood-cooling actions.

Chi Shao cools the blood and expels stasis; Dan Shen quickens the blood and dispels stasis and regulates menses and relieves pain; and Cang Zhu fortifies the spleen and dries dampness, thus counteracting the potential for digestion impairment and loose stools induced by the blood-nourishing yin-enriching medicinals. These additions complement and enhance this formula's overall blood-nourishing menstruation (blood)-regulating, blood-cooling stasis-dispelling, and yin-nourishing qi-supplementing actions. Depending on the presenting signs, symptoms, and pattern, Dr. Lee may also add Ren Shen (powder) or Ren Shen/Chuan Qi Powder.

Dr. Lee utilizes this formula's stasis-dispelling blood-cooling actions for the treatment of vascular wall pathologies such as chemotherapy-induced nephrotoxicity (e.g., interstitial nephritis), chemotherapy-induced hepatotoxicity (e.g., hepatitis), aneurysm, and retinopathy (e.g., diabetic). For the treatment of chemotherapy side effects manifesting as vascular wall pathoconditions, Dr. Lee will typically prescribe **Xiao Chai Hu Tang** combined with **Sheng Yu Tang**. **Sheng Yu Tang** is an excellent formula for providing *stable* and *lasting* effects in the promotion of blood perfusion, but it neither *controls* blood as effectively as **Blood Desiccation Formula**, nor does it *promote* blood perfusion as rapidly as **Bu Yang Huan Wu Tang**.

Shi Quan Da Bu Tang Tang (十全大補湯)

Huang Qin	2 qian
Dan Shen, Cang Zhu, Fu Ling, Gan Cao	3 qian each
Dang Gui, Chuan Xiong, Chi Shao	3 qian each
Sheng Di Huang, Gan Jiang, Fu Zi	3 qian each
Rou Gui	5 qian
Huang Qi	1 liang

This formula combines the blood-quickening blood-supplementing actions of **(Yu Sheng) Si Wu Tang** (Dang Gui, Chuan Xiong, Chi Shao, and Sheng Di Huang) and the qi-boosting spleen-fortifying actions of **(Yu Sheng) Si Jun Zi Tang** (Dan Shen, Cang Zhu, Fu Ling, and Gan Cao) adding Gan Jiang, Fu Zi, Huang Qin, and a large dose of Huang Qi. Huang Qin is added to counteract the heat of The Three Great Yang-Supplementers.

The Yu Sheng version of this formula provides enhanced blood-quickening blood-supplementing, qi-boosting spleen-fortifying, and kidney yang-supplementing actions applicable for the treatment of a broad range of dual qi and blood vacuity with yang vacuity pattern pathoconditions. In addition to other applications, Dr. Lee commonly prescribes this formula for pediatric patients with delayed growth (i.e., height and weight), cerebral palsy (congenital or acquired), and congenital developmental delay (e.g., physical, cognitive, emotional, speech and language).

Shi Zao Tang (十棗湯)
Yan Hua, Gan Sui, Da Ji, Da Zao

Si Jun Zi Tang (四君子湯)
Ren Shen, Gan Cao, Fu Ling, Bai Zhu

Si Ling Tang (四苓湯)
Fu Ling, Bai Zhu, Zhu Ling, Ze Xie, Deng Xin Cao

Si Ni Tang (四逆湯)
Gan Cao, Gan Jiang, Fu Zi

Si Shen Tang (四神湯)

Fu Ling, Qian Shi, Bai Guo, Lian Zi	3 qian each
Shan Yao	5 qian
Yi Yi Ren	1 liang
Shan Zha	2 qian

Si Miao Wan (四妙丸)
Huang Bo, Cang Zhu, Niu Xi, Yi Yi Ren

Si Wu Tang (四物湯/Four Agents Decoction)
Dang Gui, Chuan Xiong, Bai Shao, Shu Di Huang

Tao Hong Si Wu Tang (桃紅四物湯)
Dang Gui, Chuan Xiong, Bai Shao, Shu Di Huang, Tao Ren, Hong Hua

Tao Ren Cheng Qi Tang (桃仁承氣湯)
Tao Ren, Da Huang, Gui Zhi, Gan Cao, Mang Xiao

Tearing on Exposure to Wind Formula (迎風落淚方/Ying Feng Luo Lei Fang)

Ma Huang	1.5 qian
Dan Shen, Cang Zhu, Fu Ling, Gan Cao	3 qian each
Chen Pi, Ban Xia, Mu Xiang	3 qian each

Sha Ren, Xi Xin, Wu Wei Zi	3 qian each
Bai Guo	4 qian
Rou Gui	5 qian

This original Yu Sheng formula contains the qi-boosting spleen-fortifying and qi-moving phlegm-transforming actions of **Xiang Sha Liu Jun Zi Tang** and is similar to **Asthma Formula (Qi Chuan Fang)** except for the subtractions of Shan Yao and Xing Ren and the addition of Xi Xin. Xi Xin dispels wind and dissipates cold, frees the orifices and relieves pain, and warms the lung and transforms rheum; Ma Huang promotes sweating, resolves the exterior, and frees the nasal orifices; Wu Wei Zi constrains the lung and stabilizes panting; Bai Guo constrains the lung and dispels phlegm; and Rou Gui warms the kidney and supplements the spleen, resolves the exterior, and frees the channels. These medicinals complement the qi-boosting spleen-fortifying and qi-moving phlegm-transforming actions of **Xiang Sha Liu Jun Zi Tang**.

As its name indicates, this formula is specifically designed for the treatment of tearing on exposure to wind (迎風落淚 yíng fēng luò lèi), a classical TCM pathologic term that correlates with allergic rhinitis and other related pathoconditions of the sinuses. The underlying pathomechanism of tearing on exposure to wind is spleen yang vacuity with exterior pattern, which inhibits the spleen's capacity to absorb and diffuse nutrients throughout the entire body and results in a compromised immune system and inability to govern flesh. Dr. Lee explains that persistent and prolonged sneezing, nasal discharge, and post-nasal drip further irritates the lacrimal drainage system apparatus, resulting in laxity of the lacrimal ducts upstream and/or clogged lacrimal puncta downstream that leads to excessive tearing (epiphora).

Ti Gang San (提肛散)

Chuan Xiong, Dang Gui, Bai Zhu, Ren Shen, Huang Qi, Chen Pi, Gan Cao, Sheng Ma, Chai Hu, Huang Qin, Huang Lian, Bai Zhi

Tian Wang Bu Xin Dan (天王補心丹)

Tian Men Dong, Ren Shen, Fu Ling, Xuan Shen, Dan Shen, Yuan Zhi, Jie Geng, Dang Gui, Wu Wei Zi, Mai Men Dong, Bo Zi Ren, Suan Zao Ren, Sheng Di Huang

Tong Jing Fang (通經方)

Cang Zhu	4 qian
Gan Cao	5 qian
Niu Xi, Xu Duan, Gu Sui Bu, Qian Cao	8 qian each

The Yu Sheng version is designed with similar therapeutic actions as its namesake **Tong Jing Wan**, but Dr. Lee has overhauled the composition choosing other medicinals with similar and complementary actions. Niu Xi dissipates stasis and quickens the blood, frees the channels and relieves pain, and supplements the liver and kidney; Xu Duan quickens the blood, joins sinew and bones, supplements the liver and kidney, and quiets the fetus; Gu Sui Bu quickens the blood, supplements the kidney, strengthens the sinew, and settles pain; and Qian Cao cools the blood and moves the blood. Cang Zhu has the action of drying dampness and fortifying the spleen to counteract the potential of digestion impairment and loose stools resulting from the blood-nourishing yin enriching medicinals, and Gan Cao supplements the center and harmonizes the nature of medicinals. The addition of liver- and kidney-supplementing and sinew- and bone-strengthening medicinals complement the original formula's blood-breaking, channel-freeing, and pain-relieving actions.

Dr. Lee typically prescribes this formula for fractures, traumatic injuries, and osteoporosis, as well as adjuvant therapy for the side efforts of chemotherapy in bone and gynecologic cancer patients. It is also a commonly prescribed formula in Dr. Lee's cancer treatment protocol, specifically administered for malignant (or benign) tumors of the striated muscle and marrow (e.g., rhabdomyosarcoma, osteosarcoma) with its capacity to inhibit tumor-cell mediated angiogenesis and neovascularization and the proliferation of cancer stem cells.

Tong Jing Wan (通經丸)

San Leng, E Zhu, Dang Gui, Chuan Xiong, Chi Shao, Chuan Shan Jia, Yan Hua, Liu Ji Nu

Wan Ling Dan (萬靈丹) – refer to **Bao An Wan Ling Dan (保安萬靈丹)**

Wen Dan Tang (溫膽湯)

Huang Qin, Zhi Shi	3 qian each
Chen Pi, Ban Xia, Fu Ling, Gan Cao	4 qian each
Zhu Ru	3 pieces
Da Zao	4 pieces

The Yu Sheng version is virtually the same as the original formula except for the addition of Huang Qin and the subtraction of Sheng Jiang. The heat-clearing dampness-drying action of Huang Qin complements this formula's overall qi-moving, phlegm-transforming, and harmonizing the gallbladder and stomach actions, making it suitable for the treatment of phlegm-heat with repletion heat or residual heat pattern pathoconditions.

Dr. Lee prescribes variants of this formula for a broad scope of ailments such as external contraction (e.g., common cold), insomnia, rhinitis, otitis, glaucoma, infertility (both male and female), and myasthenia gravis (damp-heat pattern type).

Wen Qing Yin (溫清飲)

Dang Gui, Chuan Xiong, Bai Shao, Shu Di Huang, Huang Qin, Huang Bo, Zhi Zi, Huang Lian

Wu Lin San (五淋散)

Chi Fu Ling, Dang Gui, Chi Shao Yao, Zhi Zi, Gan Cao, Deng Xin Cao

Wu Ling San (五苓散)

Zhu Ling, Ze Xie, Bai Zhu, Fu Ling, Gui Zhi

Wu Ling San (Calculi Formula) (五苓散 (結石方))

Rou Gui	2 qian
Yan Hu Suo, Mu Xiang, Huang Bo, Gan Cao	3 qian each
Cang Zhu, Zhu Ling, Fu Ling	5 qian each
Dang Gui	8 qian
Ze Xie	1 liang

This Yu Sheng version contains the essential components of the original formula except for replacing Gui Zhi with Rou Gui and Bai Zhu with Cang Zhu, and adding Dang Gui, Yan Hu Suo, Mu Xiang, Huang Bo, and Gan Cao. This formula includes large doses of Ze Xie for its water-inhibiting dampness-percolating and heat-draining actions, and large doses of Dang Gui for its blood-supplementing blood-quickening actions—a medicinal pair that promotes smooth muscle contractions of the bile ducts, kidneys, and urinary tract, thus resulting in the dislodgement and evacuation of calculi. Mu Xiang moves qi, relieves pain, and relaxes smooth muscle; and Yan Hu Suo quickens the blood, moves qi, and functions as a strong analgesic to promote evacuation of calculi and provide relief for pain. Huang Bo drains lower burner fire, dries dampness, resolves toxin, and disinhibits the gallbladder to treat inflammation.

As its name implies, Dr. Lee has specifically designed this formula for the treatment of calculi in the kidneys (nephrolithiasis) and other sites along the urogenital tract (e.g., urethra, bladder), bile ducts (gallstones/choledocholithiasis), and the pancreatic duct (pancreatolithiasis).

Wu Ling San (Nephritis Formula) (五苓散 (腎炎方))

Dang Gui	2 qian
Gan Jiang, Fu Zi, Huang Bo	3 qian each
Zhu Ling, Fu Ling, Cang Zhu, Ze Xie, Rou Gui	5 qian each
Huang Qi	1 liang

This Yu Sheng version contains the essential components of the original formula except for Rou Gui replacing Gui Zhi, Cang Zhu replacing Bai Zhu, and the addition of Dang Gui, Huang Qi, Gan Jiang, Fu Zi, and Huang Bo. Huang Qi supplements qi, disinhibits water and disperses swelling, increases myocardial contractility, promotes passage across membranes, and functions as a broad-spectrum antimicrobial, which complements Dang Gui's actions of supplementing and quickening the blood, as these medicinals combine to improve renal blood flow and filtration through the glomeruli. Rou Gui reinforces yang, greatly supplements life gate fire, conducts medicinals throughout the entire body, and promotes blood circulation, which complements Fu Zi's actions of reinforcing yang, supplementing the kidney and life-gate fire, freeing the twelve channels, and strengthening cardiac contractility, as these medicinals combine to increase stroke volume and reduce heart rate.

This formula warms kidney yang and promotes qi transformation and disinhibits water and percolates dampness for the treatment of inhibited urination, water swelling (edema), and water-damp collecting internally. Dr. Lee commonly prescribes this formula for the treatment of post-acute and chronic pathoconditions that present with proteinuria, edema, uremia, and hypoalbuminemia (e.g., nephrotic syndrome, glomerulonephritis, chronic kidney failure); pulmonary edema (e.g., intrinsic lung disease, congestive heart failure, kidney failure); and increased intracranial pressure (ICP).

Wu Wei Yi Gong San (五味異功散)
Ren Shen, Bai Zhu, Fu Ling, Gan Cao, Chen Pi, Sheng Jiang, Da Zao

Wu Zhu Yu Tang (吳茱萸湯)
Wu Zhu Yu, Ren Shen, Sheng Jiang, Da Zao

Wu Zi Yan Zong Wan (五子衍宗丸)
Tu Si Zi, Wu Wei Zi, Gou Ji Zi, Fu Pen Zi, Che Qian Zi

Xi Ji (洗劑/Vaginal Wash/Douche)
Long Dan Cao, She Chuang Zi, Xiong Huang, Liu Huang, Lu Gan Shi

This formula composition is similar to **Sai Ji (Vaginal Suppository)** except for the subtraction of Da Huang and the addition of Long Dan Cao and Lu Gan Shi. It is used as an immersion and wash therapy prescribed for various types of infections of the vulva and vaginal opening, including bacterial vaginosis (i.e., *Gardnerella vaginalis*), yeast (candidiasis), parasites (trichomoniasis), and sexually transmitted diseases (STDs) (e.g., genital herpes, gonorrhea, Chlamydia) that present with itching, irritation, and watery or viscous vaginal discharge.

This formula is typically prescribed as part of a therapeutic regimen that includes decocted formulas taken orally such as **Long Dan Xie Gan Tang**, **Jin Suo Gu Jing Wan**, or **Bu Zhong Yi Qi Tang**.

Xi Jiao Di Huang Tang (犀角地黃湯)
Xi Jiao (or Shui Niu Jiao), Sheng Di Huang, Shao Yao, Mu Dan Pi

Xian Fang Huo Ming Yin (仙方活命飲)/aka **Zhen Ren Huo Ming Yin (真人活命飲)**

Chen Pi, Tian Hua, Jin Yin Hua, Ru Xiang	3 qian each
Mo Yao, Fang Feng, Zao Jiao Ci, Dang Gui	3 qian each
Niu Bang Zi, Chi Shao, Bai Zhi, Gan Cao	3 qian each
Cang Zhu	4 qian
Sheng Shi Gao	1 liang

The Yu Sheng version is similar to the original formula except for the exclusion of Chuan Shan Jia, an endangered animal species that is now prohibited, and Zhe Bei Mu is either taken separately or added into the formula after decoction. Instead of Chuan Shan Jia, Dr. Lee includes Niu Bang Zi for its wind-coursing heat-dissipating, papule-outthrusting toxin-resolving, and swelling-dispersing actions; Sheng Shi Gao for its heat-clearing fire-draining actions; and Cang Zhu for its dampness-drying spleen-fortifying actions. These additions complement the blood-quickening and pus-expelling swelling-dispersing actions of Zao Jiao Ci, and provide an effective alternative for Chuan Shan Jia.

In TCM classical texts this formula is classified as a "sore sage formula" for its heat-clearing toxin-resolving, swelling-dispersing hardness-breaking, and blood-quickening pain-relieving actions. It is traditionally prescribed for the treatment of acute and post-acute stage swelling and toxin of welling-abscesses (carbuncles, furuncles, boils) and sores in which there is localized redness, heat, swelling, and pain or generalized heat with mild aversion to cold. In addition to these types of external medicine pathoconditions, Dr. Lee prescribes this formula for pathoconditions such as innominate toxin swellings (both benign and malignant), cellulitis, appendicitis, postherpetic neuralgia (phantom pain), and pulmonary abscesses.

Xiang Sha Liu Jun Zi Tang (香砂六君子湯)

Dan Shen, Cang Zhu, Fu Ling	3 qian each
Gan Cao, Mu Xiang, Sha Ren	3 qian each
Chen Pi, Ban Xia	4 qian each

The Yu Sheng version is similar to the original formula except that Dan Shen replaces Ren Shen, Cang Zhu replaces Bai Zhu, and Sheng Jiang and Da Zao are subtracted. Dan Shen quickens the blood and dispels stasis; and Cang Zhu fortifies the spleen and dries dampness, which is ideal for Taiwan's humid subtropical climate. Depending on the presenting signs, symptoms, and pattern, Dr. Lee may also add Ren Shen (powder) or Ren Shen/Chuan Qi Powder; Sheng Jiang, as in the original formula, for the treatment of morning sickness during the first trimester of pregnancy; and Gan Jiang for the treatment of interior cold pattern pathoconditions.

This formula's qi-boosting spleen-fortifying and qi-moving phlegm-transforming actions are traditionally administered for pathoconditions involving spleen and stomach vacuity, dampness obstruction and qi stagnation, abdominal distention after food intake, acid reflux, and poor appetite. Some specific pathoconditions Dr. Lee typically prescribes this formula for are gastrointestinal reflux disease (GERD), gastritis, autoimmune diseases (e.g., SLE), ascites (e.g., hepatic disorders), renal disease (e.g., azotemia), and poor appetite and malnutrition during the late stages of cancer.

The qi-boosting spleen-fortifying and qi-moving phlegm-transforming actions of **Xiang Sha Liu Jun Zi Tang** form the foundation of the three formulas that treat the "allergic triad" manifestations of atopy—**Asthma Formula (Qi Chuan Fang)** treats the lung, **Atopic Dermatitis Formula (Yi Wei Xing Pi Fu Yan Fang)** treats the skin, and **Tearing on Exposure to Wind Formula (Ying Feng Luo Lei Fang)** treats the sinuses. These hyperallergic reactions may present as an inflammatory response in the upper respiratory tract (e.g., lungs, sinuses) or manifest on the skin.

In TCM theory, the spleen belongs to earth and engenders metal, governs the movement and transformation of the essence of grain and water and also governs the flesh. The lung belongs to metal and governs qi, skin and hair, opens at the nose, and has an upward and outward diffusing movement, which carries moisture and nourishment to the skin.

Xiao Ban Xia Jia Fu Ling Tang (小半夏加茯苓湯)
Ban Xia, Sheng Jiang, Fu Ling

Xiao Chai Hu Tang (小柴胡湯)

Huang Qin	3 qian
Dan Shen, Ban Xia, Gan Cao, Sheng Jiang	5 qian each
Chai Hu	6 qian
Da Zao	5 pieces

The Yu Sheng version is nearly identical to the original formula except for Dan Shen replacing Ren Shen. However, depending on the presenting signs, symptoms, and pattern, Ren Shen (powder) or Ren Shen/Chuan Qi Powder may also be included.

Traditionally, this is a commonly prescribed formula for the treatment of Shao Yang pattern pathoconditions (e.g., alternating heat and cold, fullness in the chest and rib-side, no desire for food and drink), general discomfort or pain in the hypochondriac region, heat entering the blood chamber, and pathoconditions of the liver, gallbladder, and spleen (e.g., hepatitis, cholecystitis, splenitis).

Dr. Lee's application of this formula can be classified into three broad categories: 1) Depressed heat (i.e., persistent low-grade fever) following external contraction (i.e., microbial infection), especially for pediatric patients and tuberculosis (TB) patients who have been administered antibiotic treatment; 2) Microbial infections, toxin (e.g., noxious chemicals), or autoimmune reactions leading to metabolic waste buildup that disrupts the capacity of the nervous system (specifically, the coordinated interactions of the CNS, ANS, and PNS) to regulate bodily functions and maintain homeostasis, thus resulting in dyscrasias (e.g., leukemia, hemophilia, multiple myeloma); and 3) For complex pattern pathoconditions that are difficult to diagnose and pathoconditions are in a transitional state which can be identified as half-interior half-exterior (mid-stage) pattern, this formula may be prescribed until a definitive diagnosis and/or pattern identification can be ascertained (e.g., whether a pathocondition is passing from the exterior into the interior or from the interior into the exterior).

Xiao Qing Long Tang (小青龍湯/Minor Green-Blue Dragon Decoction)

Ma Huang, Gui Zhi, Bai Shao, Gan Cao, Gan Jiang, Xi Xin, Ban Xia, Wu Wei Zi

Xiao Yao San (逍遙散)

Chai Hu, Dang Gui, Bai Shao, Bai Zhu, Fu Ling, Gan Cao, Sheng Jiang, Bo He

Xie Xin Tang (寫心湯)/aka **San Huang Xie Xin Tang (三黃瀉心湯)**

Da Huang, Huang Lian, Huang Qin

Xue Fu Zhu Yu Tang (血腹逐瘀湯)

Dang Gui, Sheng Di Huang, Tao Ren, Hong Hua, Zhi Ke, Chi Shao, Chai Hu, Gan Cao, Jie Geng, Chuan Xiong, Niu Xi

Xue Ku Fang (血枯方) – refer to **Blood Desiccation Formula**

Xun Qi Huo Xue Tang (順氣活血湯)

Su Geng, Hou Po, Zhi Ke, Sha Ren, Dang Gui, Hong Hua, Mu Xiang, Chi Shao, Tao Ren, Su Mu, Xiang Fu, Mi Jiu

Yang Dan Tang (陽但湯)

Rou Gui, Chi Shao, Sheng Cao, Sheng Jiang	5 qian each
Huang Qin	3 qian
Da Zao	5 pieces

This Yu Sheng version is virtually identical to the original formula, which is a derivative of **Gui Zhi Tang** (Gui Zhi, Bai Shao, Gan Cao, Sheng Jiang, Da Zao), except as is the case in many of Dr. Lee's other formulas Chi Shao is substituted for Bai Shao and Rou Gui for Gui Zhi.

Traditionally, this formula is prescribed for the treatment of wind strike cold damage, floating pulse, alternating heat (fever) and aversion to cold, sweating and aversion to wind, stiff neck, noisy nose (鼻鳴 bí míng) and dry retching. Its composition forms the foundation for Dr. Lee's therapeutic approach for the treatment of exterior wind-heat pattern pathoconditions of the sinuses, eyes, and skin. Dr. Lee typically does not prescribe **Gui Zhi Tang** decocting pieces for decoction on its own, but he may prescribe extract granules of this classic formula (or in combination with other formulas) for relatively mild external contraction wind-cold exterior vacuity pattern pathoconditions.

Yi Gan San (抑肝散)

Dang Gui, Bai Zhu, Fu Ling, Gou Teng, Chuan Xiong, Chai Hu, Gan Cao

Yi Qi Cong Ming Tang (益氣聰明湯)

Huang Qi, Ren Shen, Ge Gen, Man Xing Zi, Bai Shao, Huang Bo, Sheng Ma, Gan Cao

Yi Wei Xing Pi Fu Yan Fang (異位性皮膚炎方) – refer to **Atopic Dermatitis Formula**

Yin Qiao San (銀翹散)

Jin Yin Hua, Lian Qiao, Jing Jie, Dan Dou Chi, Jie Geng, Bo He, Niu Bang Zi, Gan Cao, Zhu Ye, Wei Gen

Ying Feng Luo Lei Fang (迎風落淚方) – refer to **Tearing on Exposure to Wind Formula**

You Gui Wan (右歸丸)

Shu Di Huang, Shan Yao, Gou Qi Zi, Tu Si Zi, Du Zhong, Lu Jiao Jiao, Shan Zhu Yu, Dang Gui, Fu Zi, Rou Gui

You Gui Yin (右歸飲)

Dang Gui, Fu Ling	2 qian each
Gou Qi Zi, Huang Bo, Gan Jiang	3 qian each
Sheng Di Huang, Shan Zhu Yu, Shan Yao	4 qian each
Cang Zhu, Du Zhong, Tu Si Zi	4 qian each
Fu Zi, Niu Xi, Rou Gui	5 qian each

The Yu Sheng version combines medicinals from **(Yu Sheng) Shen Qi Wan** and the original version of **You Gui Wan**, but adds medicinals to enhance its kidney yang-warming and -supplementing actions. Sheng Di Huang is included instead of Shu Di Huang, and Huang Bo, Gan Jiang, Cang Zhu, and Niu Xi are added. Along with providing blood-quickening stasis-dissipating, liver- and kidney-supplementing, and sinew- and bone-strengthening actions, Niu Xi and Du Zhong serve as channel conductors directing medicinals to the lower limbs. Huang Bo counteracts the heat of The Three Great Yang-Supplementers, and Cang Zhu dries dampness and fortifies the spleen to counteract the potential of digestion impairment and loose stools resulting from large doses of blood-nourishing yin-enriching and yang-supplementing medicinals.

Dr. Lee commonly prescribes this formula for a wide range of yang vacuity and depletion pattern pathoconditions such as lumbar and back pain (e.g., radiculopathy (sciatica) from herniated intervertebral disc, spondylolisthesis, spinal stenosis), limp knees and weak legs (e.g., various post-acute articular cartilage, ligament, and tendon injuries), congenital development disorders, and atopy (especially in male patients) (e.g., chronic stage asthma, tearing on exposure to wind, atopic dermatitis).

Yu Sheng Wan (育生丸)

Man Tuo Luo Hua	0.04 g/pill
Shan Yao	0.6 g/pill
Honey	

The principal medicinal in this pill is Man Tuo Luo Hua (aka Yang Jin Hua, Datura Flower, *Datura metel* L.), whose bioactive constituents are the anticholinergics scopolamine (hyoscine) and hyoscyamine (atropine). Shan Yao serves as a filler and diluent, and its balanced nature and qi-boosting spleen-supplementing and yin-nourishing actions provide a moderating effect on Man Tuo Luo Hua. Honey serves as a binder and preservative, and it supplements the center and moderates the nature of Man Tuo Luo Hua. Honey is boiled repeatedly until it solidifies into a gelatinous state and then the pulverized powder of these two medicinals are mixed into the honey, made into pills, and allowed to dry.

This is a commonly prescribed pill that Dr. Lee includes in the therapeutic regimen for a broad spectrum of pathoconditions. Dr. Lee explains that the underlying pharmacodynamics of this pill is its capacity to stimulate cerebral collateral circulation and rejuvenate the brain's self-regulating function. Cerebral circulation fluctuates in response to physical and mental activities and metabolic processes, and normally the brain is able to self-regulate (autoregulation) in order to maintain homeostasis. However, certain pathoconditions, as well as the process of aging, may lead to microvascular changes, decreased vascular density, and pericyte degeneration. These changes cause the brain to *misinterpret* the internal environment it holds dominion over, functioning imperceptively in a compromised state of dyshomeostasis.

Dr. Lee utilizes the actions of these properties to supplement the brain, remedy insomnia and depression, eliminate anxiety and stress, slow the degenerative process of aging and disease (e.g., dementia, Alzheimer's disease, Parkinson's disease), relieve all types of pain, check spasm, and stabilize panting (asthma). Its capacity to relax smooth muscle makes it effective for treating overactive bladder (females) and enlarged prostate (males) and for promoting the passage of urinary tract calculi and gallstones (using a large 1x dose of 4–6 pills for males and 4–8 pills for females accompanied by acupuncture). It is also prescribed as a part of Dr. Lee's cancer treatment protocol.

The efficacy of this pill is very much dose-related with large doses potentially causing side effects such as dry mouth, drowsiness, blurry vision, and confusion; thus, it is essential to limit the standard dosage to 1–3 pills per day.

Yu Zhen San (玉真散)
Tian Nan Xing, Bai Zhi, Fang Feng, Qiang Huo, Tian Ma, Bai Fu Zi

Yue Bi Tang (越婢湯/Spleen-Effusing Decoction/Maidservant from *Yue* Decoction)
Ma Huang, Shi Gao, Sheng Jiang, Gan Cao, Da Zao

Zao Fu Tang (棗附湯)
Fu Zi, Da Zao, Sheng Jiang

Zhi Bo Di Huang Tang (知柏地黄湯)

Gan Cao, Huang Bo	3 qian
Zhi Mu, Shan Zhu Yu, Shan Yao, Fu Ling	4 qian each
Mu Dan Pi, Ze Xie, Niu Xi, Cang Zhu	4 qian each
Sheng Di Huang	8 qian

The Yu Sheng version is similar to the original formula except for Sheng Di Huang replacing Shu Di Huang and the addition of Niu Xi, Cang Zhu, and Gan Cao. Niu Xi quickens the blood, strengthens the sinews and bones, and is a channel conductor leading other medicinals downward; Cang Zhu supplements the spleen and dries dampness; and Gan Cao supplements the center and harmonizes the nature of medicinals. The combination of Huang Bo, Niu Xi, and Cang Zhu forms **San Miao Wan**, a commonly prescribed heat-clearing dampness-drying formula used for pathoconditions in the lower burner and lower limbs such as genitourinary damp-heat pouring downward and arthritic ailments.

Dr. Lee typically prescribes this yin-enriching fire-downbearing formula for effulgent yin vacuity fire and steaming bone pathoconditions such as osteomyelitis, pulling of the sinews and inhibited bending and stretching (e.g., musculoskeletal sprains, strains, and tears; osteoarthritis), bone fractures, heel pain syndrome, tuberculosis, yin vacuity cough (aka dryness cough), epilepsy, diabetes, genitourinary tract disorders, seminal emission, and menopausal symptoms.

This is an essential formula for acute and sub-acute musculoskeletal injuries (e.g., arthritic, traumatic, autoimmune) manifesting in swelling and inflammation, because of its capacity to promote self-repair and prevent the potential development of further degeneration (e.g., fibrosis, enthesopathy) that may arise as a result of complications from aspiration, bleeding, or administration of anti-inflammatory agents.

Zhi Zi Bo Pi Tang (梔子柏皮湯)
Shan Zhi Zi, Huang Bo, Gan Cao

Zi Yun Gao (紫雲膏/Purple Cloud Ointment, aka **Run Ji Gao)**

Zi Cao	120g
Dang Gui	60g
Ma You (Sesame Oil)	520g
Mi La (Beeswax)	300g

Dr. Lee purchases this ointment ready-prepared from a proprietary supplier. This formula is derived from the original composition presented in the *Orthodox Manual of External Medicine.*

Zi Cao enters the blood aspect of the liver channel, cools and quickens the blood, and resolves toxin and outthrusts papules; and Dang Gui quickens and supplements the blood, moistens dryness, disperses swelling and relieves pain, and engenders flesh. Sesame Oil functions both as an extractant, extracting the lipophilic active ingredients of the principal medicinals, and as a skin-conditioner and emollient (moisturizer). Beeswax functions as an excipient, both as an emulsifier, used to blend and stabilize liquids that are not mutually soluble and to improve the bioavailability of lipid-soluble compounds, and as a bulking agent.

This ointment provides antibacterial and bactericidal actions for external injuries of the skin, promotes the growth of granulation tissue at the site of wounds, and enriches and moistens the skin. Dr. Lee will commonly prescribe this topical application for the treatment of minor burns, eczematous dry fissured skin (e.g., pompholyx, cracked heels, atopic dermatitis), erosions (have reached the epidermis, but *not* for ulcerations, which have reached the dermis), chilblains, and hemorrhoids.

Zuo Gui Yin (左歸飲)

Dang Gui	2 qian
Gou Qi Zi, Fu Ling, Gan Cao	3 qian each
Sheng Di Huang, Shan Zhu Yu, Shan Yao	4 qian each
Tu Si Zi, Du Zhong, Cang Zhu	4 qian each
Niu Xi	5 qian

The Yu Sheng version is similar to the original formula except for replacing Shu Di Huang with Sheng Di Huang and adding Niu Xi, Du Zhong, and Tu Si Zi. Niu Xi quickens the blood and frees the channels, supplements the liver and kidney, strengthens the sinews and bones, conducts fire (blood) downward, and conducts medicinals downward to the lumbus and lower limbs; Du Zhong supplements the liver and kidney, strengthens sinew and bones, and conducts medicinals downward to the lumbus and lower limbs; and Tu Si Zi supplements the kidney and secures essence. These additions enhance this formula's essence-replenishing and blood-supplementing actions and complement it with kidney yang-supplementing medicinals that target the lumbus and lower limbs.

In the early years of Dr. Lee's clinical practice, he would prescribe this formula for post-acute and chronic stage lumbar pain (e.g., degenerative disc disease) and limp knees and weak legs (e.g., articular cartilage, ligament, and tendon injuries of the lower limbs) in which heat pattern (inflammation) was still pronounced and for patients with yin vacuity constitutions. Nowadays, Dr. Lee seldom prescribes this formula, often choosing to use **Zhi Bo Di Huang Tang** variants instead.

BIBLIOGRAPHY

Bensky, Dan, Steve Clavey, Erich Stoger. *Chinese Herbal Medicine: Materia Medica* (3rd Edition). Eastland Press, 2015.

Chang, Hsian-che; Tsai, Gui-hua. *Processing of Traditional Chinese Medicine Materia Medica* [Zhong Yao Pao Zhi Xue] Second Edition (Chinese). Taichung, Taiwan (R.O.C.): China Medical University, 2003.

Chen, Shi-gong. *Orthodox Manual of External Medicine* [Wai Ke Zheng Zong] (Chinese). China: Qing Dynasty (1617).

Cheng, Wu-ji. *The Clear Rationale of Cold Damage* [Shang Han Ming Li Lun] (Chinese). China: Jin Dynasty (1156).

Chinese Materia Medica [Zhong Hua Ben Cao] (Chinese). Shanghai, China: Shanghai Science Technology Publication, 1998.

Chinese Materia Medica Grand Dictionary [Xin Bian Zhong Yao Da Ci Dian] (Chinese). Taipei, Taiwan (R.O.C.): Xin Wen Feng Publishing Co., Ltd., 1982.

Clinical Applications of Traditional Chinese Medicinals [Zhong Yao Lin Chuang Ying Yong] (Chinese). Taipei, Taiwan (R.O.C.): Cheers Books Co., 1988.

Deng, Tie-tao. *Traditional Chinese Medicine Diagnostics* [Zhong Yi Zhen Duan Xue] (Chinese). Taipei, Taiwan (R.O.C.): Jyin Publishing Co., 2003.

Fundamentals of Chinese Medicine [Zhong Yi Ji Chu Xue] (Chinese). Taipei, Taiwan (R.O.C.): Cheers Books Co., 1994.

Harrison's Principles of Internal Medicine 19th Edition. McGraw-Hill, 2015.

Hong, Zhen-hui. *Dictionary of Chinese Medicine* [Zhong Guo Yi Xue Ci Dian] (Chinese). Taipei, Taiwan (R.O.C.): Li De Publishing Co., Ltd., 1983.

Huang, Wei-san. *Science of Acupuncture and Moxibustion* [Zhen Jiu Ke Xue] (Chinese). Taipei, Taiwan (R.O.C.): Zheng Zhong Publishing Co., Ltd., 1985.

Ke Qin. *Collected Writings on the Renewal of the 'Treatise on Cold Damage'* [Shang Han Lun Su Ji] (Chinese). China: Ming Dynasty (1674).

Keisetsu, Ōtsuka, *Thirty Years of Kampo Diagnosis and Treatment* [Han Fang Zhen Liao San Shi Nian] (Chinese). Tainan, Taiwan (R.O.C.): Zheng Yan Medical Publications, 1959.

Kou, Zong-yi. *Expanded Herbal Foundation* [Ben Cao Yan Yi] (Chinese). China: Song Dynasty (1116)

Lee, Chen-yu. *Neuropathy: Traditional Chinese Herbal Treatment in a Modern Medical Environment.* tr. Daniel L. Altschuler. Taipei, Taiwan (R.O.C.): Cheers Books Co., 2005.

Lee, Chen-yu. *Traditional Chinese Medicine Treatment of Common Liver Diseases* [Chang Jian Gan Bing Zhong Yi Liao Fa] (Chinese). Taipei, Taiwan (R.O.C.): Cheers Books Co., 2001.

Li, Dong-yuan. *Treatise on the Spleen and Stomach* [Pi Wei Lun] (Chinese). China: Jin Dynasty (1249).

Li, Nian-e. *Essential Knowledge of Internal Medicine* [Nei Jing Zhi Yao] (Chinese). China: Ming Dynasty (1642).

Li, Shi-zhen. *Herbal Foundation Compendium* [Ben Cao Gang Mu] (Chinese). China: Ming Dynasty (1590).

Li, Shi-zhen. *Supplement to the Herbal Foundation* [Ben Cao Gang Mu Shi Yi] (Chinese). China: Ming Dynasty (1590).

Ma, Jian Zhong. *Chinese Medicine Internal Medicine* [Zhong Yi Nei Ke Xue] (Chinese). Taipei, Taiwan (R.O.C.): Zheng Zhong Publishing Co., Ltd., 1986.

Neal, Anthony J., Peter J. Hoskin. *Clinical Oncology Basic Principles and Practice* (Third Edition). London, UK: Arnold, 2003.

Oswald, Cyril, Frank Delaigue. *Les Hommes de l'Art* (French). You-Feng (Librairie), 2013.

Taber's Cyclopedic Medical Dictionary (23rd Edition). Philadelphia, PA (U.S.A.): F.A. Davis Company, 2017.

Tang, Zong-zai. *Treatise on Blood Syndromes* [Xue Zheng Lun] (Chinese). China: Qing Dynasty (1884).

The Divine Husbandman's Herbal Foundation Canon [Shen Nong Ben Cao Jing] (Chinese). China: est. Qin or Han Dynasty.

The Yellow Emperor's Inner Cannon [Huang Di Nei Jing] (Chinese). China: Eastern Han Dynasty.

Wang, Ang. *Medical Formulas Gathered and Explained* [Yi Fang Ji Jie] (Chinese). China: Qing Dynasty (1682).

Wang, Ang. *The Essential Herbal Foundation* [Ben Cao Bei Yao] (Chinese). China: Qing Dynasty (1694).

Wang, Qing-ren. *Correction of Errors in Medical Classics* [Yi Lin Gai Cuo] (Chinese). China: Qing Dynasty (1830).

Wiseman, Nigel and Ye, Feng. *A Practical Dictionary of Chinese Medicine* (Second Edition). Brookline, Massachusetts: Paradigm Publications, 1998.

Wu, Qian. *Essential Teachings on Acupuncture and Moxibustion* [Ci Jiu Xin Fa Yao Jue] (Chinese). China: Qing Dynasty (1742).

Wu, Qian. *Essential Teachings on Miscellaneous Diseases* [Za Bing Xin Fa] (Chinese). China: Qing Dynasty (1742).

Wu, Qian. *The Golden Mirror of Medicin*e [Yi Zong Jin Jian] (Chinese). China: Qing Dynasty (1742).

Yakazu, Dōmei. *Kampo Prescriptions Explained* [Han Fang Chu Fang Jie Shuo] (Chinese). Tainan, Taiwan (R.O.C.): Zheng Yan Medical Publications, 1966.

Yang, Ji-zhou. *The Great Compendium of Acupuncture and Moxibustion* [Zhen Jiu Da Cheng] (Chinese). China: Ming Dynasty (1601).

Young, Wei-chieh. Annotated Explanations of The Yellow Emperor's Inner Classic: Basic Questions [Huang Di Nei Jing Su Wen Yi Jie] (Chinese). Taipei, Taiwan (R.O.C.): Chih-Yuan Publishing Co., Ltd., (1994).

Young, Wei-chieh. Annotated Explanations of The Yellow Emperor's Inner Classic: The Spiritual Pivot [Huang Di Nei Jing Ling Shu Yi